ORTHOPAEDIC MANIFESTATIONS AND BONE CHANGES IN SICKLE CELL HAEMOGLOBINOPATHY

ORTHOPAEDIC MANIFESTATIONS AND BONE CHANGES IN SICKLE CELL HAEMOGLOBINOPATHY

Prof. Dr. Sudhir Babhulkar
M.S. (Orth.), D.Orth., Ph.D. Orth., F.I.C.S., F.I.C.A., F.A.C.S.
Hon. Professor of Orthopaedics, Indira Gandhi Medical College, Nagpur;
Hon. Orthopaedic Surgeon, Mayo General Hospital, Nagpur;
Director, Sushrut Hospital, Research Centre and
Postgraduate Institute of Orthopaedics, Nagpur, India

CBS

CBS PUBLISHERS & DISTRIBUTORS
4596/1 A, 11-DARYAGANJ, NEW DELHI-110002

ISBN : 81-239-0577-7

First Edition : 1997

Published by :
Satish Kumar Jain for CBS Publishers & Distributors,
4596/1-A, 11 Darya Ganj, New Delhi - 2 (India)

Production Director : Vinod Jain

Laser typesetting at :
Rafah Typesetters, Delhi - 110 032

Printed at :
Tara Art Printers, NOIDA (U.P.)

Foreword

This book is the culmination of a lifetime of pioneering work by a single physician dedicated to the study of one disease. Throughout his illustrious career, Prof. Dr. Sudhir Babhulkar has been particularly interested in the sickle cell hemoglobinopathies. His important observations on the anthropometric abnormalities ("sickler facies") were originally documented in his Ph.D. thesis. In this monograph and his previous publications, Prof. Babhulkar has created a lucid text by integrating older material with newer knowledge. This scholarly monograph significantly increases our current knowledge on this subject since it reviews 7380 patients with this genetic disorder, which is very common in the Nagpur region of central India. Since 944 of these patients with skeletal involvement have been studied, this monograph will become a classic text regarding the diagnosis, staging, and treatment of this condition.

About 1970, Prof. Babhulkar built the first hospital in Nagpur, and he named it the Sushrut Hospital and Research Centre, in honor of Sushrut, who was the first surgeon in India. His son Sushrut and daughter Sonali are also orthopedic surgeons who share their father's enthusiasm for treating these patients. Prof. Babhulkar has presented this superb work on sickle cell disorders at several meetings, and his authoritative article on sickle cell dactylitis has recently been published in the Journal of Bone and Joint Surgery. The surgical skills and workmanship of Prof. Babhulkar are also reflected in this compilation of studies, which will certainly form a foundation for future investigations in this field.

In 1994, I had the opportunity to visit the Sushrut Hospital and meet several hemoglobinopathy patients with orthopedic complications, especially those with femoral and humeral head necrosis. With sincere gratitude, I would like to personally acknowledge the support and encouragement that Prof. Babhulkar provided me in studying hemoglobinopathy patients, particularly those with intervertebral disc disease associated with vertebral end-plate necrosis. It has been a pleasure knowing this outstanding clinician and researcher, and having the opportunity to recognize his magnificent contributions.

John Paul Jones, Jr., M.D.
Past President, Association Research Circulation Osseous

Preface

During the early years of my practice in Central India, I came across numerous patients with severe skeletal manifestations and physical handicap secondary to complications of Sickle Cell Disease. Sickle Cell Haemoglobinopathy is a genetically transmitted disease resulting from a defect in beta chain of haemoglobin where glutamic acid at position six is replaced by valine. Extensive research has revealed the aetiopathogenesis of the disease and made accurate laboratory diagnosis feasible. Although different modalities of treatment have been tried including bone marrow transplantation, none has proved to be curative. Most of the morbidity and mortality associated with the disease is as a result of the complications. Hence early diagnosis and prevention of complications remains the gold standard in the management of Sickle Cell Haemoglobinopathy.

Sickle Cell Haemoglobinopathy is highly prevalent in Central India in the scheduled tribes and scheduled castes. We conducted various diagnostic camps and surveys in and around Nagpur. We had followed patients over last twenty five years studying the natural history of the disease. This monogram is the culmination of the extensive research of last two and a half decades. It deals with the historical aspects, aetiopathogenesis, radiological features, anthropological measurements and then in detail about individual skeletal involvement in Sickle Cell Haemoglobinopathy. I hope that this book will be of use to Orthopaedic Surgeons, Physicians, Paediatricians and Radiologists alike in recognising the patients, understanding the disease process and in effective management. I also want to stress on the importance of marriage and genetic counselling in prevention of the disease. The main aim of the monogram is to present a precise and concise description of all aspects of the orthopaedic manifestations of the disease that will be of help to medical professionals to offer the patients of Sickle Cell Haemoglobinopathy a better prognosis.

This monogram is the result of co-operative effort of a large number of colleagues who have helped and assisted me during the last twenty six years of research. Most of the work was carried out at Indira Gandhi Medical College, Mayo General Hospital, and Sushrut Hospital, Research Centre and Post-Graduate Institute, Nagpur. I would like to express my gratitude to my dear friend Dr. P.K. Kolwadkar, Radiologist, for his invaluable help during this work. I am also thankful to Prof. W.B. Tayade for his constant help and appreciate his active participation in the various surveys. I am grateful to the Dean, Indira Gandhi Medical College & Civil Surgeon, Mayo General Hospital, Nagpur for permitting me to conduct the study. I am thankful to Dr. Mrs. Pendharkar, Professor of Radiology Department, Indira Gandhi Medical College and Professor of Pathology for their cooperation. I would like to acknowledge the help I have received from Dr. Parchand, Professor of Anatomy for his assistance in conducting Anthropometric studies. I would also like to thank late Dr. B.S. Patil, Dr. Ashok Lawange, Dr. Sudhir Soni, Dr. Sanjiv Choudhary, Dr. Ajay Duddalwar and the Staff of Department of Orthopaedics. I must thank Dr. Santosh Somani, Research Fellow in Sushrut Hospital and Research Centre who was of immense help in completing the project. All the statistics of the study were efficiently handled by

Dr. Vijay Vaidya to whom I express my gratitude. Mr. Prashant Gupte and Mr. Surendra Gokhale, computer personnel have put in great efforts in the technical details of this book. I am thankful to Mr. Girish Shrivastav, Retina Photo Studio for his photography work.

I appreciate the efforts put in by Mr. Satish Jain and Mr. Vinod Jain, CBS Publishers & Distributors, New Delhi in editing and printing the book. Last but not the least, I would like to express my deepest gratitude to all my patients who have given me an opportunity to study the disease in detail. Without their cooperation this work would not have been possible.

Acknowledgments would be incomplete without thanks to my beloved wife Aruna whose co-operation and understanding made this work possible.

Prof. Dr. S.S. Babhulkar

Contents

1

Introduction

Sickle cell haemoglobinopathy is a genetically transmitted multisystem disease which includes a group of disorders that differ in severity of signs and symptoms. The disease is not uniformly seen everywhere but it has some topographical distribution. In India, it is frequently seen in Central India, in and around the vicinity of Nagpur. Despite the fact that Sickle cell haemoglobinopathy is infrequently observed, it has great pathological significance considering the high morbidity and mortality resulting from the disease process. The exact etiopathology at both molecular and genetic level has been extensively studied and deciphered thoroughly, yet there is no cure or established treatment regimen that will arrest the disease. Different modalities of treatment including bone marrow transplant are still in experimental stages and as today we do not have any satisfactory modality available that will be effective in treatment of this disease and its complications. Hence early diagnosis and efficient medical supervision for recognition of complications remain the gold standard in management of this inherited disorder. The risk of death from complications of Sickle cell disease is highest in children under the age of five years and it is suggested that with early detection and appropriate management the mortality in this age group can be reduced to less than five per cent.

Another important aspect as regards the prevention of Sickle cell haemoglobinopathy is genetic and marriage counselling as this being an autosomal recessive disorder and the incidence can be significantly reduced if consanguineous marriages in the susceptible community are avoided.

Skeletal manifestations resulting from this haematological disorder are seen in patients in all age groups as a result of the disease process, sequelae and its complications. Observations are based on the personal experience of more than fifteen thousand patients seen in the last three decades detected through various sickle cell centres opened in the region of Nagpur, Central India. These patients have been followed up on long term basis so as to document the various manifestations of this disease. Seven thousand three hundred and eighty patients were studied, followed and treated in last twenty five years (from January 1970 to December 95), amongst these nine hundred forty four patients (12.7%) had skeletal affection and many patients had multiple bone involvement. The patients were detected at Mayo General Hospital, Indira Gandhi Medical College, Nagpur, and Sushrut Hospital, Research Centre & Postgraduate Institute of Orthopaedics, Nagpur and during various surveys and camps especially in the vicinity of Nagpur, Central India, where the specific community of sicklers belonging to scheduled caste and tribes is thickly populated. Subsequent follow up was done at Sickle Cell Centres of Mayo General Hospital & Sushrut Hospital, Research Centre, Nagpur. Sickling was done by sickling test with sealed moist preparation as described by Daland and Castle in 1948 and diagnosis was confirmed by haemoglobin electrophoresis done with paper electrophoresis as described by Goldberg 1956. Each patient underwent a thorough clinical examination, height and weight parameters were accurately recorded, X-rays were taken and subsequently followed.

The main aim of this monogram is to present various skeletal manifestations commonly seen in patients of Sickle cell haemoglobinopathy, their pathogenesis and clinical presentations depending upon the site, time and pattern of involvement. After initial few years of various surveys, it was observed that the patients affected with this disorder had typical facies which we designated as **Sickler facies**. Anthropometrical criteria revealed a significant stunting of growth in the affected children as compared with unaffected normal identical children of same age, sex and community. These physical abnormalities are seen in patients with Sickle cell disease as well as trait and are observed much earlier than their expected time of reporting to the hospital or earlier than clinical presentation. Anthropometric study were done for the "Sickler facies" in detail with clinical photographs, X-ray of the skull and physical measurements. These facies are peculiar to Sickle cell haemoglobinopathy and can assist and be useful in the early detection of cases of Sickle cell disease.

Hence skeletal survey is an important factor in the early detection. Accordingly, apart from physical and facial anthropometry, skull X-ray, X-rays of the suspected skeletal involvement and growth measurements are important landmarks in diagnosing sicklers at the earliest amongst the specific community.

Promoting awareness regarding Sickle cell disease, its relation with socio-economic status, its presence in certain communities i.e. scheduled castes and tribes and clues to early diagnosis through mass education and encouraging frequent check up, especially in people of susceptible community will reduce the mortality and morbidity due to Sickle cell disease. Similarly observations based on personal experience, especially for early detection should assist Orthopaedic Surgeons, Radiologist, Paediatricians and Physicians in diagnosis and management of patients of Sickle cell haemoglobinopathy. Genetic and marriage counselling still remains the gold standard for prevention and dilution of disease until on effective cure is found.

2

Historical Aspects

Although Sickle cell disease has been known for years and many of its clinical features are recognised, yet some of its clinical manifestations are poorly understood. It is one of the less commonly observed diseases but of great pathological significance, that develops and can readily be identified in the early years of life.

In **1910, J.B. Herrick**, a cardiologist from Chicago first reported a case with "peculiar elongated and sickle shaped red blood corpuscles" in a case of severe anaemia. So called as "Herrick anaemia", Sickle cell anaemia affects almost all systems of the human body. It retards the growth and development, provides unequivocal evidence of impairment in various anthropometric measures e.g. height, weight, body fat, skeletal maturation, delayed puberty and skull growth. Thus Sickle cell anaemia acts as a great retarder of the human body.

Second and third cases of Sickle cell anaemia were reported by **Washburn 1911, Cook** and **Meyer 1915.** The term of "Sickle cell anaemia" was first used in **1922 by Mason**. In **1948, Daland and Castle** demonstrated a simple and rapid method for detection of sickling of red blood cells by the use of reducing agents. **Pauling 1949** found by use of electrophoresis that erythrocytes from the patient of Sickle cell trait contained approximately 60% normal haemoglobin and 40% abnormal haemoglobin. In Sickle cell anaemia patients he found 100% sickle haemoglobins. **Ingram 1959** showed that the chemical differences in haemoglobins is the substitution of valine for glutamic acid at the sixth position of Beta chain. The normal adult haemoglobin pattern is AA. In Sickle cell anaemia an abnormal adult haemoglobin, designed as haemoglobin "S" is present. The typical or homozygous Sickle cell anaemia is designated as SS. An increasing number of abnormal haemoglobins associated with Sickle cell anaemia have been identified so far and are variously labelled as SF, SC, AS etc.

According to **Ponder 1948**, sickling begins with the rim of cells becoming thicker on one side and thinner on opposite side. The thinning proceeds while continuity is broken down. Newly formed ends become separated by straightening out of the arc, which flattens biconcavity between them as the curvature decreases. The thinned and flattened out material of the biconcavative expands at its unsupported edge into a series of veil like material of the biconcavity follows the change of form of arc and its characteristic anisocyte looks like a very thin and almost invisible fringe between the sickle.

Fundamental abnormality resides in Sickle cell haemoglobin which is gene determined type of abnormal haemoglobin. In the deoxygenated state this haemoglobin 'S' is relatively insoluble, and forms needle like tactoids which destroy shape of erythrocytes producing characteristic sickle cell deformity. These sickled erythrocytes are mechanically more fragile and are phagocytosed readily and destroyed more rapidly in the circulation than are non sickled cells. This increased blood destruction is associated with jaundice—haemolytic type, hyperplasia of bone marrow, reticulosis and formation of immature cells in the peripheral blood and destruction which produces varying degree of anaemia. The clinical presentation of the patient depends on the type of crisis. The common being vascular occlusive or painful crisis. The other type of crisis is hyperhaemolytic crisis in which there is constant increase in the destruction of RBCs associated with erythroid hyperplasia in bone marrow. This hyperhaemolytic crisis is usually accompanied by bony pains, fever, anaemia, reticulosis and increased serum unconjugated bilirubin level. The Aplastic crisis is a misnomer since there is only an acute erythroblastopaenia. The word 'Crisis' was first used in association with Sickle cell anaemia in **1924** by **Sydenstricher.** However, the accepted definition and classification of Sickle cell crisis was reported by **L.W. Diggs, 1965.**

Sickle cell disease is an important cause for bone and joint pains and swelling. Skeletal changes in Sickle cell disease were observed as early as **1924 by Graham.** Association of skeletal changes with Sickle cell disease were also observed by **Caffey 1937, Golding 1959, Diggs 1965.** The effect of Sickle cell disease on skeletal system during the multiple episodes was reported by **Diggs 1965 & Handerson 1946.**

REVIEW OF LITERATURE

Skeletal changes in Sickle cell disease

Roentgenographic evidence of osseous manifestations in Sickle cell disease and in Cooley's anaemia was described in **1932 by LeWald L.T.**, who presented a most unusual and remarkable condition resulting from expansion of medullary cavity with thickening of the inner and outer tables of the skull, associated with peculiar radiating lines passing almost at right angles to the inner table of the skull. The skull was approximately 1 to 2 inches thick at the vertex, giving it a peculiar shape resembling that of tower skull. **Rose (1929)** examined skull of this type in which the blood findings that had been studied represented a Sickle cell anaemia. He described characteristic changes involving the vertex of the skull in Sickle cell anaemia, showing an enormous thickening in the form of radiating lines at right angles to the inner table of the skull.

In **1935 Grinnan A.G.** studied four cases of Sickle cell anaemia presenting roentgenological bone changes. The skull changes were characterised by thickening of the frontal, parietal, occipital, and temporal bones, with thinning of the inner tables and very thin or absent outer tables. The skull changes found in Sickle cell anaemia and erythroblastic, or Cooley's anaemia were so similar that they could not be differentiated by Roentgen examination alone. Long bone changes were found in one case of Sickle cell anaemia, consisting of cortical thinning, extension of the shafts, and medullary trabeculations. Striations found in erythroblastic anaemia occurred in the metacarpals and skull.

According to **Cooley T.B. et al. 1927, Reynolds,** in his first description of the skeletal manifestations in erythroblastic anaemia, mentioned a case of Sickle cell anaemia which showed thickening and vertical striation of the occipital bone, similar to the cranial lesions of erythroblastic anaemia. The long bones in this case were normal.

Borzell F.F. 1933, also found changes in the skull and long bones similar to those of erythroblastic anaemia. **Grinnan** examined four cases of Sickle cell anaemia - 4,5,7, and 11 years of age. The skulls in all cases showed lesions similar to those of erythroblastic anaemia.

Feingold B.F. and Case J.T. 1933 presented a careful roentgenological and haematologic investigation of a black infant, 15 months of age, with severe thickening and striation of the parietal bone. The long bone changes in this patient were negative. **Cooley and Lee** studied the skeletons of thirty cases of latent sickle cell anaemia.

Moore S. 1929 found some sickling lesions in his roentgen studies of a black, 24 years of age, with active Sickle cell anaemia. The skull showed findings identical with those of erythroblastic anaemia. The long bones, however, showed changes which were directly opposite those of erythroblastic anaemia. Moore thought that these manifestations in the long bones offered an important point in differential diagnosis between erythroblastic and Sickle cell anaemia. His roentgen findings in the long bones coincided almost exactly with the anatomic changes described by Graham. It should be emphasised that these osteosclerotic changes have never been reported in children, and they are not necessarily present in adults.

Fifteen patients, from 8 months to 15 years of age, with Sickle cell anaemia were studied by **Caffey J.** in **1937.** All these patients had splenomegaly with osseous changes.

The roentgenograms of the skull of patients with Sickle cell anaemia, which showed an increase in the thickness of the calvarium in all areas, were described by **Harden in 1937.** There was a loss of continuity of the outer table of the skull. The marrow cavity had been replaced by radially placed bone formations simulating many individual hair shafts standing erect. On gross examination the condition of the skull was classified as tower skull, with its increase in height and corresponding decrease in lateral diameter. There was also flattening of the frontal bones. The long bones of two patients described by Harden showed moderate thinning of the cortex, with diffuse coarse, irregular trabeculations of the medullary cavity, most marked near the ends of the bones.

Brandau G.M. 1932 found decreased density and splotching of the medullary portions in the tibia and fibula of a 22 year old black with Sickle cell disease. A 4 year old black girl whose "metacarpals have striations, giving the shafts a reticular structure" was described in **1935 by Grinnan A.G. Diggs L.W. et al.. 1937** reported periosteal elevation in roentgenograms of three children with Sickle cell anaemia, and in older patients with advanced osteosclerotic lesions. There were irregularities of the outer margin of the cortex and periosteal new bone formation.

Sickle cell anaemia with unusual bone changes, which occurred in a black male infant, was observed and described by **Danford E.A.** et al. in **1941.** This black infant, 8 months of age, with Sickle cell anaemia, developed symptoms of vomiting, fever and painful swollen hands. Fifteen days later, roentgenograms showed periosteal thickening and bone destruction of the metacarpals and phalanges. A marked anaemia and a high degree of sickling of the red blood cells, accompanied by otitis media, developed during the same period of time. After repeated blood transfusions, the health of the infant improved and the bone lesions disappeared entirely. The fourth metacarpal of the right hand and the second metacarpal of the left hand showed irregular areas of decreased density at the distal end involving the medullary cavity, cortex, and periosteum, a thickened periosteum along the shafts, with punched-out areas within its outline, and a cortex not abnormally widened; however, the parallel thickening of the periosteum gave each bone a rectangular appearance. The third and fourth metacarpals of the left hand were only slightly involved, but in a similar manner.

A case reported in **1947 by Kraft E. and Bertel G.** had an especially interesting feature, which was stunted growth, underdevelopment, and emaciation, observed in a 43 year old black male who had Sickle cell anaemia. Peculiar osseous texture and areas of porosis intermingled with coalescent coarse and sclerotic trabeculae were observed in the rib cage, which had generalised decalcification of the lower ribs. Ballooning of the cervical discs, with a biconcave shape of the cervical bodies, was also noticeable. Lipping and flattening, as well as sclerotic and porotic areas of vertebral bodies, were seen in the thoracic spine. Exaggerations of the lumbosacral curve were also evident.

Mushroom deformity of the femoral heads and moderate bilateral coxa vara deformity were simultaneously described. Kraft and Bertel further stated that skeletal changes at advanced age are different from those seen in early life and, because of the predominance of sclerotic bone reactions, may resemble osteoplastic carcinomatosis, Paget's disease, osteosclerotic anaemia, and leukemia and bone conditions observed on apparently healthy parents whose children are affected by Sickle cell anaemia.

A case of long standing Sickle cell anaemia associated with unusual roentgen changes involving the skull, tubular and flat bones were described by **Weil I.F. & Lerner H.H. in 1948.** The cortices were markedly thickened. The phalanges of the fingers and the metacarpal bones of the hands showed cyst-like areas within the medullary cavity, with expansion of the shafts. Both fibular and ulnar bones revealed cortical thickening. In some areas there was widening and increased trabeculations of the medullary cavity, with concomitant fending of the adjacent cortex. There was marked variation in density, suggesting cyst formation. The upper third of the left tibia showed marked overgrowth of the cortical bone, so that it encroached upon the medullary cavity. Weil and Lerner further commented that the bone changes were apparently secondary to the degree of strain placed on the hematopoietic reservoir, which would explain the rarity of bony lesions in young children.

Twenty six adults with Sickle cell anaemia were studied in detail by **Legant O. and Ball R.P. 1948** who described the most frequent abnormal finding as being cardiac enlargement. The abnormal bone finding in their group consisted of (a) generalised osseous demineralisation; (b) a biconcave deformity of the vertebral bodies, which was believed to be the result of bone softening; (c) patchy cortical thickening of the long bones, which might have been the result of infarction; (d) localised bony infarcts, five cases. Four of the twenty-six cases showed nothing abnormal on the films. One case, however, showed a patchy cortical thickening consistent with infarction.

Based on a radiological study of forty-eight cases of proven Sickle cell anaemia, **Macht S.H. and Roman D.W. 1948** concluded that the roentgen manifestations of changes in bone occurred later than the clinical findings of cardiac enlargement, heat, swelling and tenderness. These destructive bone changes are transitory and may be missed unless serial roentgen examinations are performed. Macht and Roman subdivided the skeletal changes into those caused by hyperplasia of the erythroblastic elements and those caused by thrombosis. The former lesions included irregular trabeculations,widening of the medullary spaces, and cortical thinning in the long bones, while the short and flat bones were characterised by exaggeration of trabecular markings of the iliac, scapulae, and phalanges. Cupping of vertebral bodies and widening of diploie of the skull, with thickening of the parietal and frontal bones, were also noted. Skeletal changes resulting from thrombosis were observed in the long bones, which revealed cortical thickening, narrowing of the medullary cavity, loss of bone tissue, and periosteal reaction. While the short bones were primarily affected by periosteal reaction and necrosis and resorption of bone, destruction of each first metacarpal & metatarsal bone of the hands and feet was also illustrated in a foetus born to heterozygous sicklers.

Collapse of the vertebral bodies in Sickle cell anaemia was observed by **Henkin W.A.** in **1949.** Two cases of Sickle cell anaemia, one in a black boy, age 14, with osteoporotic collapse of the thoracic and lumbar vertebral bodies, and the other in a black girl, age twelve and half, with similar changes in the lumbar vertebral bodies, were presented in detail. Coarsening of the trabecular structure was evidence of osteoblastic reaction in the weakened bone. The thoracic and lumbar vertebral bodies, composed of cancellous bone and subject to great stresses, may show a gradual reduction in height.

Sickle cell disease simulating osteomyelitis was described in **1949** by **Buchman J.** in a 5-year old black female child, roentgenograms on anteroposterior and lateral views of the left leg revealed a periosteitis involving the middle half of the fibula, with areas of rarefaction and sclerosis in the midportion of the shaft, characteristic of sequestration. The subsequent clinical course of the disease led to the belief that the lesion was caused by an aseptic necrosis of the shaft of the fibula, incidental to thrombotic and infarctive phenomenon occurring in Sickle cell disease, not as a manifestation of acute pyogenic osteomyelitis which was initially diagnosed on the basis of leukocytosis, high fever, and severe pain in the lower extremities.

In **1950 Hamburg A.E.** summarised the skeletal changes in Sickle cell anaemia and reached the conclusion that Sickle cell anaemia may be suspected from roentgenographic findings of the bones but cannot definitely be diagnosed from such evidence alone. In older patients the symptoms of bone and joint disease, rather than the anaemia, brought the patient to the attention of the physician. The essential changes of widespread thrombosis, infarction, and marrow hyperplasia account for the symptoms of the patient. The bizarre roentgenograms represented a far-advanced, long standing process, as indicated by the marked sclerosis and degenerative arthritis.

Two types of pathological changes may occur in the long bones of children with Sickle cell anaemia. A hyperplastic bone marrow represents the response to continued destruction of the erythrocytes, and this produces a wide medullary cavity and a thin cortex. The thrombosis of vessels in the marrow and bone results in abnormal areas of calcification and new bone formation producing a thick cortex and a small medullary cavity. The findings on roentgenographic examination will depend upon which of the two processes is dominant.

A 20 month-old black with Sickle cell anaemia, seen by **Almklov J.R. et al. 1950,** began at 4 months of age to have typical roentgenographic findings resulting from a hyperplastic marrow. The cortex in the femur had become so thin that a pathologic fracture resulted. According to Almklov et al. their 21 month-old black patient with sickle cell anaemia was the first reported incidence of the occurrence of a pathalogic fracture of the femur caused by excessive hyperplasia of the marrow, which resulted in a cortical thinness which was thought to be in a extreme degree.

Paratyphoid osteomyelitis caused by S.paratyphi is a comparatively rare entity. In **1934 Veal J.R.** and **McFetridge E.M.** added two cases to the eighteen which they found in the world literature. In **1949 Burch J.E.** reported a case of paratyphoid osteomyelitis complicating Sickle cell anaemia. **Wigh R.** and **Thompson H.J. in 1950,** added one more case of paratyphoid osteomyelitis in a patient with Sickle cell anaemia with unusual roentgen changes consisting of intracortical fissuring in the areas of osteomyelitis. Most authors described the osteomyelitis caused by S.paratyphi as being more frequently diaphyseal than metaphyseal in position. The cortical fissuring, however since it has not been described in instance of paratyphoid osteomyelitis occurring in otherwise normal bones, would appear to result from the underlying factor of a bony abnormality related to the Sickle cell anaemia.

Similar changes of bony lesion described hereforth were observed and confirmed in **1952** by **Ehrenpreis B.** and **Schwinger H.** who reviewed seventy two cases of Sickle cell anaemia. Aseptic necrosis involving femoral capital epiphysis, proximal epiphysis of the humerus, hair-on-end appearance of the skull, loss of vertical height, and alteration of the height-width ratio of the spine were also described. Biconcave deformity and a spotty sclerosis of the bodies of the vertebrae were considered specific changes in patients with Sickle cell anaemia.

In **1952 Robinson I.B.** and **Sarnat B.G.** first described the roentgenographic changes in the maxillary and mandibular bones in patients with Sickle cell anaemia. Eighteen of their twenty-two patients with Sickle cell anaemia showed relative degrees of osteoporosis. Robinson and Sarnat emphasised that dental roentgenograms should be taken in addition to those of the long bones and the skull, since Sickle cell anaemia is a systemic disease.

Aseptic necrosis of the femoral head was described by **Moseley J.E.** and **Manly J.B. (1953)** in patients with the Sickle cell trait. Their patient, a 38 year old male black baker, was brought to the hospital with rather severe joint pain, presenting radiographic evidence of aseptic necrosis of the hips and shoulders, with secondary degenerative arthritic changes at the weight bearing joints. There was sickling but no anaemia. Four other cases presenting aseptic necrosis of bone occurred in young black patients with Sickle cell anaemia whose ages ranged from 7 to 38 years. There was no direct correlation between the severity of the disease and the occurrence of bone necrosis. Aseptic necrosis may be present associated with osteosclerosis, with osteoporosis, or in the absence of any other osseous abnormality.

One case reported by Moseley and Manly was particularly interesting because the skeletal changes occurred in the presence of a normal blood count and hemoglobin. Aseptic necrosis of the femur, resulting from bone infarction, was characterised by marked sclerosis associated with areas of rarefaction in the head of the femur, which was misshaped and flattened on its superior aspect. Bony destruction and production in the head of the left humerus and trabeculae in the head and neck of the right humerus were also seen in all four patients with Sickle cell anaemia. Diffuse osteosclerosis in the spine and the medial aspect of the iliac bones were frequently associated with aseptic necrosis of the femoral heads as reported by Moseley and Manly. Aseptic necrosis, as seen in Sickle cell disease, may resemble the radiographic changes occurring in Caisson's disease, Legg-Perthes disease, slipped femoral epiphysis, advanced hypertrophic arthritis and necrosis following interruption of the circulation in fractures of the femoral neck, and dislocation of the femoral head.

The cases described by Moseley and Manly indicated that aseptic necrosis may occur in Sickle cell disease in a wide variety of ages, being demonstrated in patients from 7 to 38 years of age. The occurrence of aseptic necrosis apparently caused by Sickle cell disease, with a normal blood count, suggested that in the presence of clinical or radiographic findings consistent with Sickle cell disease a normal blood count does not exclude such a diagnosis.

Aseptic necrosis of bone in Caucasians with chronic haemolytic anaemia, resulting from combined sickling and thalassemia traits, was described in **1953** by **Reich R.S.** and **Rosenberg N.J.**, who observed three patients in two Caucasian families in whom both Sickle cell and Cooley's traits occurred simultaneously. Two of these patients had aseptic necrosis of the head of the femur and one of them had similar changes in the head of the humerus. Neel suggested that perhaps some of the cases reported as Sickle cell anaemia in Caucasians might rather show Sickle cell trait as well as Cooley's trait.

One patient of Reich and Rosenberg who had Sicilian parents presented evidence of Sickle cell trait as well as Cooley's trait, with roentgenographic changes in the heads of the femur and the humerus. The second patient was a 12 year old boy whose mother and father were both Sicilian. The aseptic necrosis exhibited in roentgenograms was confined to the head of the left femur and had been indistinguishable from Perthes disease. It has been observed that the skeletal changes in Sickle cell anaemia are more common in weight bearing bones and among older age groups. In thirty nine patients studied at necropsy by Diggs et al. only one was over the age of 31.

Smith 1953, described two cases of salmonella like osteomyelitis occurring in two patients with Sickle cell anaemia.

A case of thalassemia with Sickle cell anaemia in a patient who developed S. enteritidis septicemia and osteomyelitis was presented by **Goldenberg I.S. 1955** who described an 11 year old boy of Sicilian parents. Thalassemia major with sickling had been demonstrated at age 7. A solitary, localised destructive process was present in the midportion of the shaft of the right fibula, slightly above the midpoint. The destruction was symmetrical about the cortex, associated with slight periosteal new bone formation.

According to **Golding** in his article 'The Bone Changes in Sickle Cell Anaemia' there were about one million Africans south of the Sahara with Sickle cell anaemia in **1956.** Earlier, Raper had reported that the incidence of Sickle cell anaemia varied from tribe to tribe between 0.25 and 45 per cent, with an overall incidence of about 20 per cent, yet Sickle cell anaemia was a rare diagnosis. Golding continued by stating that patients with Sickle cell anaemia are usually small with a short trunk and comparatively long, thin limbs and "spider" fingers. There is often mild kyphosis and lordosis. The chest tends to be hoop-shaped. In children the abdomen is protuberant. Chronic ulcers over the lower third of the legs are quite frequent. The most common form for the crisis to take is to simulate some bone or joint disease. A crisis has been described as early as in a 19 day old infant.

The twenty skull radiographs in Golding's series showed marked changes in six cases and mild but definite changes in an additional six cases. The most common radiographic change was a loss of trabecular definition giving a ground glass appearance to the skull. The outer table appeared thin and partly absorbed, as suggested by **Cole in 1955.** The classical hair on end appearance was not common in Sickle cell anaemia and was more likely to be seen in thalassemia. The peculiar result of erythroid hypertrophy in the diploic marrow accounted for the tower skull deformity, which was characteristic. The parietal bones were usually symmetrically affected according to Hamburg (1950). In the long bones as the medulla hypertrophied, the cortex was thinned on its inner surface. The diaphyseal extremities widened and, as osteoporosis proceeded, the metaphysis appeared relatively denser.

The flat bones, pelvis, scapula, and particularly the ribs showed these changes very well. Thus the ribs showed wide trabeculae, osteoporosis, a thin cortex, and sometimes patchy erosion or sclerosis if the process of infarction had been superimposed. This was a most useful finding, for these changes were often visible on the chest film. Golding stated that these hyperplastic changes were of more interest to the clinician in making the diagnosis than anything else, for they do not cause symptoms.

Although avascular necrosis, causing death of complete bone, was not seen in Golding's series, it has been described in the wrist and tarsal navicular as well as in the lumbar spine. Death of a whole segment of shaft was seen in a child of 15 months, who was admitted to a hospital with a history of pain and swelling in the lower part of the buttocks, which had been present for the previous three weeks. The patient was shown to have Sickle cell anaemia; both parents had the trait. The child was uncooperative and miserable, according to Golding, and there was slight pyrexia. The upper part of both thighs was intensely painful, and there was pseudoparalysis of both legs. A radiograph showed that the upper one third of both femoral shafts was symmetrically expanded and that within a shell of subperiosteal new bone formation the shaft was infarcted and crumbling. There was an obvious pathological fracture on the right side and possibly a healing fracture on the left, accounting for the new bone formation. This was at first thought to be an unusual type of osteomyelitis, but as there was a negative blood culture and the fever rapidly settled, the diagnosis was revised. In four weeks the structure of the bone could be seen to be returning to normal, and the tenderness had completely disappeared. Five weeks after admission the patient again became miserable and the temperature rose to 102 . Six months after discharge from the hospital, the patient had tenderness and swelling of the left ankle, which settled without trouble. There were no X-ray changes in the ankle. At this time the femoral shafts were seen to be enlarged, but the bone structure had returned to normal.

According to Golding, at the children's Hospital in Los Angeles, three case of Salmonella osteomyelitis and two cases of osteomyelitis caused by *H. influenzae* B were demonstrated in children who very often had no history of intestinal infection but who were found to have Sickle cell anaemia. Golding stated that this remarkable association of two rather rare conditions, as far as the United States is concerned, is not understood. Two factors would seem to play a part in this association :

1. Certainly before the advent of antibiotics, and possibly still, a number of Sickle cell children must have succumbed to the overwhelming force of an attack of staphylococcal osteomyelitis.
2. Most of the literature was written in pre-penicillin days.

Since the introduction of antimicrobial agents, the incidence of osteomyelitis has decreased in the general population, except for children under the age of 1 **(Blanche 1952).** However, the incidence of osteomyelitis in patients with haemoglobinopathies is greater than in the general population with osteomyelitis of etiology other than Salmonella in proven Sickle cell hemoglobin C disease **(Lohmuller and Marshall 1958).** The pathogenesis of osteomyelitis in Sickle cell disease has been described by many authors **(Curtis 1959, Green et al. 1956, Henriques 1958, Hook et al. 1957, Silver et al. 1957, Trueta 1953, Turek 1959, Widen and Cardon 1961).** It has been shown that minute capillary thrombosis occur throughout the body as a result of the sickling phenomenon. These may permit entrance of bacteria to the blood from nonsterile foci, such as the gastrointestinal tract, or from foci of infection, such as the genitourinary tract.

As a result of this bacteremia, organisms lodge in areas of bone which have undergone localized ischaemia, devitalization, infarction, and necrosis and which provide fertile areas for bacterial growth, and osteomyelitis results. In keeping with this hypothesis, most of the cases of osteomyelitis in patients with homozygous S disease are in young children, but most cases with the heterozygous disease are in older children and young adults, according to Widen and Cardon. This age distribution of osteomyelitis corresponds to the ages at which symptoms of thrombosis and crisis first occur in Sickle cell haemoglobinopathies.

In patients with haematogenous osteomyelitis in the general population whose primary site of infection is the genitourinary tract, E.coli is the most frequent cause of the osteomyelitis **(Brandt et al. 1956, Henriques 1958, Keefer 1941, Spittel et al. 1954).**

The diagnosis of acute haematogenous osteomyelitis is particularly difficult to establish in patients with haemoglobinopathy. Both conditions exhibit similar bone changes resulting from multiple small thrombosis. Those associated with haemoglobinopathy include generalized osteoporosis, increased trabecular markings, irregular thickening of the cortex,with areas of localized rarefaction, abnormal new bone formation, irregularly margined medullary cavities, with narrowing and occasional obliteration, small areas of sclerosis, mild to moderate fish mouth appearance of the intervertebral margins, with cupping or biconcave deformity, and small areas suggestive of infarction. Any or all of these changes may be present, but generally they are less marked in the heterozygous than in the homozygous haemoglobinopathies. These changes are quite similar to those seen in acute haematogenous osteomyelitis. Nevertheless, osteomyelitis of the long bones in patient with hemoglobin disorders is limited almost exclusively to the diaphysis whereas it is a metaphyseal juxtaepiphyseal process in patient with normal hemoglobin constitution. An aid in detecting the presence of infection is the finding of longitudinal intracortical fissuring; this considered by some to be pathognomonic of osteomyelitis in patients with Sickle cell haemoglobinopathies (Hook et al.).

Clinically, patients with haemoglobinopathies have repeated bouts of bone pain, tenderness, fever, leukocytosis, and toxicity. The bone pain in crisis, as in osteomyelitis, may be unilateral, migratory, juxta articular, or in the bone shaft, and of comparable severity. A history of gradual onset of deep bone pain, accentuated at night in the recumbent position, is important in suspecting an underlying osteomyelitis. Therefore, one must be alert to the possibility of superimposed osteomyelitis in sickle haemoglobinopathies and not simply attribute the pain or other manifestations of toxicity to crisis per se. Careful roentgen-ray examination to uncover this masked but treatable complication is mandatory.

Carroll D.S. 1957 observed rather frequently thrombosis and aseptic necrosis involving an entire ossification center, such as an epiphysis. There were nine cases of aseptic necrosis of the capital femoral epiphysis among the patients with Sickle cell disease. One patient had aseptic necrosis of the head of the humerus, one had aseptic necrosis of the primary centers of ossification for the bodies of the ninth and tenth thoracic vertebrae, and one had aseptic necrosis of the patella. Since the incidence of epiphysitis or aseptic necrosis in Sickle cell disease is so high (10 percent of Carroll's cases) it is probably wise to exclude Sickle cell disease in all black patients.

Four of Carroll's patients with Sickle cell disease had an associated Salmonella osteomyelitis. The reason for this increased incidence of Salmonella osteomyelitis in sicklers was not definitely known, but it could possibly have been caused by thrombosis in the wall of the gut, allowing enteric organisms to enter the bloodstream. All of the patients with Salmonella osteomyelitis showed involvement of multiple bones, and infection was quite severe. Periosteal proliferation was the first sign, followed by widespread areas of bone destruction, extending throughout the shaft of the bone. Destruction was sometimes severe enough to be associated with pathologic fractures. In none of Carroll's cases had the infection crossed the epiphyseal line. Cortical fissuring was frequently seen, and it was thought that this was due to the fact that in Sickle cell anaemia the haversian canals were quite wide and permitted easy extension of the infection into the cortex of the bone. The combination of rapidly destructive osteomyelitis involving several bones, together with cortical fissuring, was such a typical clinical picture in black patients that one should suspect the combination of Salmonella osteomyelitis and Sickle cell disease.

Extensive bone destruction with marked periosteal reaction, occurring in the small bones of the hands of children with Sickle cell anaemia, was illustrated by **Victor** and **Imperiale 1957,** who described two black children, ages 7 months and 13 months respectively. Roentgenographs of the hands showed multiple areas of rarefaction in the bones, with marked widening and periosteal proliferation which were most evident in the first, fourth, and fifth metacarpals of the hands. The Orthopedic consultant's diagnosis was tuberculous dactylitis.

Ivy R.E and **Howard F.H. 1953** reported a black girl age 1, who developed swelling, tenderness, and increased warmth in the hands and feet on the fifteenth day of illness. On X-ray there were radiolucent areas in the distal metaphysis of the radial and ulnar bones, as well as in the metacarpals and phalanges; these areas were both subperiosteal and intramedullary. There was also medullary expansion in the phalanges. In **1954 Tori G.** described another case with destruction and periosteal reaction of the metacarpal bones of both hands. Custer noted the occurrence of fibrous patches and areas of new bone formation, particularly in the marrow of the long bones, and felt that they probably mark the site of intramedullary thrombosis or haemorrhages.

Many have suggested that capillary thrombosis in the gastrointestinal tract might lower the resistance of patients with Sickle cell anaemia to invasion of the body by intestinal organism. **Hook E.W. et al. 1957** pointed out that the general debility and disease of the spleen associated with Sickle cell anaemia might well interfere with the general defense mechanisms after the body has been invaded by Salmonella. Once the organism has entered the bloodstream, it may find favourable conditions in areas of ischaemia and necrosis which result from the blockage of small vessels by sickled cells.

The recognition of salmonella infection of the bones can be difficult in Sickle cell anaemia. Fever, pain and swelling of the limbs and joints are found in many cases of infarction and osteomyelitis. On X-ray examination the bone infarction of Sickle cell anaemia and of osteomyelitis look very much alike. Even if the diagnosis of osteomyelitis is made, it is difficult to decide whether the infection is streptococcal or staphylococcal. Hook et al. emphasized the need for aspiration of the infected bone if the diagnosis is in doubt. The most effective treatment of Salmonella osteitis is chloromphenical and surgical drainage. However, the results are not dramatic. Hodges and Holt found drug sensitive organisms to persist in the tissue for months in one patient, and in another they noted a recurrence of the osteomyelitis two years after the apparent healing of a previous infection.

Sherman M. 1959 suggested that the minority of patients having Sickle cell anaemia live long enough to have permanent damage to joints, usually the hips. It appeared that the damage to the joint and head of the femur was related to pathologic changes in the small vessels and attendant focal haemorrhage. Sherman further postulated that the breakdown of the hip joint in patients with Sickle cell disease appeared to depend upon several mechanisms, all of which were secondary to local damage to extremely small vessels. There may be complete interruption of the circulation to the head, perhaps caused by damage to the vasa vasorum; focal haemorrhage in the soft tissues; and inflammatory changes. This may be followed by the classic picture of creeping replacement and late pathologic fracture at the advancing margins of revascularisation. Chronic synovitis, also caused by focal haemorrhage, activated the synovial membrane to grow across the articular surface as a pannus and destroy the cartilage from above.

Golding J.S.R. et al. **1959** redescribed the bone changes in fifty one cases of Sickle cell anaemia, nineteen cases of Sickle cell hemoglobin C disease, and two cases of Sickle cell thalassemia. Avascular necrosis of the head of femur has been found in all three types of Sickle cell disease. The changes found in six cases of Perthes disease in the blacks were compared with the damage in avascular necrosis of the head of the femur in Sickle cell disease, Hyperplastic bone changes were only seen in two cases of sickle cell anaemia and in none on the variants. In Sickle cell anaemia the erythroid hyperplasia affects the bony trabeculae and causes absorption, osteoporosis, softening, and change in shape; this is well illustrated in the vertebrae, which are affected in about 70 percent of cases.

Reduction of the vertebral height and broadening of its transverse diameter, with biconcave plate impressions, was mentioned in **1959 by Deibert** who emphasized that in an average adult a correlation exists between the vertical height and transverse breadth of a lumbar vertebra. The average height width ratio of a lumbar vertebra is 1:1.8; in the case of Sickle cell anaemia it was 1:2.8, confirming the observations by Golding et al..

Dunnagan W.A. 1960 studied three cases of Salmonella osteomyelitis, two of which were complications of Sickle cell anaemia. The skeletal changes occurring in these cases gave further support to the opinion that children with Sickle cell anaemia have a predisposition to osteomyelitis and that there is a striking tendency for paratyphoid organisms to be the offending agent. The roentgen characteristics of polyosteotic involvement, particularly of the upper extremities, diaphyseal predilection, extensive periosteal proliferation, and longitudinal fissuring of the cortex of tubular bones were further substantiated.

The combination of osteomyelitis, Salmonella infection, and Sickle cell anaemia was described in three patients, ages 8, 19 and 33, by **de Torregrosa M.V. et al. 1960.** The infecting organism was identified as S.typhi, S.st.paul, and S.typhimurium, respectively, in the three patients. One patient had been treated with penicillin for two years without success. It is important to identify the organism and to recognize the nature of the anaemia in cases of this sort, for open, suppurating lesions that discharge Salmonella are dangerous to attendants, and antibiotics are of no avail unless they are adapted to the causative organism. Murphy in 1916, found an incidence of 0.82 percent of osteomyelitis among 18,840 patients with typhoid fever. The figures for osteomyelitis after *S. paratyphi A, S. paratyphi B*, and other *Salmonella*-produced septicemia are also low. By contrast the association of *Salmonella* caused osteomyelitis with Sickle cell disease is frequent. In Los Angeles Country Hospital, among 865 children with osteomyelitis, only three had *Salmonella* as the offending agent, and all three had Sickle cell anaemia (**Roberts A.R.** and **Hilburg L.E. 1958**). It was suggested that there is danger of the spread of *Salmonella* infections from patients with open, suppurative lesions.

According to **Pollen A.G. 1981** and **Cockshott W.P. 1958** radiological bone changes in Sickle cell hemoglobin C disease may be divided into three groups: (a) changes associated with erythropoietic marrow hyperplasia, the result of a chronic haemolytic anaemia; (b) changes resulting from bone infarction;

(c) changes associated with bone infection. These patients seem peculiarly prone to develop Salmonella osteomyelitis, and they may show lesions typical of chronic osteomyelitis. Bone changes in Sickle cell haemoglobin C disease were also observed in detail by **Barton** and **Cockshott** in **1962.**

The development of these lesions has been well described and illustrated by **Sherman 1959 and Bobechko** and **Harris 1960.** The hip joints are most often involved, and next in order of frequency are the shoulders, but other joints can be implicated. In Nigeria, according to Barton and Cockshott, Sickle cell hemoglobin C disease is responsible for hip changes far more than is the homozygous disease. The high infant mortality in true Sickle cell anaemia in Africa means that many children do not live long enough to develop hip disease. The changes in the hip joints present at a later age than in Perthes disease, and the two types of avascular hip changes can usually be differentiated by roentgenography. The avascular process is often multifocal in Sickle cell hemoglobin C disease, rather than affecting the whole of the capital epiphysis, as in Perthes disease.

Three types of roentogenographic changes which may be noted in the hips in this disease are as follows:

1. Coarse osteoporotic trabeculations and a degree of coxa vara.
2. A focal area of hip disintegration caused by involvement of sector of the femoral head, consequent on vascular thrombosis. (This is really a form of osteochondritis dissecans. As a rule, fragment of the femoral articular surface will be found to have become depressed following the collapse of the underlying subchondral bone).
3. Generalized narrowing of joint space resulting from multiple vascular focal lesions.

Among the antenatal patients of Barton and Cockshott, three were found who had dactylitis, and one patient showed active bone infection. The hand roentgenograms of two of the seven blood donors showed evidence of previous dactylitis. In the clinical group, as is to be expected since there were more children, the incidence of active bone infection or infarction was far higher. Twenty-eight percent showed evidence of one or another of these conditions and in 24 per cent the lesions were in an active stage when first seen. Five patients all children under the age of 10 had active dactylitis. Three others were incidentally noted to have a shortened digit, consequent on previous infarction of other long bones involved, the humerus was implicated seven times, the femora four times, and the ulnae, tibiae, and radii three times, other sites affected include the clavicle, pubis, and ilium. Salmonella bone infection frequently follows bone infarction in the sickle haemoglobinopathies.

Hendrickse R.G. and **Collard P. 1960** in their series, found four proven instances of bone infarction, including an acute arthritis affecting a hip joint. In three patients with backache, changes were noted in the lumbar vertebral bodies. **Becker J.A. 1962** stated that the osseous manifestations seen in Sickle cell haemoglobin C disease are the same as Sickle cell anaemia, the sequelae being marrow hyperplasia and bone infarction.

Smith E.W. and **Conley C.L. 1954** felt that the finding of aseptic necrosis is almost indicative of a diagnosis of Sickle cell hemoglobin C disease in a patient demonstrating sickle cells; however, this aseptic necrosis can also be found in Sickle cell anaemia patients. A case of osteomyelitis in the extremities in Sickle cell hemoglobin C disease was described by **Sackner M.A. 1959 et al.**, but the etiology was not Salmonella.

Various osseous alteration described repeatedly were readily demonstrable in our series, ranging from massive erythropoietic hyperplasia to ischaemic infarction with absorption and aseptic necrosis of the femoral head. No "fish vertebra" however, was observed in our cases.

In **1963 Burko H. et al.** reviewed the roentgenograms of 126 children with Sickle cell disease in a period of over five years (1956-1961) at Kings County Hospital Center in New York, and disclosed several unusual skeletal changes resulting from infarction. The bony abnormalities in Sickle cell disease were caused by marrow hyperplasia, infarction, and osteomyelitis. The hand-foot syndrome was caused by infarction of the short tubular bones of the hands and feet. The bony changes were related to absorption of infarcted areas and hyperaemic stimulation of the adjacent periosteum. This syndrome occurred in twenty one children (17 percent) usually in the first two years of life. Bilateral symmetrical scapular infarcts, which have been reported previously, were evident in two children. Infarction of an entire long tubular bone was also an unusual event and was noted to involve the fibula in one case. This single instance of associated *Salmonella* infection was a Salmonella chondritis.

In **1964 Hewett B.V.** and **Nice C.M.** summarised the radiographic changes occurring in sickle cell subjects. Generalized deossification was the most common radiographic finding in the skeletal system. Widening of the diploe and thinning of the outer table result in a thickened skull that may appear granular on the radiograph. The classic hair on end appearance resulting from radiostriations of the prominent diploic trabeculae in children was a rare finding, prominence of the trabecular pattern of alveolar bone was greatest between the roots of the teeth. Deossification occurred, and the trabecular pattern was accentuated in the spine and the pelvis. There was also cortical thinning and a decrease of the vertical height of the vertebral bodies. There may be biconcave end plates secondary to prolonged pressure from the nucleus pulposus or collapse of the vertebral body; less frequently there may be localized osteosclerosis secondary to infarction.

Watson J. and **Burko H. 1963** designated "Hand-foot syndrome" a common initial manifestation of Sickle cell disease is usually seen in children and is referred to a condition in which there is dactylitis resulting from symmetrical involvement of metacarpals and metatarsal bones. It is manifested by painful swelling of dorsum of hands and feet. Painful crisis involving joints and extremities usually is seen in early childhood. Pain may be due to infarction of long bones and bone marrow or involvement of periarticular tissue. Painful abdominal crisis are due to infarction of areas of liver, spleen and lymph nodes. Pain is usually attributed to stretching of the capsules of these structures. The first case of dactylitis in a child with Sickle cell anaemia was reported by **Danford and associates** in **1941.** In **1960 Smith** used the term "Hand-foot syndrome" in describing this acute swelling in hands and feet of children with Sickle cell disease.

Leg ulcerations are infrequently seen in this disease as chronic presentation over both malleoli in adolescents or in adults but are uncommonly seen in children.

There are various types of medical manifestations which is beyond the scope of this book.

REVIEW OF LITERATURE ON ANTHROPOMETRY

Sickle cell trait is usually considered to be a clinically benign condition **(M.K. McCormack et al. 1975)**. However there is increasing evidence to indicate the contrary, that is, the clinical pathophysiology is variable, ranging from benign condition in most cases, to relatively few cases of severe pathological involvement. Although it is generally agreed that gross anatomical lesions are rarely seen in Sickle cell trait, current data indicate that sickle cell carriers may be susceptible to some of the pathophysiological symptoms commonly seen in Sickle cell anaemics. Even in Sickle cell trait many complications have been reported at both high altitude and at sea level, including Pulmonary infarction, Splenic infarction, Massive haematuria, Renal papillary necrosis, Renal failure, retroperitoneal fibrosis, Osteomyelitis, Leg ulcerations, retinal artery occlusion and death. It is rather a condition which clinically ranges from no effects, in most cases to delayed physical growth and development and in rare cases, even to severe clinical manifestation and sometimes death. Persons with Sickle cell trait lead relatively normal life but those with disease seldom live past forty years and usually presents with variety of clinical manifestations, i.e.

Fatigue and weakness.
Pains in long bones and joints
Pains in hands and feet
Cardiomegaly and systolic murmur
Chronic leg ulcerations and osteomyelitis
Severe abdominal pain and sickling crisis
Icteric sclera and epistaxis
Bone deformities like tower-shaped skull, kyphosis, scoliosis
Spleno/hepatomegaly
Variety of orthopaedic manifestations

Despite the several studies the effect of homozygous Sickle cell disease on the growth of young children is not clear. Normal weight but subnormal height was reported by **Winsor T & Burch J E. 1944**, a normal height but subnormal weight was reported by **Scott R B et al. 1955 and Gray R H 1971**. Both height and weight were subnormal **(Whitten C F 1961, Jiminez C T et al. 1966, Dicker L M K et al. 1976).**

Sickle cell trait children show significant decreased skeletal age, total body height and biacromial breadth **(Mc Cormack M K et al. 1976).** When compared with normal children, SS children have smaller body measurements and lower skeletal age, total body height and biacromial breadth (**Mc Cormack M.K. et al. 1976). Booker et al. 1964** noted that retardation in weight began as early as 6 months, but was not noted in new born infants & neonates (**M.S. Krammer 1980).** This is because the blood of newborn infants with Sickle cell disease contain only 10-20% of HbS and physiological evidence of sickling does not begin until diminution of Haemoglobin F concentration after 5-6 months of life. Longitudinal data is necessary to assess children with expected delay in somatic and sexual development. In children two hormones are essential to growth, growth hormone (GH) and thyroid hormones. G.H. is secreted directly from the pituitary and works in conjunction with somatomedin. Samatomedin is a "growth hormone dependent plasma factor" which affects the growth of cartilage, as well as the metabolism of adipose tissues, muscles and other tissues. The thyroid hormones T3-T4 have profound effects on growth by action on messenger RNA transcriptase, as well as on the rate at which the body produces energy.

Low weight for height appears to persist throughout life and is one of the most characteristic anthropometric features of adult with S S disease (**Ashcroft M.T.** and **Sergeant G.R. 1972).** Changes of height with age are more complex. Height for age in this study differs little from standards upto 13 years but thereafter (**Ashcroft M.T., Sergeant G.R.** and **Desai P. 1972**) falls behind. This lag is probably associated with delay in the puberty (**Jiminez C.T. et al. 1966)** but the growth spurt occurs later so that the final height of S S adults is similar to that of normal (**Ashcroft M.T.** and **Sergeant G.R. 1972).**

The growth failure which was observed in subjects with Sickle Cell anaemia at ages 11 to 16 years. is consistent with prior deficiency of gonadal steroid secretion necessary for optimal growth. The observation of subnormal height in S.S. children coupled with finding of normal adult height in patients with this disorder indicates that the growth failure of adolescent S S subjects is temporary (**Ashcroft M.T. 1972** and **Sergeant G.R. 1986).**

Ashcroft & Sergeant 1972 study showed that the average height of younger S S subjects was less than controls but this was not observed at later ages. This evidence suggests that the increase in stature during the adolescent period is greater in the S S children than normals, and may be associated with the delay in skeletal maturation. This could possibly result in longer legs and above average heights seen in S S adults (**Ashcroft M.T. 1972).** In adolescence there is marked acceleration of linear growth as well as the onset of sexual maturation. During adolescence the velocity of linear growth doubles. Trunk length, muscle mass and cortical bones all increase, while fat decreases. This adolescent growth spurt is accompanied by and related to the occurrence of sexual maturation. **Winsor T. & Burch G.E. 1944** described subnormal heights and weights in the adults. These patients had short trunk, long limbs and evidence of gonadal hypofunction as demonstrated by diminution in facial and body hair and absolute & relative sterility.

In India only **Dr. B.R. Kate's 1967,** publication could be traced regarding the Anthropometric studies in patients of Sickle Cell anaemia. He studied only 25 patients of proved Sickle cell anaemia, by 30 various measurements and 10 indices were calculated and compared with normal values. The results showed overall subnormal growth of cranium. Various other measurements were smaller than normal except facial length and frontal breadth.

3

Epidemiology and Pathological Aspects

Sickle cell haemoglobinopathies represent a family of related molecular disorder. These related types of Sickle cell diseases are grouped under one heading of "Sickle Cell Haemoglobinopathies" which includes Sickle cell anaemia (homozygous SS), Sickle cell trait (heterozygous SA), Sickle cell haemoglobin C disease, Sickle cell Thalassemia, Sickle cell haemoglobin D & G disorder and Sickle cell hereditary spherocytosis. Commonly we came across Sickle cell trait (SA) and Sickle cell anaemia (SS) in this area of Central India. Patients of Sickle cell trait leads relatively normal life since it is a benign state except under grossly unphysiological condition, and in that situation it can behave exactly like the patients of Sickle cell anaemia whereas patients of Sickle cell anaemia seldom live past forty. There is still no cure for this painful disabling disease.

Normal adult human haemoglobin is actually composed of two different haemoglobins which can readily be separated by electrophoresis. The major portion of haemoglobin molecules is called haemoglobin A; the minor portion is called haemoglobin A_2. The haemoglobin A molecule, besides the haem group, contains a total of 574 amino acids. All of the amino acids except isoleucine are present. These aminoacids are joined in peptide bonds and form two pairs of two different polypeptide chains, alpha and beta chains. There are two alpha chains and two beta chains in each molecule, and these are coiled in helical fashion in the intact molecule. Each alpha chain contains 141 amino acids; each beta chain contains 146. Analysis of haemoglobin A_2 shows that it is similar to haemoglobin A and contains two alpha chains and two other chains that are designated as S chains which are distinct from alpha and beta chains.

Haemoglobin of a human foetus or a newborn baby contains still a different haemoglobin named F. Hemoglobin F is characteristic of the human foetus and is replaced by adult haemoglobin A in normal individuals within the first 2 months after birth. Hemoglobin F consists of two alpha chains, the same as those found in haemoglobin A, and two others which are distinct, designated as γ chains. The γ chains contain all twenty amino acids including isoleucine. Large segments of alpha, beta and γ (and S) chains contain homologous or invariant sequences, that is, the order of the amino acids is identical in many portions of the chains.

SICKLE CELL HAEMOGLOBINS

One of the most interesting mutant human haemoglobins has been designated haemoglobin S. The mutation affects the beta chain. Haemoglobin S may be separated and distinguished from haemoglobin A by means of starch-gel or paper electrophoresis. Haemoglobin S may be demonstrated by performing a sickling test on fresh blood. When the red cells are placed in an atmosphere from which oxygen has been excluded, then the reduced oxygen tension leads to the crinkling of red cells into sickle shapes when they contain

HbS. Individuals whose red cells do this are called sicklers, and the disease is called Sickle cell anemia or sicklemia. The Sickle cell trait is inherited as if it were a nondominant autosomal allele. Both heterozygotes and homozygotes have anaemia of varying degrees of severity. The red cells from both genotypes sickle in an oxygen-free atmosphere; the sickling of red cells of heterozygotes is less severe, and the sickling of red cells of homozygotes is more severe. The homozygous individuals are severely affected and usually die before reaching maturity. The presence of the Sickle cell gene, as the allele is often named, produces a large number of clinical symptoms, among which are enlarged spleen, rheumatism, impaired mental functions, and the aforementioned anaemia and various skeletal manifestations. The consequences of this mutation are dramatic.

The observation that haemoglobin S and haemoglobin A are electrophoretically different (the two haemoglobins do not migrate the same distance on paper or starch) immediately suggests that there is a difference between the two in amino acid composition and primary structure. It has already been proved the difference lies in the beta chain, and a demonstration of the specific biochemical defect in haemoglobin S was made when Ingram 1956 performed his famous "fingerprint" experiments and paper electrophoresis.

Skeletal changes in Sickle cell haemoglobinopathies

In this paragraph the Pathology and Biochemistry of Sickle cell haemoglobinopathies is described along with salient features.

1. Pathology

Bone changes in Sickle cell disease occur mainly because of hyperplasia of bone marrow and because of vascular insufficiency resulting into thrombosis and infarction. Associated bone infection is quite common leading to osteomyelitis and sequestration. Because of hyperplasia the multiple erythrocyte causes increase in blood viscosity, stasis, capillary thrombosis and finally infarction of bone. The initial infarcts occur in the most distal portion of bones (i.e. femoral head), in the subchondral area, where there is maximum sickling and where the circulation through collaterals is very poor and limited. The blood supply is reduced to the cartilage and bone & it shows the dead bone which is avascular and impaired. Continuation of the weight bearing on this femoral head leads to the flattening and irregularities in the contour of femoral head. In later stages proliferative arthritic changes appear in the hip joints. In addition to the femoral head necrosis, there are changes in other bones also. Changes are seen in long bones, skull, vertebrae, short bones of the hand and feet, ribs and scapulae. Changes due to vascular insufficiency like avascular necrosis are seen in patient's humeral head also. Roentgen findings in skull includes - thickening of the outer table, "hair on end" appearance and marked osteoporosis. In long bones there is marked thinning and irregularity of cortex, prominent trabeculations, expansion of medullary cavity. All these changes are mainly because of hyperplastic bone marrow.

2. Biochemistry

Haemoglobin is a conjugated protein containing 4 haeme and a globin with a molecular weight of 66,7000. "Pauling 1949 and co-workers" showed the difference in electrical charges causing the Sickle cell haemoglobins to move differently from normal, Hb. in an electric field and is explained by difference in the aminoacid composition of globin content of normal and sickle cell. Globin is a polypeptide chain of 28 short Amino acids. "Ingram " 1956 showed the change of Hb A - Glutamyl in Hb A is replaced by Valine in HbS and this change occurs at Beta chain only.

There are many varieties of Sickle cell disease and its genetic variants - depending upon the abnormal Hb - SS, SAF, SF, SC Sickle cell trait etc. The changes are more in SS, SF & SC because of severity of Sickling which results in the early death from occlusive disease before skeletal maturity.

Pain in the musculoskeletal system prompts the affected to seek orthopaedic assistance. Therefore, Orthopaedist may be the first physician to see patients of Sickle cell disease. Early diagnosis and treatment of the disease may not correct the condition completely but would certainly go a long way in arresting its disabling consequences and complications. Assessing and predicting the rate of recovery is obviously a concern of both the orthopaedist and patients and their relatives.

Though severity and type of Sickle cell haemoglobinopathies may be a primary factor in determining the chances and speed of recovery, it may not be the sole factor. Other factors that may count in the recovery of patients may be genetic involvement, age, sex, personality make up, socio-economic status and, of course, the quality of treatment. Each of these factors by itself and possibly with interaction with other factors may count in the rate of recovery. The primary interest of this book is to spread awareness about the contribution of some selected factors individually and through their interaction with other factors, to the process of recovery in Sickle cell haemoglobinopathies.

MOLECULAR BASIS OF SICKLING

Basic defect in haemoglobin "S" is substitution of valine in place of glutamic acid at 6th position on "β" chain. Difference being glutamic acid is hydrophilic, while valine is hydrophobic, with acidosis and hypoxia decreasing the distance between 2 Hb "S" molecules (Fig. 3.1). Ultimately instead of one normal hydrophobic amino acid at "N" terminal sickle haemoglobin has two hydrophobic amino acids in "Beta" chain.

The chain assumes importance that when sickling process is initiated by acidosis and hypoxia two "HbS" molecule are brought together which in turn leads to hydrophobic bonding. The crystallization of two "Hb-S" molecules leads to formation of one anciomorphic molecule of Hb-S which has tendency for parallel alignment along the cell wall, making cell wall weak. This progresses to tactoids formation and red blood cell gradually assumes, the shape of "sickle" to be called as sickled red blood cell. While flowing through capillaries and small sized blood vessels there is, mechanical entanglement which leads to stasis, invoking vasospasm, liberation of coagulation factors, which adds to vaso-occlusion so the involved vascular territory suffers ischaemia and ultimately infarction. These episodes are responsible for ischaemic "pains" which characterise the course of disease. The vaso-occlusive crisis is most characteristic and dramatic phenomenon and is diagnostic hall mark of Sickle cell disease. The vaso-occlusive crisis is most common type of presentation of Sickle cell disease.

Unconjugated hyperbilirubinaemia, increased reticulocyte count, erythroid hyperplasia in bone marrow and shortened life span of erythrocytes are parameters indicative of haemolytic process in Sickle cell anaemia

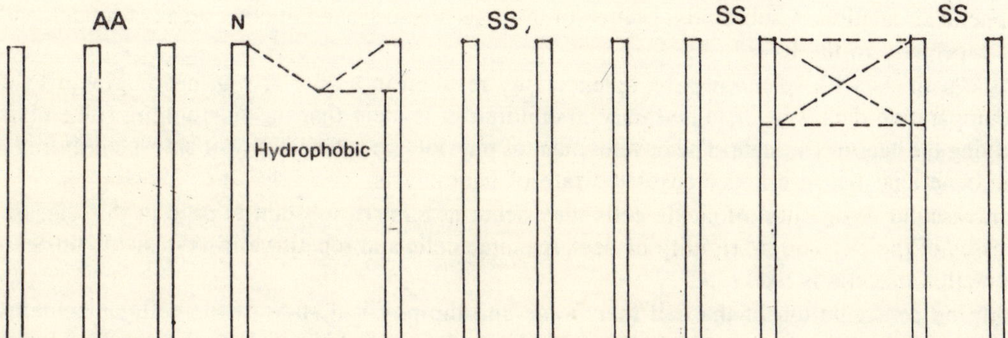

Fig. 3.1. Diagram showing hydrophobic binding, crystallization and parallel alignment of haemoglobin which results in formation of sickled RBCs.

where sickle cell ultimately die is not entirely clear but both intravascular and extravascular haemolysis occurs. Intravascular destruction of sickle cells may occur at a fairly substantial pace in this disease. There is hydrophobic bonding, crystallisation, parallel alignment which results in formation of sickled RBCs.

Sherman's (1940) observation of birefringence in sickled RBCs proposed that certain surface region of deoxygenated molecules bear sufficient configurational similarity to each other so that one molecule can fit closely against another molecule much like the fitting of antigen to antibodies. Deoxygenated molecules of Hb "S" according to this concept would aggregate to form aligned structers of sufficient rigidity to distort RBC membranes into sickled shapes.

Some other observations suggested, loss of oxygen lowered the solubility of Sickle haemoglobin and that the insoluble polymers taking on needle like configurations formed bundles of sufficient rigidity to sickle the cell.

ULTRASTRUCTURAL FEATURES OF ERYTHROCYTE AND HAEMOGLOBIN SICKLING

Haemoglobin polymerisation develops from process of condensation, interaction, aggregation and assembly. Molecular organisation of structures formed during polymerisation depends on the type of haemoglobin, its specific defect and its state of oxygenation. Sickling exemplifies haemoglobin polymerisation in the reduced state. Sickle haemoglobin (Hb"S") alone or in combination with other haemoglobin undergoes condensation, aggregation and assembly into long rod-like structures. Oxygenated or red normal and abnormal haemoglobins and oxy-Hbs also polymerise, they form aggregates microtubules or rods but molecular reorganisation of earlier structures into a new lattice is required. Thus Sickling is due to sol-gel transformation rather than crystallisation and polymers of Hb "S" are unique because they differ in molecular organisation from haemoglobin aggregates, microtubules and crystals. Normally in capillaries bigonal erythrocyte flow centrally with plasma lined on both sides thereby linear flow is smooth. Sickled erythrocytes get mechanical entanglement leading to sluggish flow. There is increase in viscosity, liberation of local factors ultimately leads to partial or total obstruction so that particular vascular region suffers ischaemia or infarcts. Here "pain" starts. This phenomenon can occur anywhere in body and thus "pains" and "aches" characterises the course of the disease.

HAEMOLYSIS IN SICKLE CELL DISEASE

Unconjugated hyperbilirubinaemia, increased reticulocyte count, erythroid hyperplasia in bone marrow and shortened life span of erythrocyte are parameters indicative of hyperhaemolytic process in Sickle cell anaemia. Where sickle cells ultimately die is not entirely clear, but both intravascular and extravascular haemolysis occurs. Increased number of cells in the sickled shape are encountered in the spleen as compared to peripheral circulation. A substantial portion of the cells are destroyed in other areas of reticuloendothelial system especially in the liver.

In the patients with splenomegaly, splenectomy resulted in a 43% rise in haemoglobin value while these comparative data were obtained only in children, it is clear that the functioning spleen has role in intensifying the haemolytic state. The development of physiologic splenectomy or autosplenectomy in adults may be beneficial because it decreases the rate of haemolysis.

Intravascular destruction of sickle cells may occur at a fairly substantial pace in this disease. Given the stresses of the circulation, rigidity of deoxygenated cells and repetitive in vivo sickle unsickle cycle, fragmentation of cells is likely.

Both the configuration of the cell membrane and the physical state of the cellular contents play a role in haemolysis. Documentation of increased plasma haemoglobin levels during the first few hours of painful crisis has recently been reported as evidence of accelerated haemolysis. Biochemical interaction that may accelerate haemolysis in "SS" patients is the associated defect of glucose-6-phosphate dehydrogenase deficiency. This has been shown to produce hyperhaemolytic crisis.

EPIDEMIOLOGY OF SICKLE CELL GENE IN INDIA

The origin of the sickle cell gene is unclear. There are two principal theories, one that a single ancestral mutation occurred and then spread to occupy the present geographical distribution, and the other theory favouring the multiple mutations in different areas.

The chief proponent of the first hypothesis was Professor Hermann Lehman who proposed that a single ancestral mutation in the area of Mesopotamia could have been followed by migration of the gene down into equatorial Africa, to the eastern province of Saudi Arabia, across to India and North-wards to Mediterranean region. Lately the multiple mutation theory has received more support, deriving partly from the recognition of other abnormal haemoglobins arising as new mutation but also from work on the polymorphisms of DNA surrounding the beta-globin gene complex.

Studies in Africa indicated that the Hb "S" gene was observed on genes with atleast two different polymorphisms when examined by the restriction enzyme HpaI. Further studies in the Carribean have indicated atleast 10 different patterns of polymorphism that, these data are possible because polymorphism could have arisen, secondary to the Hb "S" mutation or may have preceded it. However, it is considered most likely that the Hb "S" mutation occurred on a variety of chromosomes bearing different polymorphic sites and probably in different areas.

Regardless of the mechanism involved, the abnormal Hb "S" gene was selected because of the advantages conferred in malarious areas. This resulted in high prevalence of the sickle gene, throughout equatorial Africa reaching prevalence upto 40 % in parts of East Africa (Fig. 3.2). Throughout West Africa, the sickle cell trait occurs in 15.25 % of most populations. It is from this area that the black population was carried to the Carribean area and North America. The sickle cell gene now occur in 10 % of black population in the Carribeans and in 7 % of those in the United States. From the Carribean there has been a secondary migration to Europe.

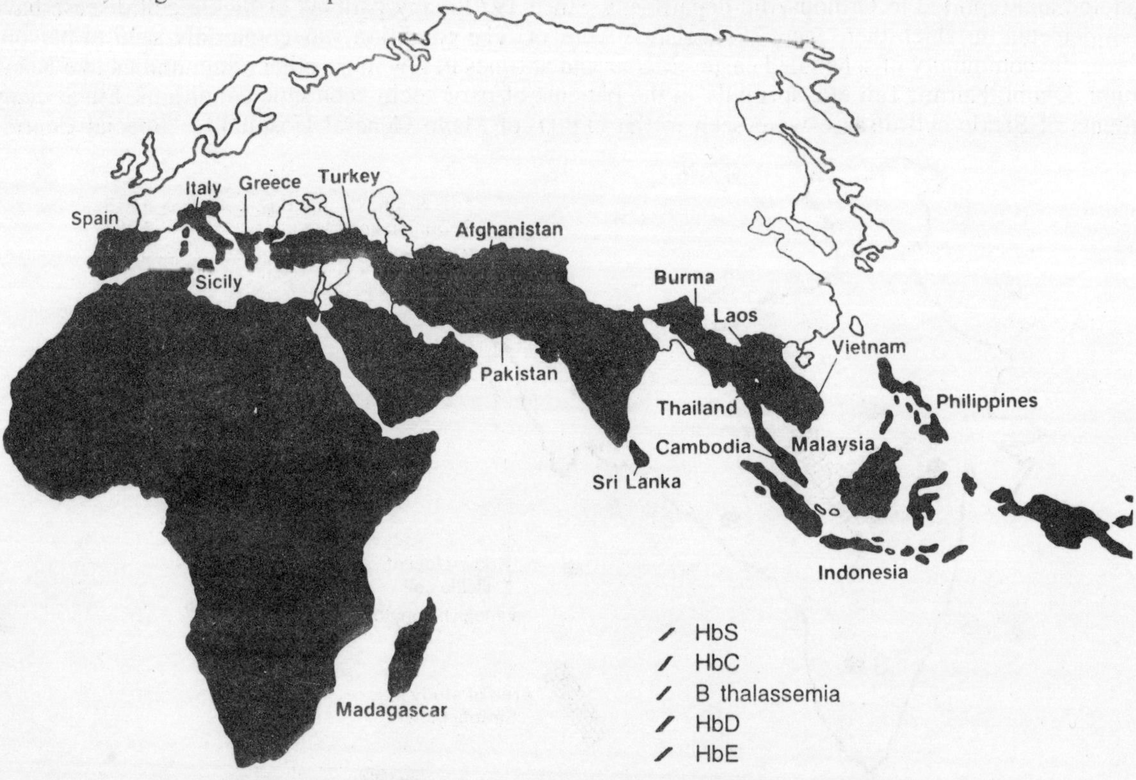

Fig. 3.2. Map of the world showing prevalence of different types of Sickle cell haemoglobinopathy. HbS types of Sickle cell disease is commonest in India.

The gene also occurs in Mediterranean areas characterised by a history of malaria including Sicily and southern Italy, the south coast of Turkey and northern Greece where some villages in the Chalkidhiki Peninsula have trait rates as high as 30%. Another important focus occurs in the Eastern province of Saudi Arabia where the sickle cell trait occurs in 20-25% inhabitants of Qatif and Al-Hasa. The gene is also well recognised in the Indian subcontinent.

The homozygous condition for Hb "S" obviously also occurs in all these areas but displays marked geographical variation in both clinical and haematological features. This variation results from the interaction of the disease with other genetic and environmental factors, the elucidation of which will teach us much about the mechanisms of sickle cell disease.

Sickle cell traits were first reported in India by Lehman and Cutbush (1952) among the aboriginal tribes of South India. Since then it has been reported in tribes of Western India, tribal population of Orrisa and Bihar. Workers in tea-gardens in Assam, in the tribal population of Uttar Pradesh,and also among the Hindi-Marathi speaking population belonging to low socio-economic group (Mahars, Telis and Kunbis) of Maharashtra in and around Nagpur.

Many cases of Sickle cell haemoglobinopathies have been reported in India (Dunlop & Mazumdar 1952, Lehman & Cutbush 1952 & Tyagi 1954). The existence of Sickle cell disease (Sickle cell anaemia & Sickle cell trait) in this area of Vidarbha and surrounding Nagpur (Central India) is well known. The first article from the region of Nagpur (Shukla & Parande) appeared in 1956 and subsequently many articles are published from this region on the topic of Sickle cell disease (1958) (Fig. 3.3 and 3.4). Dunlop and Mazumdar (1952) reported presumptive cases of Sickle cell anaemia from tea-garden labourers of Assam. R.N. Shukla and B.R. Solanki (1958) examined 1010 adult labourers of different caste for the Sickle cell trait. In Mahars, Kunbis and Telis its incidence ranged from 9.4% to 22.2%.

The interest in this disease was developed when many patients of this genetic disorder involved the skeleton and reported to Orthopaedic department. Since 1970 many patients of Sickle cell disease have been detected in which there were skeletal involvement. The condition was commonly seen in persons of specific community of scheduled caste - Mahar and at times in few more other communities like Kosti, Kunbi, Dhobi, Kurmi, Teli etc, specially in the patients of poor socio-economic conditions. Since many patients of Sickle cell disease were seen in the O.P.D. of Mayo General Hospital, a "Special Centre"

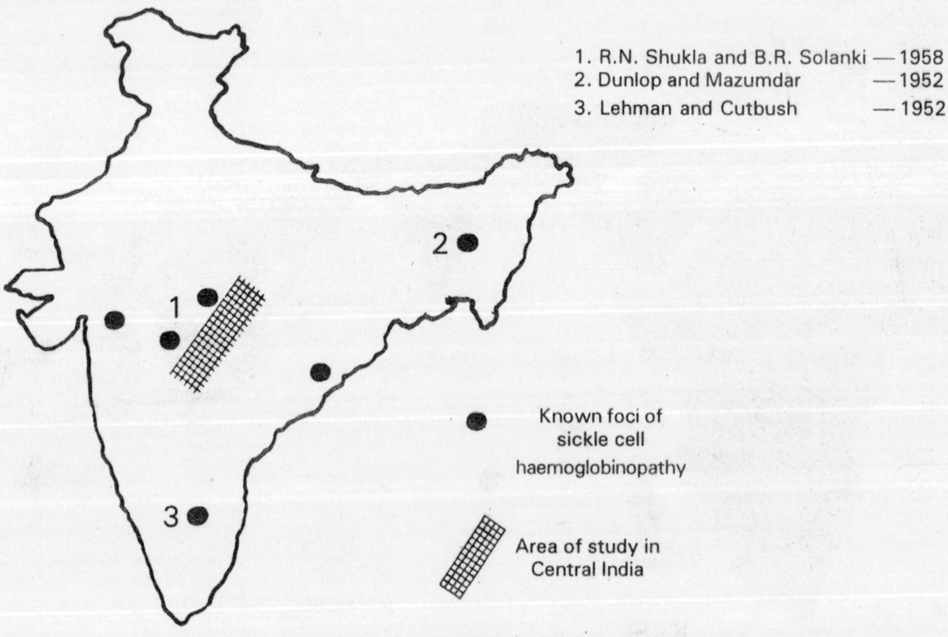

Fig. 3.3. Map of India showing the different sites from where the work on Sickle cell haemoglobinopathy is published or carried out.

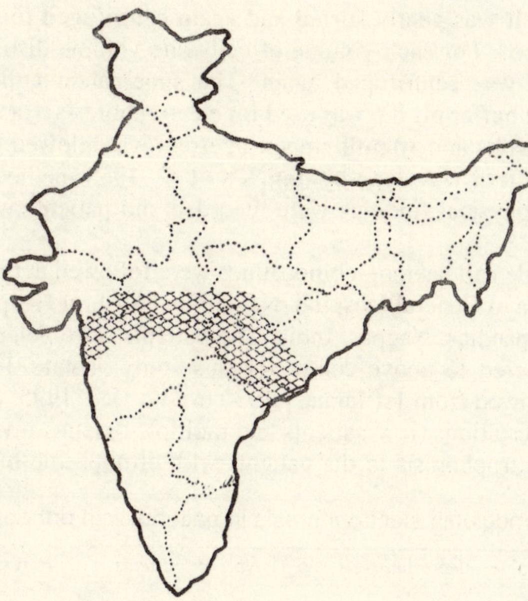

Fig. 3.4. Map of India showing the belt of Sickle cell along the border of the states of Gujarat, Madhya Pradesh, Maharashtra, Orissa and Andhra Pradesh.

was opened only for the patients of Sickle cell disease. In the year 1977-78 more than five hundred patients of Sickle cell disease were screened and diagnosed which were inhabitants of specific areas in the region of Nagpur, mostly the slums. Most of the patients were very poor and illiterate who did not seek the medical advice, hence camps were taken in these areas for screening of Sickle cell disease. (Random survey was carried out in such areas).

ANTHROPOMETRIC MEASURES

To study in detail each patient of Sickle cell haemoglobinopathy certain anthropometric measures were decided to find out exact criterion for identification of these sicklers amongst the community. As stated earlier face has been chosen as prime criteria to detect the faces of the sicklers among the known community in whom the affection of Sickle cell haemoglobinopathies is very common. Certain anatomical points were fixed to measure the positive findings for these sickler faces. Few more anatomical points were also chosen like pelvis, long bones - tibia and femur for the anthropometric measures in these patients of Sickle cell haemoglobinopathies.

The subjects (children, adolescents and adults) were measured wearing light clothing, without any footwear. Height was measured by using Anthropometer with the subject standing erect and heels touching together and against the vertical bar of height scale. Weight was measured by the same weighing machine for all the subjects by the same person.

Sickling was done in all patients by sealed moist preparation described by Daland & Castle 1948. Freshly prepared 2 per cent solution of sodium meta-bi-sulphite was used as reducing agent. The erythrocytes were observed immediately after 15 minutes and after 24 hours for delayed sickling (Fig. 5.1, 5.2, 5.3)

The haemoglobin electrophoresis was done by either paper electrophoresis as described by Goldberg 1957 or by other described methods. Haemolysite was prepared by placing 5 cc of oxalated blood into centrifugal tube. It was centrifuged for 10 minutes. The supernatant was withdrawn & 10 cc normal saline was added to the packed cells. It was gently stirred and again centrifuged for 10 mts. Supernatant was withdrawn and cells were washed. For each volume of cells one volume distilled water was added and was shaked vigorously and it was centrifuged again. The supernatant collected now was used for electrophoresis. Sodium barbital buffer pH 8.6 was used for electrophoresis. Haemolysite was applied over Whatman No. 3 paper and 250 volts and 10 milliamperes current was allowed to pass for 12 to 16 hours. The staining electrophoresis pattern was done by **Jenck's et al. 1955** method.

In every patient's history, physical findings were recorded and patients were X-rayed according to the clinical proforma.

All the proved cases of Sickle cell haemoglobinopathies were followed at the Sickle cell centre, Indira Gandhi Medical College and Mayo General Hospital, Nagpur and Sushrut Hospital, Research Centre, and Postgraduate Institute of Orthopaedics, Nagpur, India. The patients were detected in various camps and different OPD's and were referred to above centre for this study. Total 7380 patients of Sickle cell haemoglobinopathies were followed from 1st January 1970 to 31st Dec. 1995. Out of these 7380 Sicklers 944 patients had skeletal manifestations (few patients had multiple osseous involvement). Following was the pattern of haemoglobin electrophoresis in the patients with orthopaedic manifestations.

Table 3.1. Pattern of haemoglobin electrophoresis in patients with orthopaedic manifestations

Sl. No.	*Type of haemoglobin electrophoresis*	*No. of patients*	*Percentage*
1.	S S Pattern	333	35.27%
2.	A S Pattern	441	46.71%
3.	S F Pattern	88	9.32%
4.	A S F Pattern	82	8.68%
	Total No. of Patients	944	

Sickle cell traits (A.S.) was observed in almost 50 % of these patients. Out of these 944 patients only about 60 % patients required frequent hospitalisation. The hospitalisation was mainly required for crisis or infection of bone, chest & Urinary tract (like osteomyelitis) and those patients requiring surgical treatment.

All these patients mainly reported for the pain in bones and joints, swelling and frequent recurrent infections. Few patients reported for inability to walk and painful limp, and growth retardation. All these patients were thoroughly examined and investigated in detail.

Crisis was mainly seen in patients with SS haemoglobin and required medical treatment every now and then. Both the group of patients of Sickle cell disease and Sickle cell trait were followed in the centre irrespective of whether they had symptoms or they required any treatment. Following was the profile of osseous involvement and their age-sex incidence.

Table 3.2 showing details of Age and Sex in 944 patients of Sickle cell haemoglobinopathies with skeletal involvement in this clinical study.

Table 3.2. Age and sex distribution

Age Group	*No. of Patients*	*Male*	*Female*
00-05	208	112	96
06-10	323	187	136
11-15	279	153	126
16 & above	134	79	55
Total	944	531	413

PATHOPHYSIOLOGY OF SKELETAL CHANGES

The fundamental abnormality in hereditary Sickle cell disease resides in the abnormal structure of the globin portion of the haemoglobin molecule. Sickle cell haemoglobin (Hb S) differs from the normal adult haemoglobin (Hb A) in that valine is substituted for glutamic acid in the 6th amino acid position in each of the 2 beta polypeptide chains. This change in the structure of the haemoglobin molecule alters the net electrical charge and allows electrophoretic separation. Hb S is much less soluble than Hb A when in the deoxygenated state. In the erythrocytes, the insoluble haemoglobin molecule aggregate in elongated direction and needle like polymers (tactoids), which distort the shape of the red cells, producing characteristic sickle cell deformity.

Blood containing long, multipointed, curved and rigid sickled cells is more viscid and flows less readily through terminal vessels. Utilisation of oxygen by living blood cells and by endothelial and tissue cells favours an exaggeration of sickling. Chronic stasis of blood in capillaries and defective oxygenation leads to infarction in various tissues. Sickle cells are mechanically more fragile, are phagocytosed more readily and are subject to haemolysis in the circulating blood. The imbalance between blood destruction and formation leads to chronic haemolytic anaemia, the degree of anaemia depending on the type of disease.

Skeletal changes in Sickle cell haemoglobinopathies occur mainly because of hyperplasia of bone marrow and vascular insufficiency resulting in thrombosis and infarction. Associated bone infection is quite common leading to osteomyelitis and sequestration. Because of hyperplasia of erythrocytes there is increase in blood viscosity, stasis, capillary thrombosis and finally infarction of bone. The bone marrow which is hyperplastic tends to expand at the expense of trabecular and cortical bone producing osteoporosis. These changes are more marked in the flat bones of skull, trunk and cancellous ends of the long bones. The specific changes are discussed under different headings in subsequent chapters.

Skeletal changes in Sickle Cell haemoglobinopathy develop as a result of two pathological processes:

(i) Chronic haemolytic anaemia, secondary to spontaneous erythrocyte sickling and premature cell death, leading to bone marrow hyperplasia.

(ii) Sickling resulting in tissue ischaemia and bone infarction secondary to small vessel thrombosis. Osteonecrosis of the femoral head is very common presentation of Sickle cell disease. The high incidence can be explained on the peculiar vascular supply of femoral head where single vessel - the ascending branch of lateral femoral circumflex artery or one of its branches if affected can lead to osteonecrosis of the femoral head. The detailed skeletal and orthopaedic manifestations are discussed in individual chapters.

4

Clinico-Radiological Aspects

The patients of Sickle cell haemoglobinopathy may present with specific symptoms pertaining to skeletal region involved or may have vague presentation of haemolytic disorder. Pathological changes are seen in the bones which are basically secondary to haemolytic anaemia which results into bone marrow hyperplasia, congestion, thrombosis with resultant infarction, necrosis and at times infection. These skeletal changes vary in different individuals depending upon the severity of the disease and may present in different stages. Changes can be grouped either into early or late changes or depending upon the region involved (Johnston et al. 1966).

The first report of a pathologic study of bone changes in Sickle cell anaemia was by Graham in 1924. He described the condition consisting essentially of chronic infection or toxic injury to the marrow and medullary bones with subsequent repair process and compensatory hyperplasia. Among his observation was focal necrosis, destroying soft tissues and injuring trabeculae. In 1953 Reich and Rosenberg described the pathophysiology of bone changes occurring in Sickle cell anaemia.

The exact mechanism by which infarction develops remain obscure. Some investigators consider it a sequelae to emboli. Others feel it is a vasospasm which leads to chronic inflammation and intense osteoblastic activity indicated by new bone formation. Radiological changes may lag 2 to 3 weeks behind the onset of clinical signs and symptoms.

In the normal tubular bone, the compact cortex is responsible for most of the density seen on the radiograph. Since the shadow cast by normal bone spongiosa is relatively faint, it seems apparent that severe changes may develop here before being detected on roentgenograms. Macht and Roman (1948) noted a time difference in the appearance of symptoms and radiographic findings as great as 21 days.

EARLY CHANGES

1. **Hyperplastic bone marrow**- due to increased demand of blood there is an increase in the volume caused by the formation and growth of new cells.
2. **Osteoporosis** - due to erythroid hyperplasia of bone marrow displacing normal bone structure and resorption of bone.
3. **Thinning of cortex** - due to resorption of bone and increased volume of marrow cavity - compensation of the cortex occurs.
4. **Jelly-like marrow** - due to increased viscosity of the red cells as a result of the compensated action of the marrow.

LATE CHANGES

1. **Thickening of cortex** - due to thrombosis of the vessels in bone causing necrosis, haemorrhage, fibrosis and new bone formation in the form of linear trabeculae or concentric layers of lamellated bone adjacent to cortex.
2. **Osteoblastic hyperplasia** - due to ischaemia, an area of necrotic bone is produced and is surrounded by hyperaemia which promotes bone forming process.
3. **Narrowing of medullary cavity** - due to new bone formation in the form of linear trabeculae or concentric layers of lamellated bone adjacent to the cortex resulting in the widening of the cortex at the expense of medullary cavity.
4. **Normal Calcification** - due to deposits of calcium which stimulate the local formation of fibroblasts to osteoblasts with bone formation.
5. **Softening and changes in bone shape.**
6. **Bone infarcts and irregular bony thickening of cortex.**

SKELETAL CHANGES

While the signs produced in bone are not all uniquely indicative of the disease, many are distinctive, and some of those produced by the ischaemia are almost pathognomonic. When such changes are detected in multiple sites, the roentgenographic diagnosis of Sickle cell haemoglobinopathy is virtually assured.

Compensatory marrow hyperplasia is not a prominent roentgenographic feature of the disease except as it affects the skull, and even in this site, changes are frequently subtle and often absent. The notorious "hair standing on end" pattern frequently cited in the older literature as a characteristic of Sickle cell anaemia is actually rather rare. The usual finding consists of simple thickening of the diploe with thinning of the outer table of calvarium in the frontal and parietal regions.This response to chronic anaemia can be detected in about fifty percent of those with SS disease.

The expansion of erythropoietic tissue in the spine, pelvis, and ribs may cause the elimination of finer trabaculae and cortical thinning. In some patients, the effects of this are manifested in the axial skeleton by moderate osteoporosis and a coarse reticular pattern produced by the remaining trabeculae, which appear prominent. However, these changes in the texture and quality are usually subtle and difficult to assess. Their interpretation can be largely subjective, and therefore, their diagnostic value is limited.

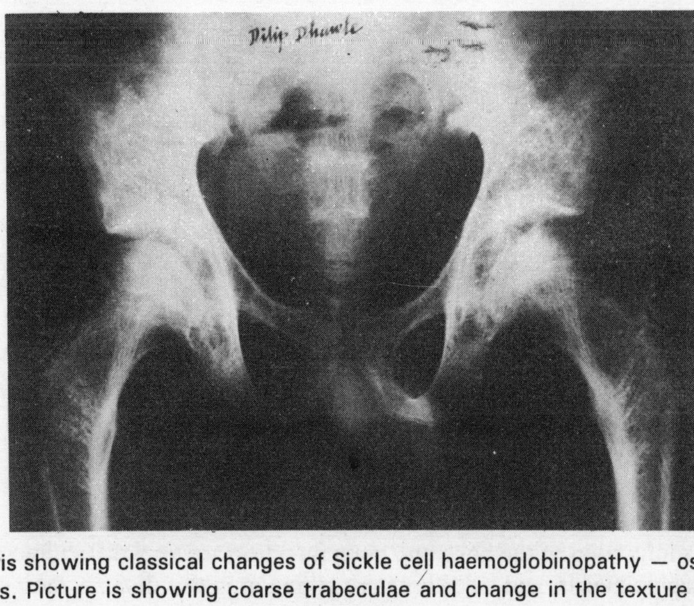

Fig. 4.1. X-ray of pelvis showing classical changes of Sickle cell haemoglobinopathy — osteoporosis, rarefaction and at places sclerosis. Picture is showing coarse trabeculae and change in the texture and quality of bone.

In contrast, the effects of focal ischaemia commonly produce dramatic radiological changes in the bone. Although massive infarcts do occur to produce large destructive lesions, most of the roentogenographic signs of ischaemic necrosis evolve slowly from the cumulative effects of recurrent, small episodes of infarction within the spongiosa. Initially the infarct produces no visible change, but with repair, new bone is laid down on the dead trabeculae, with resultant increase in roentgenographic density. Eventually, these small, sclerotic foci coalesce to produce, by the second or third decade, larger areas of dense bone. The roentgenographic features of these ischaemic lesions vary with their location within the skeleton, and they are best discussed according to their anatomic region.

In the long bone shafts, two different patterns are encountered. The most common consists of small, poorly marginated, mottled and strand like zones of increased density that are randomly distributed within the medullary bone. The femurs, the tibias and the humeri are most frequently involved and the changes are usually bilateral. This is one of the most common radiological stigmas of Sickle cell haemoglobinopathies. Occasionally in older patients, extensive mottled bony sclerosis is seen to involve the axial skeleton as well.

The other pattern encountered in the diaphysis is less common but very distinctive. It consists of a layer of dense bone near the periphery of the medullary canal but separated from the inner aspect of the cortex by a narrow lucent zone. Although less compact than cortical bone, it resembles a cortex within the cortex, and the unique sign is of great diagnostic value. It usually involves the femurs and humeri bilaterally.

The tubular bones of the hands and feet in children are susceptible to massive infarction, which may involve the entire shaft. Such lesions are most common between 6 and 24 months of age, when these bones are the site of accelerated erythropoiesis. It is more common in the hands and metacarpals bilaterally. This "Hand-Foot Syndrome" produces pain and swelling, and it is difficult to distinguish from osteomyelitis, both clinically and roentgenographically. Initially, no bony changes are evident, but about two weeks after infarction, periosteal new bone formation becomes visible about the afflicted shaft and this may last for six or eight weeks. Major bony destruction and prominent deformities are not common, but occasionally there is enough ischaemic damage to cause growth arrest.

Bone infarcts seen in Sickle cell haemoglobinopathy produces striking roentgenographic picture of extreme bone destruction and rapid new bone formation and rapid rebuilding. First kind of such infarcts was published by Diggs et al. in 1937 who stated that patients with this disease were subjected to attacks of severe bone pain with localised tenderness, fever and leucocytosis leading to a false diagnosis of osteomyelitis and subsequent unrequired surgery. On opening of bones in such patients no exudate was encountered and marrow cultures were sterile. The phenomenon of bone infarcts in Sickle cell disease has long been recognised and aseptic necrosis resulting into infarction pathologically has been described virtually in every organ and tissue of the body.

It is observed that many cases of bone infarction in individuals with Sickle cell anaemia go unrecognised either because no films are made, or because of an insufficient interval between the onset of symptoms and roentgen examination. Cases in which bone lesions are discovered, on the other hand, may be mistakenly diagnosed as osteomyelitis when the lesions in reality were uncomplicated bone infarcts.

The earliest radiological sign is nonspecific swelling of soft tissue and obliteration of the fat planes which may lag behind the clinical presentation. The radiological development of destruction of bone at the site of necrosis and infection requires approximately 30% to 50% of demineralisation before the lytic process can be appreciated (Dana Majid et al. 1984). This lytic process is the earliest change in the bone with new bone formation appearing afterwards.

In their early stages infarction of the bone and bone infection are very difficult to distinguish by either clinical or roentgenographic means, and since both are common in this disease, their correct identification is frequently the source of diagnostic dilemmas. Fortunately, however, recent publication in nuclear medicine have described differences in the scintigraphic patterns of these entities that should make their early and accurate diagnosis possible at times and hence clinical findings and its assessment is important for the exact diagnosis.

Bone infarcts present in a variety of changes ranging from homogeneous increase in the density to a bizzare mottled destruction and collapse. Medullary infarcts usually appear as a localised lucent area surrounded by reactive osteosclerosis or calcification. In adults common long bone changes are diffuse thickening of inner aspect of the cortex with narrowing of medullary space. Thus new bone may be separated from the inner cortex by a thin lucent line presenting what has been described as "Bone within Bone " appearance or the thickened cortex may remain uninterrupted and show a single thick compact layer of bone.This pattern is due to prolonged chronic anoxia which produces medullary infarcts that may be separated from the normal cortical endosteum by a thin radiolucent line or interface. This sort of longitudinal intra-cortical diaphyseal fissuring and overabundant new bone formation in volume is characteristic of Sickle cell disease.

In its symptomatic form it is characterised by chronic anaemia, episodes of jaundice, hepatosplenomegaly and recurrent bouts of pain in the extremities and the back.

Jack Reynolds 1973 observed distinctive radiological changes in the skeleton and the pattern was conveniently arranged into four categories.

1. Diaphyseal lesions of long bones

Small patchy amorphous areas of increased density. Mottled appearance caused by repair of acute infarcts deep in the spongiosa. Infarcts are probably produced by chronic anoxia. It evolves slowly to form a thin layer of dense bone near the periphery of medullary canal, but separated from the inner aspect of the cortex by a narrow lucent cleft which resembles cortex within cortex.

2. Epiphyseal lesions of long bones

Proximal epiphyses of Humerus and head of Femur are particularly susceptible to damage by regional ischaemia. The pathological changes usually evolve slowly as a result of chronic anoxia, but in sudden massive ischaemic necrosis, chalky appearance is produced by ischaemic damage with diffuse sclerosis.

3. Vertebral changes

- Increased translucency.
- Coarsening of trabecular pattern.
- Biconcave vertebral deformity.
- Prominent cup-like depression.
- Intramedullary infarct—mottled areas of increased density.

4. Skull changes

- Massive thickening of diploe
- Fine vertical striations—''Hair on end'' appearance
- Marrow hyperplasia showing alterations in the contour of the skull which is manifested by bilateral bossing in the posterosuperior parietal region.

In this series amongst this vast study 944 patients had skeletal affection which are enumerated in detail in the Table 4.1.

Table 4.1. Details of different presentations seen in patients of Sickle cell haemoglobinopathy when reported for the first time.

Presentation	No. of patients
1. Osteonecrosis femoral head	224
2. Osteonecrosis humeral head	178
3. Osteonecrosis of vertebral end plates	036
4. Osteomyelitis (378 Bones)	192
- Tibia	138
- Fibula	84
- Femur	63
- Humerus	33
- Radius ulna	51
- Lumbar spine	3
- Iliac bone	3
- Calcaneum	3
5. Hand-Foot Syndrome	46
6. Changes in Vertebrae	48
7. Pathological Fractures	46
8. Growth disturbances	76
9. Changes in Skull	16
10. Associated Osteoarticular Tuberculosis	24
11. Multiple affection of bones including sickle cell arthropathy, ulcerations etc	58
Total No. of Patients with skeletal affection	944

Edward O'Hara (1967) has described that bony changes in Sickle cell anaemia and its variants are reflected by one or combination of the following:

1. Reactive marrow hyperplasia
2. Infarction.
3. Disturbances in growth.
4. Infection
5. Fractures.

Marrow hyperplasia is thought to occur as a result of hypoxia due to extensive haemolysis of abnormal and fragile red cells. The resultant cellular increase produces resorption of some of the bony trabeculations of spongiosa and a thinning of cortex, thus resulting in a widening of marrow cavity yielding the roentgenographic findings of osteoporosis.

When sickling occurs in a sufficient amount, sequestration of cells is produced. Stasis, congestion and anoxia ensue, which brings more sickling and a vicious cycle is set up. Infarction develops in end organ. Bone infarction clinically presents with local bone pain, soft tissue swelling, fever, leucocytosis. As a result of vascular obstruction produced by accumulation of sickled cells, death and necrosis occurs with destruction followed by repair. The initial roentgen picture is that of a patchy area of bone destruction of spongiosa and cortex and periosteal reaction. Such changes may be indistinguishable from osteomyelitis and have to be correlated with clinical findings. When aseptic necrosis involves the epiphysis like the femoral head, the changes may closely resemble osteochondritis.

The severity of clinical and roentgenographic manifestations of Sickle cell disease varies greatly among the individuals with this disorder. Some patients suffer a painful, debilitating illness which seems almost identical to the syndrome seen in homozygous "SS" Sickle cell disease, however some patients experience no overt disease and like most individuals with simple heterozygous condition "AS" Sickle cell trait, remain unaware about their haematological disorder.

The measure of the severity of the disease can be roughly predicted on certain criteria.

1. Frequency of painful crises.
2. Nature of gene—homozygous or heterozygous.
3. Early presentation of crisis and severity of crisis.
4. Clinical evidence of hepatosplenomegaly.
5. Incidence of haemolytic crisis.
6. Associated physiological conditions like pregnancy or unphysiological conditions of any illness.
7. Haemolytic crisis.

Haemolytic crisis is commonly seen in pregnancy with Sickle cell disease. It is associated with very high percentage of maternal deaths. Incidence of life-threatening complications are very high in gravid patients. Maternal dyscrasia also leads to high percentage of foetal loss. Sudden complications like severe anaemia, pulmonary infarction and other infections are seen.

Since Sickle cell - beta thalassaemia can be absolutely distinguished from other forms of Sickle cell haemoglobinopathy only by elaborate physiochemical techniques, diagnostic information provided by the roentgen signs might seem to be of little value, particularly in patients with typical symptoms. However, in many patients with this genotype, the disease is clinically occult and virtually indistinguishable from Sickle cell trait, and under such circumstances, the radiologist can play a key role. For some of these patients, despite of their mild clinical course, may exhibit distinctive osseous stigmata which are known to occur only in the morbid forms of sicklemia. Thus roentgen signs can provide the initial clue which indicates the potentially serious nature of the patients disorder. Greater diagnostic precision by roentgenologic means, is not often possible, for the roentgen features of Sickle cell - beta thalassaemia are those which are common to all forms of symptomatic Sickle cell haemoglobinopathy, and therefore a specific diagnosis in terms of the genotype cannot be advanced. Occasionally, however, by noting the co-existence of unique skeletal changes and certain visceral abnormalities, it is possible to differentiate with reasonable accuracy between homozygous Sickle cell anaemia, and the heterozygous variants. Although further diagnostic refinement by roentgenological means alone is not feasible, the knowledge that the patient has a variant form of disease can be important in his future medical management.

Visceral changes were also seen as a result of intravascular Sickling and circulatory stasis. Prominent organs involved are described under the following headings.

1. Lungs

Increased susceptibility to pulmonary infarction and pneumonia. Lung changes are caused by pulmonary vascular occlusion.

Roentgen signs of pulmonary infarction were observed. Pulmonary circulatory stasis, pulmonary vascular blockade by embolus is probably the more common cause of acute infarction. Such emboli consist of bits of bone marrow which enter the circulation from the foci of ischaemic necrosis in the spine or extremities.

2. Spleen

Splenomegaly is a constant feature. Enlargement is primarily due to the fact that sickled RBC's cannot pass freely through small, tortuous vascular channels and the organ becomes engorged with the red cells sequestrated within the sinusoids. The size of spleen in response to systemic and local conditions which control the tendency of circulating erythrocytes to become destroyed. Massive sequestration causes rapid enlargement and circulatory stasis—the state which is conducive for splenic infarction. Focal ischaemic changes are pronounced. The condition which favours splenic fibrosis occurs more frequently. The tendency towards autosplenectomy is quite high. There might be splenic calcification.

3. Liver and gall bladder

Transient episodes of hepatomegaly are frequently noticed. Enlargement occurs during the crisis or during intermittent bouts of other illness. Focal parenchymal damage occurs due to intravascular sickling.

Biliary calculus:Incidence of radiolucent gall stones is high, demonstrated by radiography and specialised radiological investigations.

4. Heart

Cor pulmonale and cardiomegaly are frequently observed. Changes in the contour of the heart, typical of cor pulmonale may develop as a complication of pulmonary vascular occlusion. Moderate, generalised cardiomegaly is common. It is produced by the effects of severe anaemia on circulatory dynamics.

5. Renal changes

The changes occur because of sickling. Corpuscles containing sickled RBC's when exposed to an environment of high osmolarity and low oxygen tension, as exists in the renal medulla, results into increase in blood viscosity which impedes the flow of blood through this region and the process may lead to complete circulatory stasis and cause ischaemic necrosis of renal papilla. Such a patient manifests with haematuria.This form of Sickle cell nephropathy which causes renal papillary necrosis is frequently seen. Necrosis occurs in the central portion of the papilla. Necrotic material might slough out to leave defect in the papilla. With repair the lesion becomes less destructive and the changes cannot be easily distinguished from changes of pyelonephritis. The incidence of pyelonephritis is very high.

RADIOLOGICAL DIAGNOSIS

In order to evaluate the efficiency of radiological examination as a diagnostic method in Sickle cell disease, reliance was placed on skeletal changes and 3 anatomical regions were observed in which the signs of greatest specificity occur more frequently.

A. Long bones - Cortex within Cortex pattern in the long bones.
B. Cup-like deformity of end plates of vertebrae because of osteonecrosis.
C. Sclerosis, fragmentation with or without collapse because of osteonecrosis of humeral or femoral head.

Based on the presence of at least one sign it was possible to make roentgenographic diagnosis of Sickle cell haemoglobinopathy.

A positive correlation between the sickle haemoglobin values and the severity of clinical and roentgen manifestations were found to exist only in those patients in whom concentration of haemoglobin S differed markedly from the mean value. The amount of haemoglobin S varied from 58% to 91% (Average:73.6%). All patients with haemoglobin S value excess of 77% exhibited characteristic skeletal lesions and in all individuals with concentrations of haemoglobin S below 67% bone lesions was rarely observed.

5

Clinical Diagnosis

HOW TO SUSPECT SICKLE CELL HAEMOGLOBINOPATHY?

The patients of Sickle cell haemoglobinopathy may present with variety of symptoms, not necessarily pertaining to skeletal involvement. The gravity of manifestations mainly depends on whether the patients has Sickle cell trait or Sickle cell disease. Commonly patients present for generalised symptoms of vague pain, malaise, weakness, fatigue, frequent recurrent episodes of Infection (Respiratory - Genito Urinary), Osteomyelitis, severe anaemia and symptoms pertaining to skeletal affection. In this area of Central India the disorder is commonly seen in specific community of Scheduled Caste & Scheduled Tribes. The clinician should be aware about these genetic disorder which is commonly seen in this area amongst Mahars, Kunbis, Gonds, Kurmis, Telis, Tribals, Adivasis and Neo-Buddhists. This genetic disorder commonly presents with multisystem affection and if all the clinical features are coupled together it is very easy to suspect Sickle cell haemoglobinopathy. Our studies have given us guidelines on how to detect Sickle cell haemoglobinopathy patient on the analysis of anthropometric studies. They present with typical Sickle cell facies and physique. The details of which are given in chapter of Anthropometry. There are many Orthopaedic manifestations, the symptoms of which are discussed in individual topics. Once you suspect the possibility of Sickle cell haemoglobinopathy the clinician should proceed with simple bed side investigations of Solubility test or Sickling Test (Daland & Castle 1948). Few drops of blood if mixed with freshly prepared solution of Sodium metabisulphite, it will show you Sickling of RBC's either immediate or within 24 hours (Early & late Sickling). This test is possible anywhere in remote area including the villages. After the confirmation of Sickling test the patient may be investigated in detail by various haematological tests, especially to find out the exact pattern of haemoglobin by electrophoresis and to predict the prognosis.

Simultaneously the skeletal survey should be done to find out the bony changes. The patients of Sickle cell haemoglobinopathy shows classical radiological changes depending upon the site of involvement, which is discussed in individual chapters. Patient may have obvious orthopaedic manifestations, but commonly the features are hidden and clinician has to search for skeletal affection depending upon the site of bone & joint involvement. In advanced cases the diagnosis is very obvious but every clinician is expected to diagnose when the changes are minimal and further progress can be arrested or minimised. Prevention of Sickle cell disease by carrier detection and marriage counselling is relatively difficult. In majority of cases the couple at risk is detected only after the birth of diseased child Hence a method is standardised to detect sickle cell mutation prenatally using Polymerase Chain Reaction (PCR) at the molecular level.

PRENATAL DIAGNOSIS OF SICKLE-CELL ANAEMIA

PCR is a recently developed procedure for the rapid in-vitro amplification of DNA sequences and it has a profound impact on various branches of biochemical sciences including the field of clinical diagnosis

(Banker M.P., Kate, S.L. et al. 1993). In the case of sickle cell haemoglobin in mutation in 6th codon, eliminates the MstII restriction site. Using PCR technique and restriction digestion it is possible to diagnose antenatally single gene mutation. For this no radioactive material or any external probe is used. The diagnosis is possible on second day after the biopsy and it can be performed in the first trimester of pregnancy. Whenever prenatal diagnosis is confirmed medical termination of pregnancy can be recommended.

PCR product from each reaction is digested with 10 units of MstII restriction enzyme for 1 hour at 37°C and analysed by agarose gel electrophoresis (1.5%), stained with ethidium bromide, visualised and photographed on a ultraviolet transilluminator. A marker was also electrophoresed alongwith the digested product.

MstII digestion products of normal, trait and homozygous for sickle cell haemoglobin revealed a pattern of 192 and 107 bp; 299, 192 and 107 bp; and 299 bp, respectively. The amplified and restriction digested samples of foetal DNA showed that one of them is heterozygous for sickle cell mutation while the other is normal.

LABORATORY INVESTIGATIONS

The laboratory diagnosis of Sickle cell disorder is confirmed by the following haematological tests.

1. Sickling test

A. Cover slip method of sickling test (Fig. 5.1-5.3)

It is based on the fact that when RBC containing sickle cell haemoglobin are exposed to low oxygen tension they assume the characteristic sickle shape because of crinkling. A freshly prepared blood slide

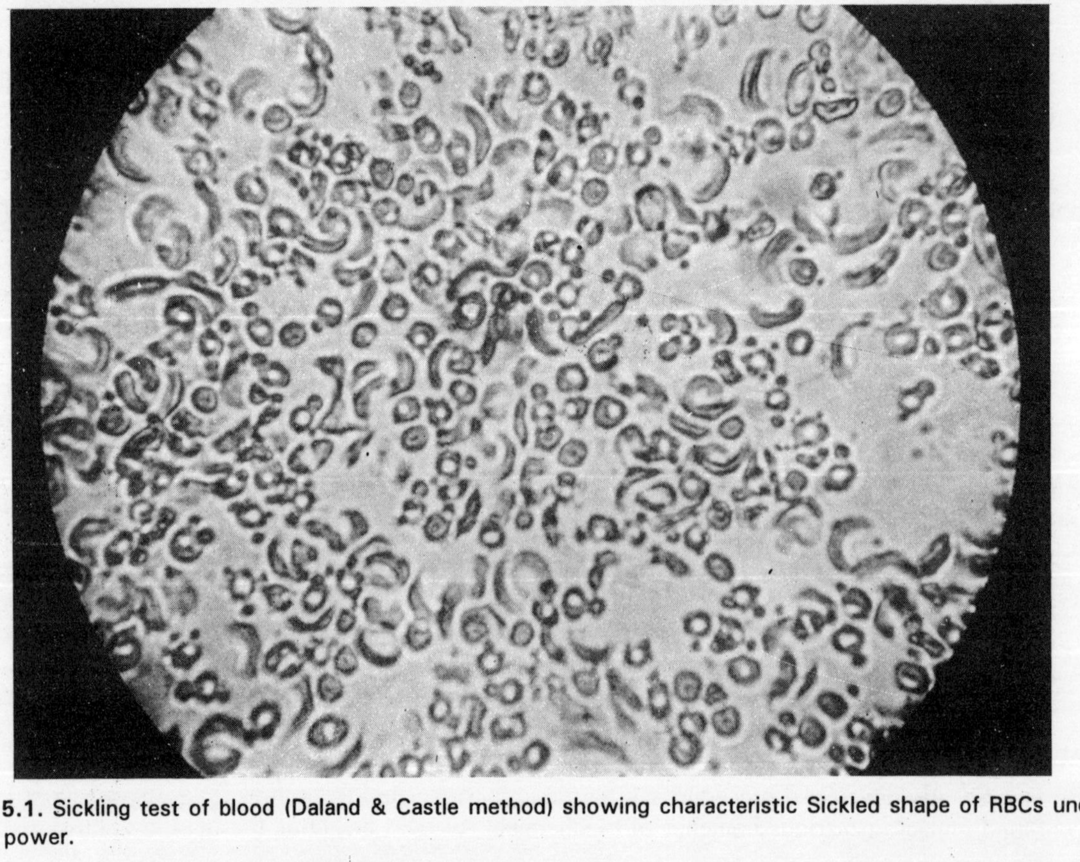

Fig. 5.1. Sickling test of blood (Daland & Castle method) showing characteristic Sickled shape of RBCs under low power.

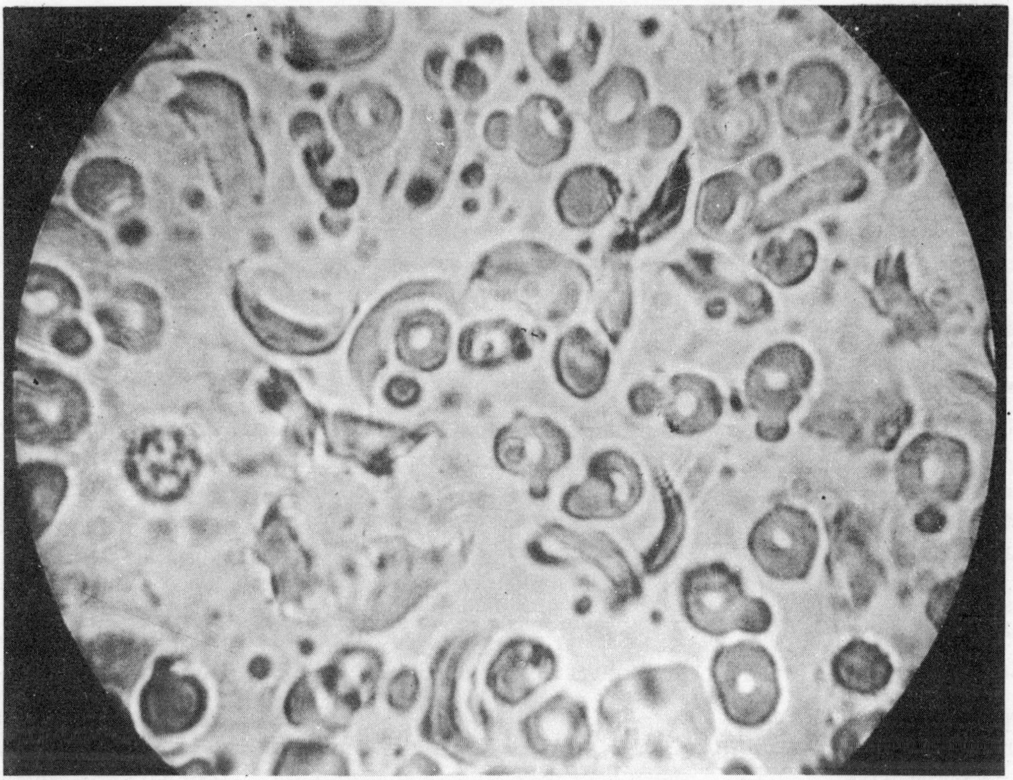

Fig. 5.2. Sickling test of blood. Peripheral smear under high power showing positive sickling of few of the RBCs.

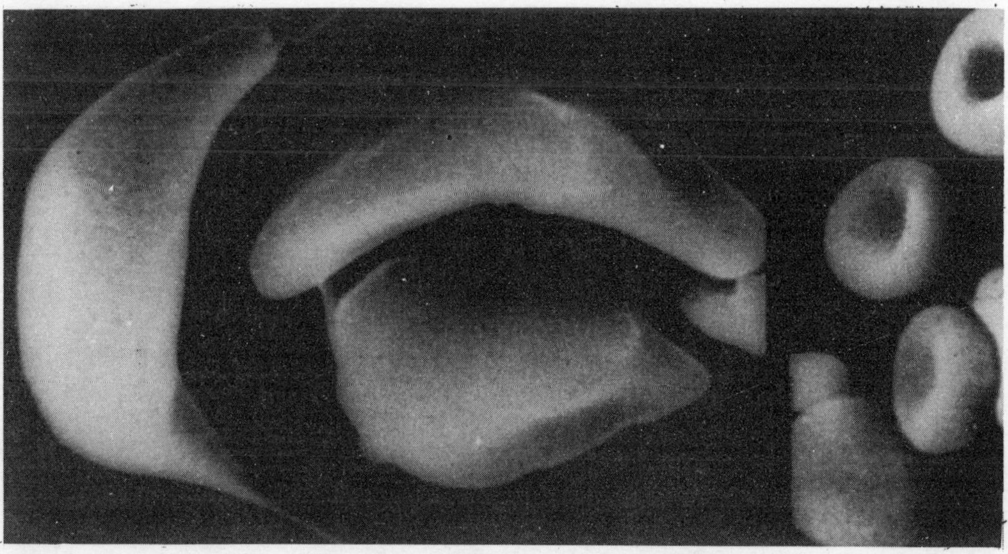

Fig. 5.3. RBCs after sickling seen under electron microscope. Typical doughnut shape of RBCs (on right side) is changed into typical Sickled shape.

is covered with coverslip and is immediately made air-tight by vaseline around the slide. Sickling of RBC's is seen under microscope, in many cases (Early). It is then kept for 24 hours and is seen under microscope again (Late). It reflects both the homozygous and heterozygous for the sickle gene. Usually in Sickle cell disease early sickling is positive whereas in Sickle cell trait it is seen as late sickling.

B. Metabisulphite method of Daland and Castle (1948)

A drop of blood on a microscope slide is mixed with two drops of freshly prepared 2% sodium metabisulphite. The preparation is covered with a cover slip which is sealed with paraffin wax, cells containing 15% or more Hb-S will sickle. Sickling of red cells is usually obvious in SS blood within 15 minutes and in AS blood within one hour, but apparently negative results should be examined again at 24 hours.

But the method does not distinguish between homozygous & heterozygous state.

2. Electrophoresis method

After the initial blood film examination haemoglobin electrophoresis should be performed to find out whether patient has Sickle cell disease or Sickle cell trait. This technique separates protein on the basis of their electrical charge when in solution. The rate of migration of a protein in an electrical field is dependent not only on the charge but also its size, molecular weight and structure, the pH and ionic strength of the buffer, the type of supporting media used and voltage applied.

Various methods of Haemoglobin electrophoresis are available to confirm the diagnosis of Sickle cell haemoglobinopathy and identify the exact pattern of haemoglobin (Fig. 5.4).

A. Cellular acetate membrane electrophoresis

For the diagnosis of Sickle cell disorder, cellular acetate membrane and paper are the commonest supportive media used for the initial electrophoretic analysis in alkaline buffers. Paper has the advantage of being simple and cheap but it requires a longer time to seperate and absorption is considerable. Cellular acetate on the other hand requires a much shorter peiod of electrophoresis, absorbs haemoglobin only minimaly and can be adopted when for use of very small volumes of blood are available. This makes it especially

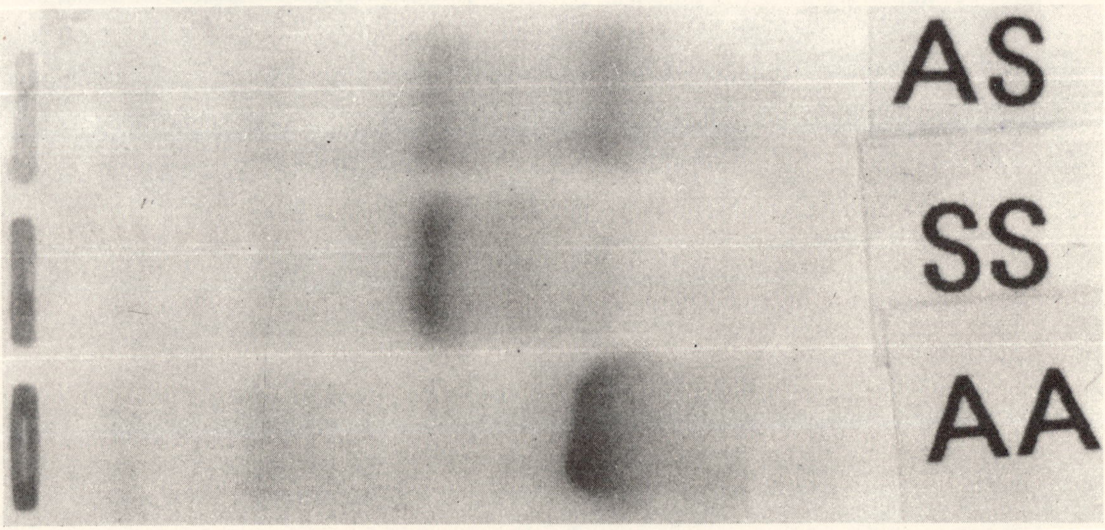

Fig. 5.4. Haemoglobin electroph‹ resis by cellular membrane method showing pattern of Hb in Sickle cell trait, Sickle cell disease and normal individual.

suitable for screening purposes and it is the recommended method. The haemoglobin are identified by their position on the electrophoretogram, for example Hb-A and Hb-C move more slowly and are nearer to the origin, HbS, HbF and HbA move faster and are further (distal) from the origin in that order. Hb-B, Hb-H and Hb-I move faster than Hb-A and it is useful to include a sample of known blood as a "control" when electrophoresis is made.

The final identification of Hb-S cannot be said to have been completed, with electrophoresis because other haemoglobin though less common, appear in the same position (area) as Hb-S on electrophoretogram in alkaline buffer. These include Hb-D and Hb Philadelphia and in most instances the Hb-S solubility tests will confirm that the abnormal Hb is in fact Hb-S, but if this test gives a negative result electrophoresis on citrate agar will be necessary.

B. Citrate agar electrophoresis

This test always provide valuable confirmation and additional evidence. Although a little more difficult and time consuming than cellulose acetate, this, at acid pH 6.1 has the advantage of clearly differentiating between HbF, A,S, SC thus making the method the procedure of choice in screening cord blood or samples from young infants. Hb-D also separates clearly from Hb-S in this system, migrating with Hb-D from Hb-S which give the same band in cellulose acetate electrophoresis (CAE) and also HbC HbO Arab is differentiated clearly.

3. Haemoglobin solubility test (Dithionite tube turbidity test)

This is simple, rapid and reliable screening test for Sickle haemoglobin (HbS). It is based on the original work done by Itano and Muraya, where they showed that HbS has low solubility in a reduced state in hypertonic buffer.

The basis of this solubility test for detection of HbS is the relative insolubility of reduced HbS in concentrated phosphate buffer, in practice the haemoglobin is added to a solution of Sodium dithionate, a reducing agent in phosphate buffer. If HbS is present the solution becomes turbid and those without HbS remains clear.

METHOD

Initially the solution is prepared by following procedure:

(a) Stock buffer is preapered from anhydrous potassium di hydrogen phosphate. Anhydrous di potassium hydrogen phosphate with white saponian and distilled water.

Reagent

1. 2.20 M. Phosphate buffer (pH 7) with Saponin

KH_2PO_4	125 gms.
K_2HPO_4	217 gms.
Saponin	2.5 gms.
Merthiolet (Preservative)	0.25 gms.
Water to make	1.0 Litre

2. Sodium Dithionite ($Na_2S_2O_4$)

(b) Working solution is freshly prepared immediately before performing the test by sodium metabisulphite 10 mg. with stock buffer 1 ml.

Collect few drops of blood by finger prick and add to 1 ml of working solution in a glass tube 3" × ½" (containing few drops of EDTA solution as a anticoagulant) and mixed thoroughly which is then centrifused at 3000 r/min for five minutes. Discard the supernatant to avoid false positive results because of plasma proteins. Take about 1 ml of reagent in 3" × ½" glass tube add small quantity (about 10 mg) of sodium dithionite powder and shake well to dissolve it. Add 0.02 ml packed red cells and mix well to produce a light pinkish violet colour and read the test after 2-3 minutes.

The tube is removed gently so as not to disturb flocculations or precipitated haemoglobin and examined. A test is read as positive if the turbidity impairs the visibility of dark, bold lines on a white paper held against a bright source of light at 1 inch distance. A negative test is indicated by clear pinkish violet solution, through which the dark lines are easily seen.

Blood of normal indvidual, known Sickle cell disease & Sickle cell trait if available is tested at the same time as the known sample, so as to provide control for comparison.

Samples that show a pattern migrating like Hb-S are subjected to the solubility test. This permits the simple detection of other abnormal haemoglobin which though migrating with Hb-S, will show normal solubility.

4. Haemoglobin A quantitation

Determination of the proportions of the total haemoglobin which is Hb-A is an important diagnostic test, when Beta thal trait is suspected. Patient with B-thal trait usually have Hb-A raised over 4 percent. The Hb are first separated by electrophoresis on cellulose acetate membrane. The portions containing the various fractions are in front and eluted into small volumes of buffers. By comparing the optical densities at 4.5 mm the relative proportions can be determined. This method has the disadvantage that it cannot be used in the presence of Hb-C which migrates with HbA.

5. Haemoglobin F quantitation (A.D. test)

The quantitation of foetal haemoglobin is based on its known property of resistance to denaturation by alkali. The one minute denaturation test of Singer or two minute denaturation test of Betke are the common methods used.The former is more accurate with larger amounts of Hb-F, while the latter is more acceptable with lower amounts.

The presence of red cells containing Hb-F can be detected by the elution technique or Kleihauer and Betke which depends on the observation that normal adult haemoglobin and other variants are soluble in Ureteric acid phosphate in pH 3.3, whereas foetal haemoglobin is not. Cells containing Hb-F appear red, whereas cells not containing Hb-F show as ghosts after counter-staining with haematoxylin.

6

Osteonecrosis of Femoral Head

Osteonecrosis of femoral head is commonly seen in young adults of Sickle cell haemoglobinopathy, which is frequently bilateral (Figs. 6.6, 6.7, 6.8, 6.9) and in high percentage of patients, it results in severely disabling, painful, stiff hip. Pathophysiology of Sickle cell disease causing osteonecrosis along with importance of surgical treatment is discussed. This study includes follow up of osteonecrosis of 352 Femoral heads in 224 patients in a duration of Twenty five years (128 patients had bilateral affection) diagnosed amongst 7380 patients of Sickle cell haemoglobinopathy.

Early diagnosis is the key to the success of head preserving operations, but once there is collapse of head with involvement of more than 60% of the weight bearing surface, and especially when associated with arthritic changes it is necessary to perform total hip replacement of hip joint so as to rehabilitate these disabled patients and provide good to excellent quality of life to these sicklers.

Lately it has been observed that the incidence of osteonecrosis of femoral head is steadily increasing amongst the patients of Sickle cell haemoglobinopathies. The clinical entity is more important since commonly it is seen in young adults between the ages of 20-40 years in the region of Nagpur - Central India and is frequently bilateral. The disease most of the time results in severely disabling painful stiff hip in the most crucial time of life when individual's career is supposed to be at the peak. The syndrome of osteonecrosis of femoral head seen in Sickle cell patients initially causes minimal pain and discomfort, and is not noticed in many cases until deformity of femoral head has already occurred (Fig.6.3-6.5).

CLINICAL MATERIAL AND METHOD

Osteonecrosis is essentially a vascular disease. The ischaemia is either due to occlusion of arteries or obstruction to venous drainage. Interruption of arterial supply or occlusion of venous drainage results in stasis and oxygen starvation. This results in bone cell death which occurs because of disparity between oxygen need of the bone cell and inability of local circulation to meet the need and demand. In the said duration we have treated these 224 patients of osteonecrosis in Sickle cell disease, 55 patients were treated conservatively and 169 patients were operated requiring 252 surgeries. There were 136 males and 88 female patients in the age group of 10-40 years with about 45% patients in the young age group of 20-30 years (Table 6.1). In 94 patients 164 head preserving surgeries were performed. In 60 patients 68 Total hip replacements were done and in 15 patients 20 hips were operated for other procedures (Table 6.2-6.5).

Most of the patients of osteonecrosis in Sickle cell disease presented with complaints of deep throbbing pain in groin and hip - initially intermittently, later more severe. Subsequently these patients had complaints of painful limited movements of the hip. Few patients had radiating pain from groin to the thigh and knee, radiating alongwith the medial aspect. In some patients the only complaint was discomfort and limp during weight bearing. In later stages almost all patients had painful stiff hips with grossly restricted movements restricting squatting and sitting cross-legged (Figs. 6.1, 6.2, 6.3).

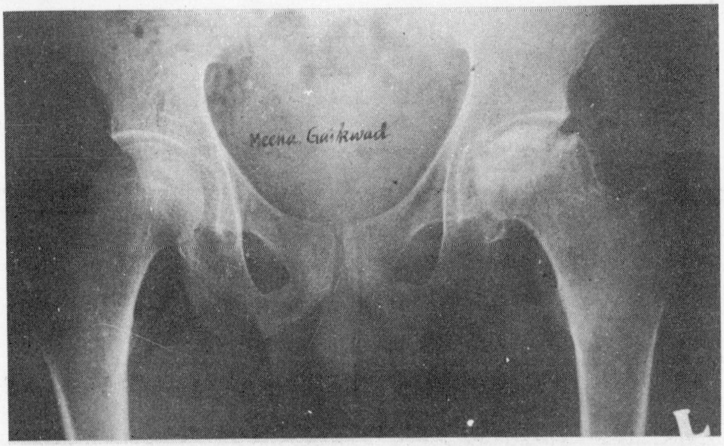

Fig. 6.1

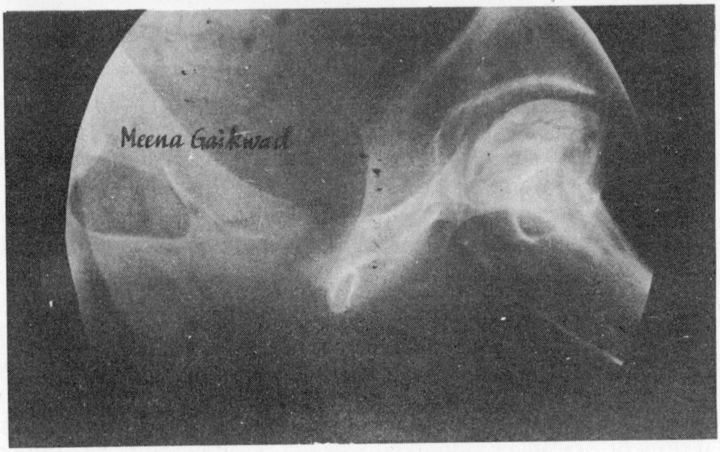

Fig. 6.2

Fig. 6.1 and 6.2. X-ray Pelvis A.P. of young female patient of 21½ years showing osteonecrosis of femoral head with fragmentation and collapse on left side. Lateral view showing classical crescent sign.

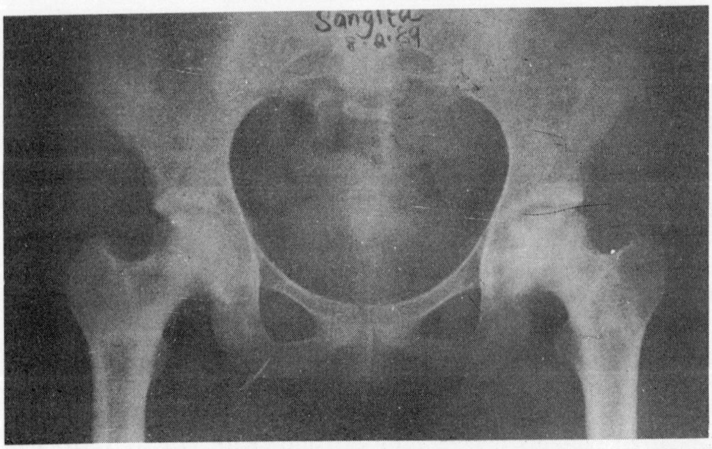

Fig. 6.3. X-ray pelvis A.P.of 22 yrs. female showing advance osteonecrosis, with fragmentation and affection of articular surface.

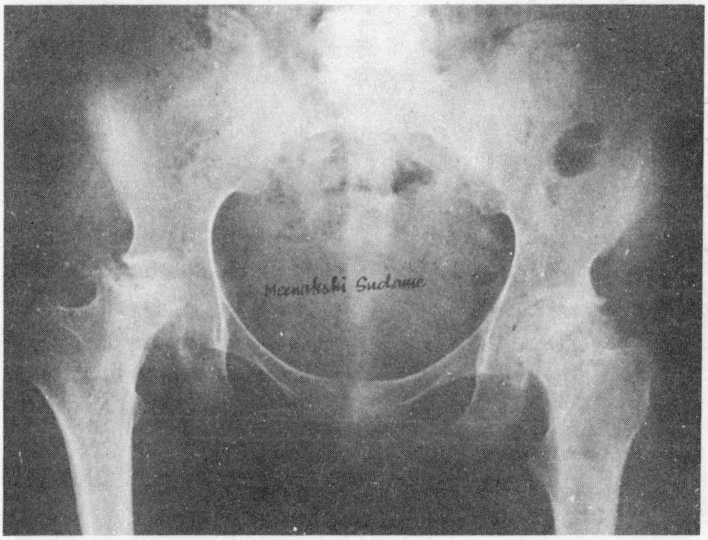

Fig. 6.4. X-ray pelvis A.P. showing advanced changes of osteonecrosis both hips with early osteoarthritic changes.

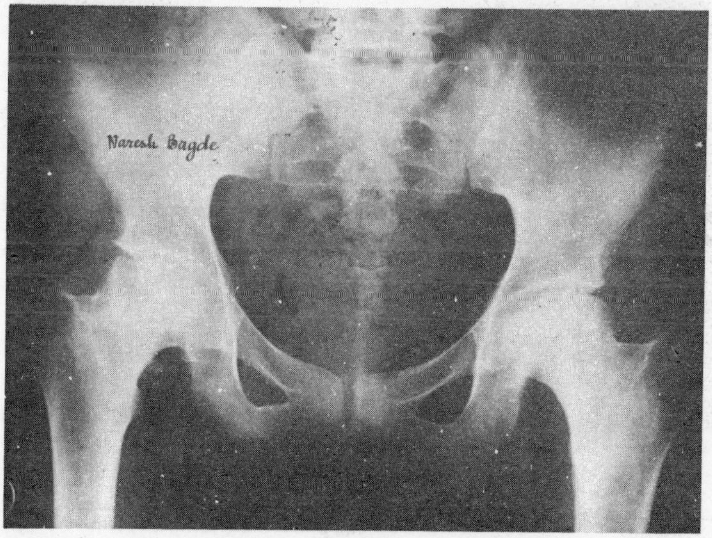

Fig. 6.5. X-ray pelvis young 18 years boy showing advanced osteonecrosis with secondary osteoarthritis in right hip and osteonecrosis and deformation of left femoral head.

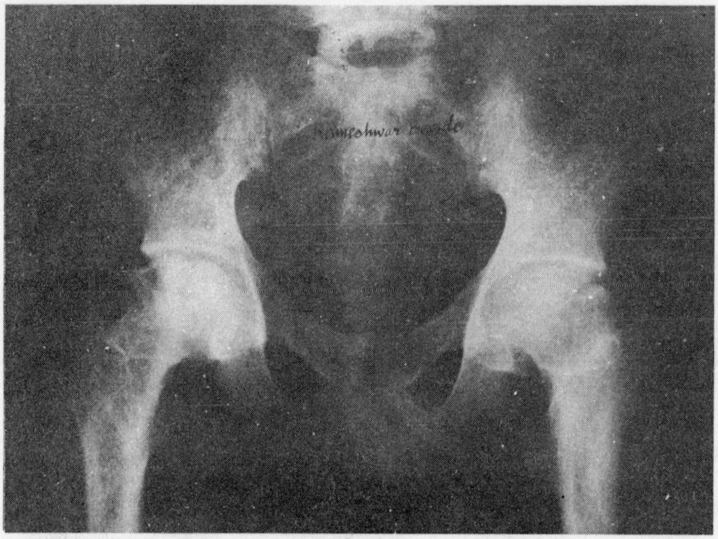

Fig. 6.6

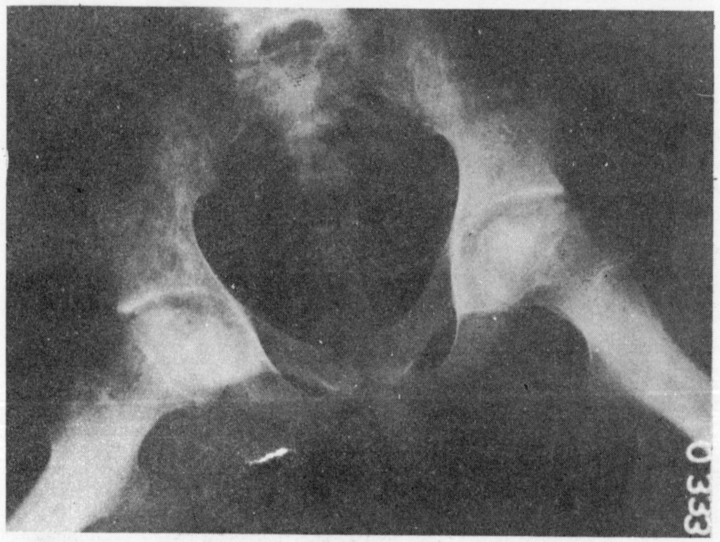

Fig. 6.7

Fig. 6.6 and 6.7. X-ray pelvis A.P. & Dunn's view of a young patient 22 years showing osteonecrosis of both heads with fairly advanced changes of arthritis.

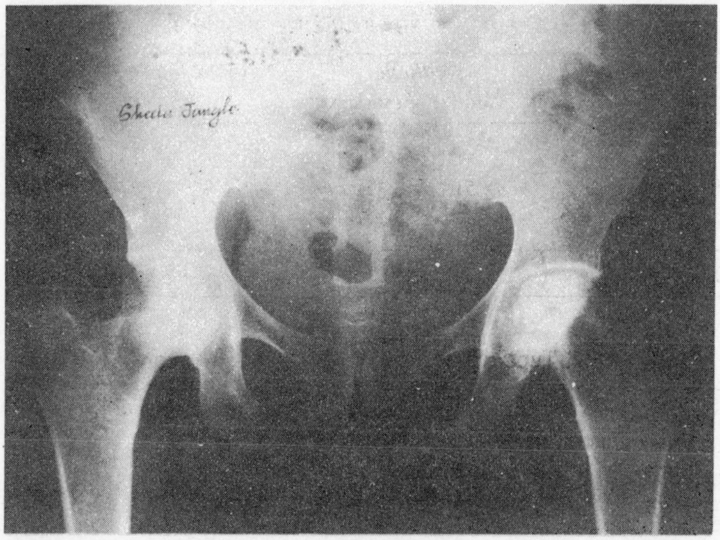

Fig. 6.8

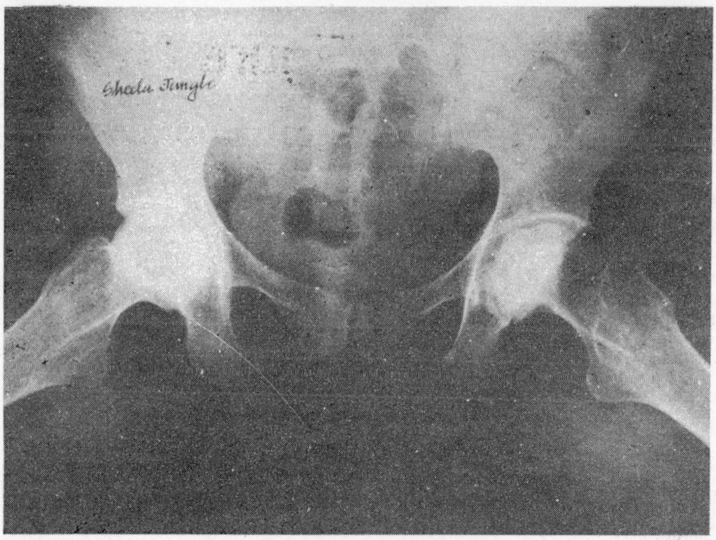

Fig. 6.9

Fig. 6.8 and 6.9. X-ray pelvis of young patient 28 years showing osteonecrosis of left femoral head with fragmentation without any collapse and early changes of osteonecrosis on right side.

Table 6.1. Age and sex incidence in osteonecrosis

Age Group	*Total No. of patients*	*Sex Ratio Males*	*Females*	*Unilateral*	*Bilateral*	*Total N/o femoral heads*
10-20	51	38	13			
21-30	99	54	45	96	128	352
31-40	74	44	30			
Total	224	136	88			

Table 6.2. Type and number of surgeries in osteonecrosis

Type of Operation	*No. of patients*	*No. of surgeries*
1. Head preserving operations	94	164
2. Total hip replacements	60	68
3. Other operations (Bipolar, AMP, Girdlestone, Arthrodesis)	15	20
Total	169	252

Table 6.3. Head preserving surgeries in osteonecrosis in Sickle cell disease

Name of operations.	*Total procedures*
I. Core decompression with bone grafting	**88**
(a) Vascular Pedicle iliac graft	18
(b) Phemister (Fibular) graft	26
(c) Cancellous iliac graft	14
(d) Meyer's muscle pedicle graft	18
(e) Sartorius muscle pedicle graft	12
II. Osteotomy	**76**
(a) Ventral rotation Osteotomy	42
(b) Flexion Osteotomy	16
(c) Valgus/Varus osteotomy	13
(d) McMurray's Osteotomy	05
Total head preserving operations	164

The activity of patients of Sickle cell disease may be impaired by factors other than the hip, therefore other joints that are affected by the disease and other systemic associated conditions must be looked for final treatment, assessment and evaluation.There is usually association of biliary duct disease, pulmonary insufficiency, osteomyelitis, cardiac abnormalities etc. (Fig. 6.10). The evaluation of hip was done by clinical and radiological assessment. Assessment was done by asking detailed history of symptoms, level of activity. The clinical examination included function of hips and final outcome which included range of motion of hip, Trendelenberg test and measurement of limb length discrepancy (Table 6.8).

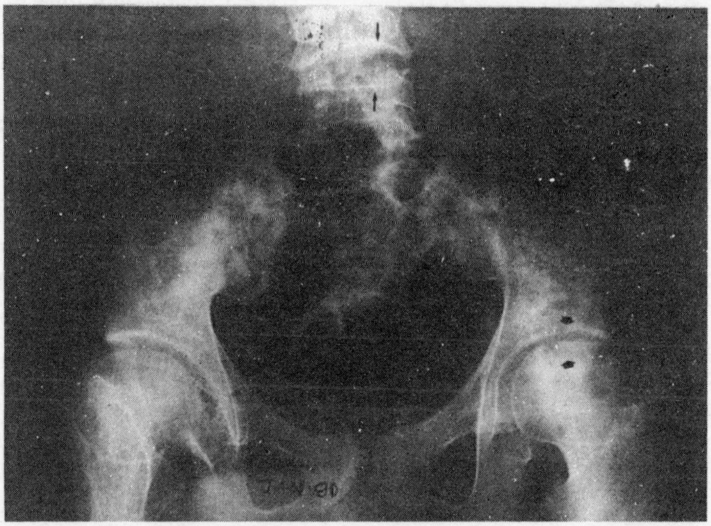

Fig. 6.10. X-ray pelvis A.P. showing increased density at the periphery in superolateral segment, but the contour of femoral head is well preserved on left side with classical radiological changes of haemoglobinopathy in pelvis and spine.

Table 6.4. Total hip replacements in Sickle cell disease

Name of procedure	*Total number of patients*	*Total surgeries hip*
1. Charnley's Total Hip	36	42
2. Isoelastic Hips	24	26
Total	60	68

Table 6.5. Other surgeries - head sacrificing

Name of surgery	*Number of patients*	*Total number of procedures*
1. Bipolar Hip replacement	06	09
2. Hemiarthroplasty AMP	03	03
3. Girdlestone excision arthroplasty	03	05
4. Arthrodesis	03	03
Total head sacrificing surgeries	15	20

ETIOPATHOLOGY

The concept of pathology and etiology must be separated since many factors are involved in the causation. It is observed that anterolateral segments of femoral head superiorly undergoes necrosis first and quickly. This is obviously because of occlusion of posterolateral retinacular vessels or by emboli from various sources finding their way through the microcirculation into the subchondral zone of femoral head.

There are various theories for causation of thromboembolic phenómenon resulting in osteonecrosis. However etiology in Sickle cell disease is proved beyond doubt.

Bony changes in Sickle cell diseases occur mainly because of hyperplasia of bone marrow and because of vascular insufficiency resulting into thrombosis and infarction. These circulatory changes results in high intraosseous pressure and the femoral head functions as a closed compartment and the eventual infarction of weight bearing bone is the end stage of progressive compartment syndrome produced by increased intraosseous pressure. Because of hyperplasia the multiple erythrocytes cause increase in blood viscosity, stasis, capillary thrombosis and finally infarction of bone. The initial infarcts occur in the most distal portion of the bone (i.e.femoral head), in the subchondral area, where there is maximum sickling and where the circulation through collaterals is very poor and limited. The blood supply to the cartilage is poor, it is impaired and there is death of bone cells. Continuation of weight bearing on this femoral head leads to the flattening and irregularities in the contour of the femoral head. Such changes results into weakening of trabecular structure leading to multiple micro-fractures and finally collapse in weight bearing portion of the femoral head. In later stages proliferative arthritic changes appear in the hip joints.

Osteonecrosis occurs with greatest frequency in classic homozygous Sickle cell anaemia in the SS and S-Thal disorders, as well as in heterozygous Sickle cell haemoglobinopathy - Sickle cell trait (SA).

Alterations in the amino acids of haemoglobin S results in confirmational changes in the haemoglobin molecule in the deoxygenated state. Molecular stacking occurs, and hollow, rigid rods or "tactoids" are formed due to regular aggregation of the molecules in the individual cells. Initially these events are reversible when the blood is re-oxygenated. However, the red cells eventually become damaged from repeated sickling and unsickling, and the sickling becomes irreversible. Cells which are sickled have difficulty in traversing the small capillaries and it increases the blood viscosity. If a sufficient number of sickled cells come together, they block blood vessels. This sets up a vicious cycle by increasing local hypoxia and promoting further sickling. Eventually, these sickle cells interfere with the blood supply to a small or large area of an organ or tissue, including bone. Such events results in the most common feature of the sickling disorder, the painful vaso-occlusive episode. If these conditions persist, they can lead to infarction and necrosis. The lesions resulting from osteonecrosis are usually accompanied by pain and may cause permanent destruction of articular cartilage, resulting in disability.

It is said that ischaemia provokes bone marrow oedema and fibrosis elevating bone marrow pressure which further decreases the bone blood flow.This cycle of ischaemia, oedema and increased pressure culminates in bone cell death. The mechanical failure and continued weight bearing results eventually in collapse of femoral head and osteoarthritic changes.

EARLY DIAGNOSIS

Since 1983 at our centre functional bone investigations were being routinely done but from the year 1993 MRI and CT has replaced this invasive procedure. Early diagnosis is important prior to the appearance of radiological changes. Any patient of Sickle cell disorder if complains of pain in the hip, is thoroughly investigated by Functional bone investigation or bone scan (Ficat R.P. 1985; Hungerford D.S. & Dennis W. Lennox 1985). Similarly in patient of osteonecrosis of femoral head the opposite hip is regarded as "high risk" patient and close watch is kept on such patient for atleast one year.

Functional Bone Investigation and Bone Scanning are of great value if the X-rays are negative in patients of high index of suspicion for osteonecrosis of femoral head. All the investigations are unnecessary if the X-rays are positive. Although X-ray examination is of limited value in making early diagnosis, it has considerable value in staging (Marcus N.B., Eneking W.F., Massam R.A. 1973; Steinberg M.E. & Brighton C.I. & others, 1984; Ficat and Arlet 1985). Bone marrow pressure study and core decompression if required was routinely done in cases where osteonecrosis of femoral head, was strongly suspected till 1985. Only haemodynamic phase of functional bone investigation was carried out at our centre and routinely venogram, oxygen saturation or temperature measurements were not done since the procedure is cumbersome. If haemodynamic phase is negative, bone scan studies are done routinely in such at high risk patients subsequently at regular intervals. If suspicion is very high even with negative bone scan, core decompression and biopsy used to be routine procedure but with the availability of MRI, these patients are closely observed and one should avoid invasive procedure. There was plenty of opportunity to study asymptomatic, radiologically negative contralateral hip in patients presenting with unilateral osteonecrosis of femoral head. Bone marrow pressure and stress test was positive in eight symptomatic hips and fifteen of asymptomatic contralateral hips in a known patient of osteonecosis of femoral head. But now the philosophy is changed and these patients of extremely high risk category are closely monitored by sequential MRI studies.

Commonly the patients present after radiographic changes are seen and at times with advanced osteoarthritic changes. If the deformity occurs because of involvement of subchondral bone or even early collapse of supportive cancellous bone which is evident radiologically, the prognosis is very poor.

CLASSIFICATION - STAGING

1. Neel Marcus et al. (1973): System involved both radiographic changes and clinical signs & symptoms. Since the association between radiographic appearance and clinical findings is often poor, this system is not widely used.
2. Steinberg et al. (1984)
   - Expanded 6 stages - mild < 15
     - moderate 15-30
     - severe > 30
3. Ficat & Arlet (1985) -I-IV
4. Hungerford & Lennox modifications of Ficat & Arlet
   - Added 'O' after MRI
5. Japanese Investigation Committee & Ohzono et al.
   A - medial & rarely progressive
   B - central with intermediate prognosis
   C - Lateral with worst prognosis
6. ARCO's Classification (1991)
   - Combination of - Ficat & Arlet
   - Quantification of Steinberg
   - Location as Japanese Inv. Committee

The success of treatment in osteonecrosis is related to, at which stage the disorder is initiated. Description of the methods used to make an accurate diagnosis early in the disease process (Diagnostic modalities currently available).

- Radiography
  - Scintigraphy
  - FBI
  - MRI
  - CT
- Histopathology

HISTORY AND CLINICAL EXAMINATION

- Pain
- Painful range of movements, especially on forced internal rotation.
- H/O associated risk factor
- High Index of suspicion

The contralateral hip in a patient of unilateral osteonecrosis must be carefully evaluated since the bilateral prevalence is reported to be 50-80%.

RADIOLOGY

Osteonecrosis of femoral head generally affects anterolateral segment which is placed superiorly in femoral head. Cancellous bone placed posteriorly is also projected in this area in AP view. It is therefore difficult to diagnose osteonecrosis of femoral head on AP view, when changes are minimal. Routinely Dunn's view in addition to AP & Lateral Views are done whenever osteonecrosis of femoral head is suspected. However tangential radiographs would delineate the entire femoral head nicely for more accurate assessment of the size of necrotic segment. Initial X-rays made earlier and latest X rays during the follow-up periods were used for the assessment of deformity of the hip, abnormalities of the growth of the proximal part of the femur and osteoarthritis. Both Ficat and Arlet Classification and ARCO's Classification for osteonecrosis of femoral head was used for clinical assessment and planning the treatment.

In early stages (pre-radiological) X-ray will not reveal any findings and diagnosis can only be done by functional bone investigation, if one suspects osteonecrosis of femoral head especially in high risk patients. (Hungerford D.S., 1979; Ficat R.P. 1983; Hungerford D.S. et al. 1985; Camp J.F. et al. 1986). The earliest changes on X-ray are diffuse or spotty osteonecrosis, sclerosis or mixed picture. At times the mixture of osteoporosis, sclerosis and cystic changes are seen. Subsequently small infarct occurs as a rim of increased density at the periphery while the contour is still maintained. This band of increased density results from the repair process. Then the femoral head appears subtly flattened and at this stage crescent sign appears which is caused by fractures through the dead subchondral bone. The fracture is caused by weakening of bone in this region when the rate of bone of resorption exceeds the rate of repair. Subsequently there is fissuring and collapse of the necrotic segment changing the contour of the femoral head with a definite step at the margins of the infarcted zones (Fig. 6.13). Finally osteoarthritic changes are seen, initially in femoral head and subsequently even in acetabular side (Fig. 6.14-6.17).

Kerboul et al. (1974) attempted to evaluate the extent of necrosis by measuring the arc of involvement on AP & Lateral radiograph. The extent was considered large when the sum of the area was 200° or small when 160° or less. He reported that when the combined angle is more than 200° the clinical outcome is poorer than when combined angle is smaller.

Osteonecrotic changes are most frequent and severe in weight bearing portion, especially in the femoral head. These changes can be subdivided into 3 groups on the basis of their roentgenographic appearance.

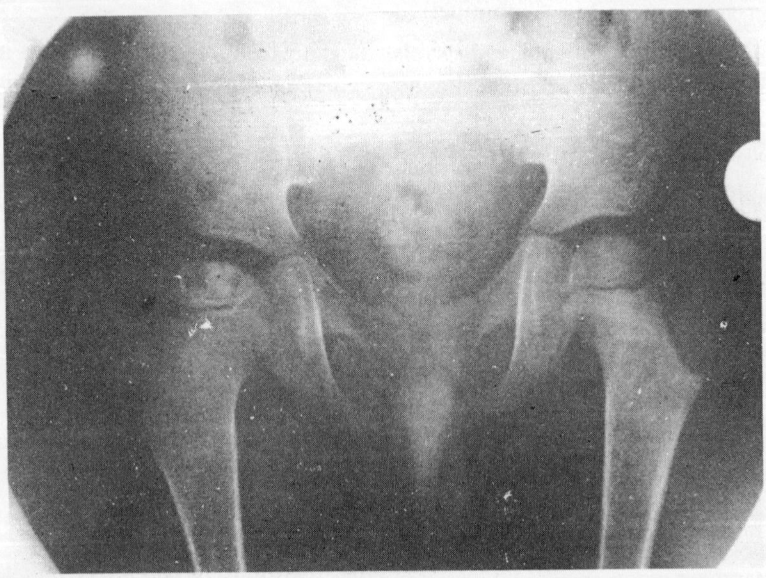

Fig. 6.11. X-ray pelvis of young boy of 8 yrs. showing sclerosis and cavitation in the epiphyseal nucleus without any collapse.

GROUP I (LEGG-CALVE-PERTHES TYPE)

Lesions are found in children 8 years old or less and are similar to those found in Legg-Calve-Perthes disease (Fig. 6.11, 6.12). They usually regenerate without producing significant disability. In teenagers from 13 to 18 years old, X-rays may show necrosis involving the entire epiphysis or only a sharply defined, segmental area in the anterosuperior epiphysis. No matter whether the epiphysis is completely or partially involved, the metaphysis is usually spared. The prognosis is not good in older adolescents with extensive epiphyseal involvement, but in younger adolescents spontaneous healing may occur if the epiphysis is only partially involved.

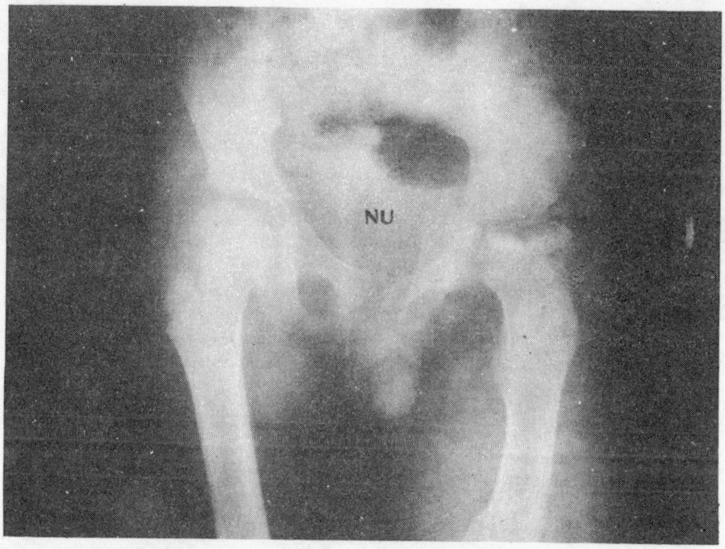

Fig. 6.12. X-ray pelvis showing osteonecrosis. Femoral head on left side is flattened . The centre of femoral nucleus is affected which is cystic and sclerotic. The patient also had osteomyelitis of same sided femur with growth disturbance.

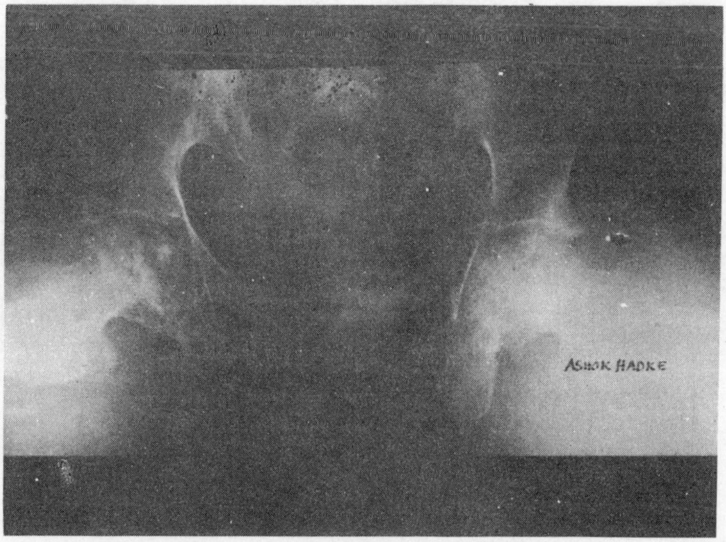

Fig. 6.13. X-ray Dunn's view of pelvis showing fissuring and collapse in a necrotic femoral head of both hips with classical changes of osteonecrosis in young sickler of 24 yrs.

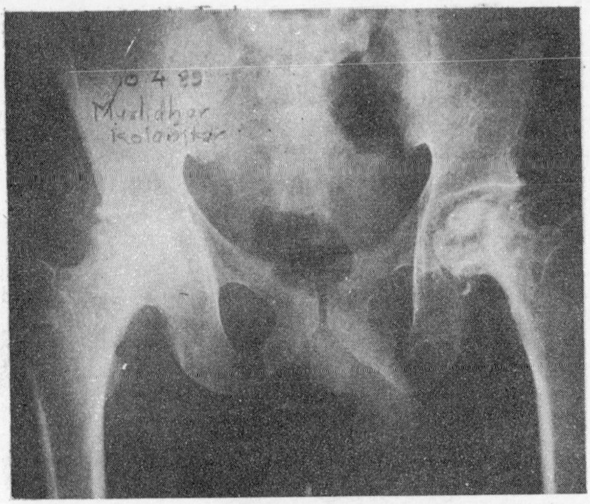

Fig. 6.14

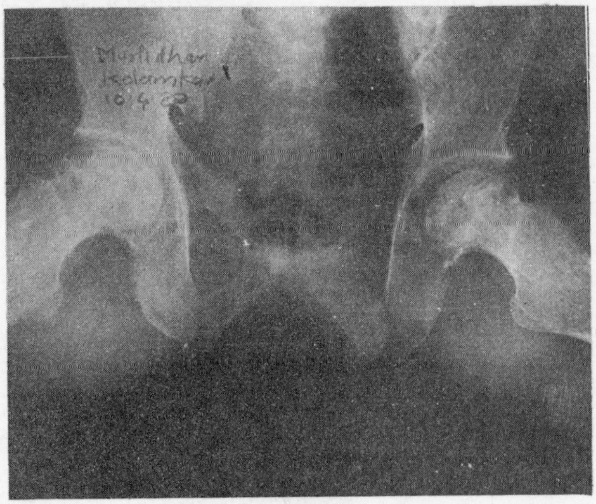

Fig. 6.15

Fig. 6.14 and 6.15. X-ray pelvis A.P. & Dunn's view showing bilateral avascular necrosis of femoral head in young 25yrs. sickler. The contour of the femoral head is well maintained on right side but lot of fragmentation, collapse of femoral head on left side with arthritic changes.

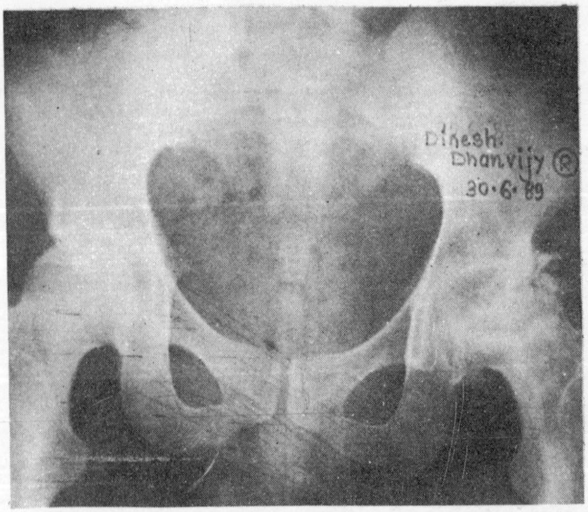

Fig. 6.16

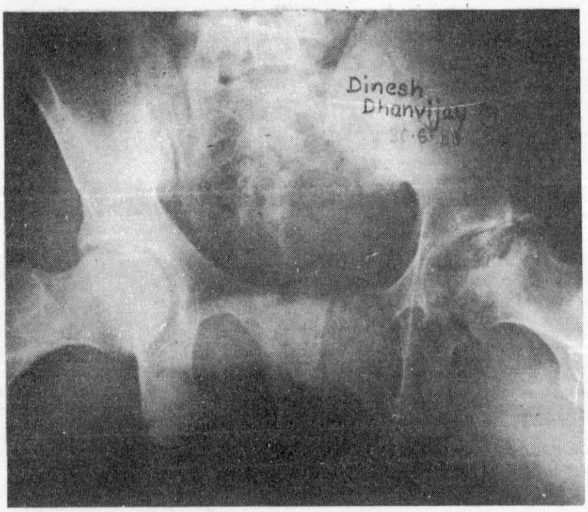

Fig. 6.17

Fig. 6.16 and 6.17. X-ray pelvis A.P. & Dunn's view in 28 years old Sickler with advanced changes of osteonecrosis and osteoarthritis.

GROUP II (OSTEOCHONDRITIS DISSECANS TYPE)

Lesions resemble those in osteochondritis dissecans. This type of lesion, which is observed in only one teenager and one adult, is restricted to a smaller area of the superior femoral head and, unlike Group I changes in adolescents, does not extend as far as the epiphyseal plate. This type of lesion did not heal spontaneously in either case.

GROUP III (DEGENERATIVE TYPE)

Lesions are characterized by massive necrosis and are restricted to adult patients. X-rays show severe distortion and flattening of the femoral head. The femoral head collapse and, as in younger patients, distortion occurs in the area above the site of the fused growth plate. This suggests persistence of the separation between vascular territories supplying the epiphysis and metaphysis.

Scintigraphy with Tc 99m diphosphonate has proven very effective for early detection of osteonecrosis when the routine roentgenograms appeared within normal limits. By obtaining the bone and bone marrow scan in the first several days after the onset of crisis, it is possible to differentiate between osteonecrosis and osteomyelitis. In the latter condition the bone scan becomes positive within few days after the onset of the symptoms. The combination of the large defect on the bone marrow scan and the smaller negative effect on the bone scan appears to be a typical finding in patients with osteonecrosis.

However M.R.I. has replaced all the investigations for early diagnosis of osteonecrosis of femoral head. MRI has been successful in detecting early osteonecrosis of femoral head in number of conditions (Totty et al. 1984, Mitchell et al. 1987). Osteonecrosis in Sickle cell disease usually begins in adolescence and in adult life and as such is rare before the age of 6-7 years. Eventually the entire femoral head collapses and it may subluxate, the joint space narrows, the head flattens, and neck becomes wide. Cysts may form in acetabulum or femoral head.

The shape of the femoral head and its flattening was evaluated by means of template with concentric circles.To be classified as spherical (Normal) surface of femoral head on AP & Lat X-rays must follow the circle on template with variation less than 2 mm. When the variation was more than 2 mm, head was considered non-spherical but as having Coxa Plana. Coxa Plana was divided into three categories. Round, Flat and Irregular depending upon the shape and regularity of the surface.The changes were labelled as Coxa Magna when femoral head was bigger in size by at least 5 mm.

Acetabular dysplasia and protrusion was diagnosed using the criteria for coverage of femoral head by CE angle of Wiberg and criteria of Armbuster et al. ~~for~~ prosthesis. Lateral subluxation of femoral head was diagnosed when the distance between acetabulum and medial surface of femoral head at the most distal point was more than 10 mm. Superior subluxation was suspected when there was break in the Shenton's line, measured by drawing the lines by projecting the inferior surface of femoral neck and relating it to the obturator foramina & distance was considered abnormal when it was more than 5 mm. For the assessment of abnormalities of growth. The X-rays were looked for Coxa vara, broadening and shortening of the neck.

Osteonecrosis of femoral head can also be divided in two categories:

A. Affection of Immature femoral head

* Flattening (widened flattened epiphysis)
* Epiphyseo-metaphyseal overlap.
* Metaphyseal lucency with sclerotic border.
* Wide femoral neck.
* Mushroom deformity of femoral head with intact cortex.
* Joint space and articular surface well preserved.
* No disability.

B. Affection of mature femoral head

* Segmental involvement, commonly Antero superior.
* Collapse of femoral head.
* Collapse & Disruption of articular surface.
* Sequestration.
* Short cortical discontinuity.
* Upward projection of lateral part of femoral head.
* Lateral Subluxation.
* Lucent subcortical line.
* Lytic defect.
* Osteophytosis & Secondary osteoarthritic changes.

Patchy sclerosis in addition to dense solid shadows, dense layers & rings with lucent centres and osteoporosis was observed in the medulla.

Immature femoral head changes are similar to those seen in Perthe's disease. Radiologically these two lesions are so similar that differentiation is based on other criteria such as younger age of onset in Perthes, negative sickling test and absence of abnormal haemoglobins.

Osteonecrosis of mature femoral head is typically segmental and frequently affects AP part of femoral head. An early radiological sign of this lesion may be lucent subcortical line described by Norman and Bullough in 1963 in Dysbaric Osteonecrosis (crescent sign). This is thought to result from subarticular trabecular fracture & resorption preceding collapse of articular surface.

After collapse there is subluxation of femoral head & medial part may result in projection lying lateral to acetabular roof and limiting abduction. It is this anterolateral subluxating portion which may bring the patient to surgical attention. Early involvement of femoral head is not painful but once the medial portion begins to collapse the lower extremity is pushed in adduction and a limp due to apparent shortening develops rapidly. Following disruption of articular surface, clinical outcome depends on the site & degree of destruction of femoral head and on the development of secondary osteoarthritis.

NON-INVASIVE TECHNIQUE

Noninvasive technique like bone scan, CT scan and MRI are useful mainly for screening high risk patients. However these investigations offer a unique opportunity (before radiological changes are evident) to diagnose osteonecrosis of femoral head in its early form.

Bone Scanning

Technetium 99 methylene-di-phosphate bone scanning is a useful technique. In general, the reactivity of bone around the infarcted segment shows a increased uptake of isotopes on the delayed image. This represents a accumulation of the radionuclide in the area of increased bone turnover at the junction of dead & reactive bone.

Although increased uptake alone can be seen in reflex sympathetic dystrophy, transient osteoporosis, infarction, tumours etc; a photopenic area surrounded by an area of the increase activity is most consistent with a diagnosis of osteonecrosis.

Since bone scan is a low cost investigation its use is recommended in patients who has a negative radiograph for osteonecrosis, no risk factors and unilateral symptoms. If the bone scan is negative patient should be observed & followed.

MRI

MRI is the most accurate imaging modality for the diagnosis of osteonecrosis. The earliest finding of osteonecrosis is single density line (a low intensity signal) on T1 generated image that presumably represents the separation of normal and ischaemic bone. Double line on T2 generated image a signal including line represents hypervascular granulation tissue. MRI is used to outline the area of involvement. It can show the revascularisation front and can provide objective evidence of changes in the tissues in response to treatment. It also allows sequential evaluation of asymptomatic lesions which are not seen on plain radiograph.

Rarely histopathological examination reveals the changes of osteonecrosis in patients who had negative MRI.

MRI is more sensitive and accurate than plain radiography. The extent as measured on an AP radiograph is not the same as in a mid coronal MRI and that in lateral radiograph does not correspond to a a mid saggital MRI. The extent of necrotic portion at the initial MRI scan predicts the risk of collapse of Femoral Head. Quantifying the extent of osteonecrosis of femoral head can be a major predictor of future collapse which can be clinically useful in the management of early stage osteonecrosis of femoral head (K.H. Koo & R. Kim 1995).

The mid coronal (A) & mid sagittal (B) sections which showed the largest diameter of femoral head were used for the measurement.

$$\frac{A}{180} \times \frac{B}{180} = \text{index of necrotic segment}$$

A = small necrosis < 33
B = medium necrosis 34-66
C = large necrosis 67-100

CT

It is expensive and exposes the patient to a considerable amount of radiation and it is usually unnecessary for establishing the diagnosis of osteonecrosis.

TREATMENT

The patient with proven osteonecrosis of femoral head should be observed closely since 50% to 80% of the patients develop bilateral affection.(Merle D'Aubingne R. Postel M. et al. 1965; Boettcher W.G. et al., 1970; Ficat R.P., 1983). Any symptoms if it develops in untreated contralateral hip should be taken as high risk and suspicious of osteonecrosis of femoral head, especially when seen in disorders which are known to cause osteonecrosis.

Rationale for the treatment of osteonecrosis of femoral head requires a lot of consideration. Prime importance in this is the age of patients, whether both hips are affected, etiopathology and type of the associated Sickle cell disease, demands and requirement of the patients and the stage of the disease when the patient presents for the treatment is equally important. (The treatment was planned according to ARCO's classification) (Table 6.6).

Non-weight-bearing conservative management of ischaemic necrosis has not been proved to be beneficial and hence various operative procedures are done depending upon the stage of necrosis of femoral head. Though maximum efforts were taken in performing head preserving surgeries, on many occasions patient required Total hip replacement in these young sicklers. It is believed that once crescent sign appears and there is a collapse of necrotic bone segment, even if it is minimal on x-ray, further collapse is inevitable and hip joints is likely to degenerate (Kenzora J.E. and Glimcher M.J., 1985). Any procedure like core decompression and bone grafting which is likely to revascularise the dead segment is not going to be useful once the collapse of segment occurs. Hence in this stage III the attempts to change the weight bearing portions by different osteotomies are performed. (Sugioka Y. 1978, 1980, Kempt I et al. 1984), though in some percentage of patients it may fail.

Chung, Alavi & Russel 1978 reported the evidence to suggest that osteonecrosis in Sickle cell disease in early stages the changes are reversible and they reported several patients of osteonecrosis treated by strict non weight bearing gained both symptomatic and radiographic impairment. Once the changes have advanced to stage 3 or more has developed, there is little chance of improvement and surgery is the only option. Amongst the surgery for osteonecrosis of femoral head the patients were graded according to stages and divided in two groups:

I. Those requiring head preserving surgery (Early Stage)
II. Those requiring head sacrificing surgery (Advanced Stage)

I. Those requiring head preserving Surgeries — Early Stage

Head preserving surgeries were done in stage I, II, III & sometime in stage IV which included core decompression and bone grafting and various osteotomies (Table 6.6). Aim of the treatment at this stage is to reduce the ischaemia, intraosseous tension and perform the procedure which will cause early revascularisation of ischaemic head. Only core decompression which was done earlier was always coupled with bone grafting as an additional procedure even in all those cases (core decompression - bone grafting was done) who had asymptomatic contralateral hip in a known patient of osteonecrosis of femoral head without any radiological changes and the diagnosis was established by functional bone investigations or MRI & Scan. An additional fibular graft was always inserted to protect the core tract similar to the patients where the changes were evident radiologically before the collapse.

Table 6.6. Details of Number of Surgical procedures according to the ARCO's Classification.

Type of procedure	*Total number of procedures*	*0 & I*	*II*	*III*	*IV*
Core decompression and Bone grafting	88				
Vascular Pedicle Graft	18	04	11	03	Nil
Phemister Fibular Graft	26	06	12	08	Nil
Cancellous Iliac Graft	14	Nil	08	06	Nil
Muscle Ped.Graft	30	Nil	08	18	04
Intertrochantric osteotomy	76				
Ventral Rot.Osteotomy	42	—	08	34	Nil
Flexion Osteotomy	16	—	03	13	—
Valgus/Varus Osteotomy	13	—	01	12	—
McMurray's Osteotomy	05	—	—	04	01

A. Prophylactic treatment (Stage 0 and I)

Whenever possible one must prevent the disease from occurring altogether. This can be very well achieved partially in the cases of osteonecrosis of femoral head following alcohol abuse, dysbarism and by avoiding the use of corticosteroids in conditions i.e. renal transplantations, skin manifestations, ulcerative colitis etc., whereas the situation is different in Sickle cell disorder. Sickle cell patients are monitored closely and at the earliest hint of a crisis they are hydrated and oxygenated properly and acidosis is corrected. The patient with proven unilateral osteonecrosis of femoral head should be observed closely since 50% to 80% of the patients develop bilateral affection (Merle D'Aubingne R., Postel M. et al. 1965; Boettcher W.G. et al. 1970; Ficat R.P. 1983). Any symptoms if it develops in untreated hip should be taken as high risk suspicious of osteonecrosis of femoral head.

Wherever there are no radiographic changes, functional bone investigation or bone scanning should be done. If the bone scan is negative, patient should be closely observed and followed. May be sequential MRI has a place in this group of patients for early diagnosis.

B. Treatment in early stages (Before Collapse, Stage II & III)

Aim of the treatment at this stage is to reduce the intraosseous tension and perform the procedure which will cause early revascularisation of ischaemic head. In all these patients the changes were evident radiologically before the collapse (II & III). Core decompression and Phemister bone grafting by using long cortical graft from fibula was done on 26 occasions (In six cases on both sides) (Figs. 6.19-6.28) in twenty patients. Core decompression and bone grafting using cancellous bone graft from iliac crest of the same side was done on fourteen occasions where as vascular pedicle grafting was done on 18 occasions. It is said that cortical graft adds both to the biomechanical and biological advantages during the process of revascularisation. Whenever the crescent sign had appeared without any collapse, it was taken as the indication of vascular or muscle pedicle grafting in addition to core decompression. On 18 occasions Meyer's (Quadratus femoris muscle pedicle graft) procedure by posterolateral approach was done (Figs. 6.34-6.40) primarily and on twelve occasions - Sartorius muscle pedicle grafting by anterolateral approach in addition to forage was done (Figs. 6.41-6.43). Use of vascularised pedicle graft is more advantageous since high percentage of marrow and osteogenic cells survive within a living graft which helps for early vascularisation. This was done by anterior approach on 18 occasions using part of iliac crest with deep circumflex iliac vessels.Vascular pedicle is raised from iliac crest with deep circumflex iliac vessels which lie above the inguinal ligament opposite the inferior epigastric artery, a branch from external iliac artery. After making the desired length & width of free vascular graft from iliac crest the bone graft is swung to the hip region and the graft is tunnelled through intermuscular plane between the Rectus femoris & Pectineus. Subsequently a window is made in the neck at the intertrochanteric line and thorough curettage of the necrosed femoral head is done and the graft is trapped and made stable without kinking of vessels (Figs. 6.29-6.33).

C. Treatment following collapse (Stage IV)

It is believed that once crescent sign appears and there is a collapse of necrotic bone segment, even if it is minimal on x-rays, further collapse is inevitable and hip joint is likely to degenerate. (Kenzora J.E. and Glimcher M.J. 1985). Any procedure like core decompression and bone grafting which is likely to revascularise the dead segment is not going to be useful once the collapse of segment occurs. Hence at this Stage IV the procedure to change the weight bearing necrotic segment to nonweight bearing portion by different osteotomies, is performed. (Sugioka Y. 1978, 1980; Kempt et al. 1984).

In our centre 37 transtrochanteric ventral rotational osteotomies (Sugioka Y. 1978, 1984) were done primarily in cases with collapse of femoral head without any degenerative changes (Figs. 6.44-6.49) and on 5 occasions secondarily (Total 42 operations). On sixteen occasions flexion osteotomies were done (Figs. 6.50, 6.51). Basically in both these osteotomies the weight bearing superolateral segment is rotated anteromedially in non weight bearing region. Valgus osteotomy was done on five occasions and varus osteotomy was done on eight (Figs. 6.52-6.56). McMurray osteotomy frequently done in earlier days was not considered presently as suitable operation for osteonecrosis of femoral head though it was done in 5 cases in very early days. In all these operated patients early mobilisation was done but non-weight bearing was maintained for 4-5 months.

II. Those requiring head sacrificing surgeries—Advanced Stage

In this second group the femoral head was so badly affected, collapsed and fragmented with secondary arthritic changes, where, to achieve painless, mobile, stable hip was not possible (Figs. 6.57-6.59). In this group again there were options for three types of surgeries :

A. Girdlestone
B. Arthrodesis
C. Replacement Surgery

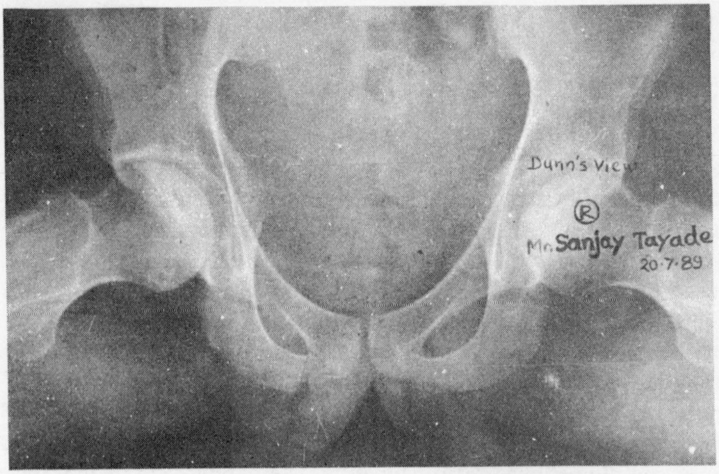

Fig. 6.18. X-ray pelvis Dunn's view showing bilateral osteonecrosis without any collapse but with subtle flattening of right femoral head in a young 20 years male with sickle cell trait.

Fig. 6.19

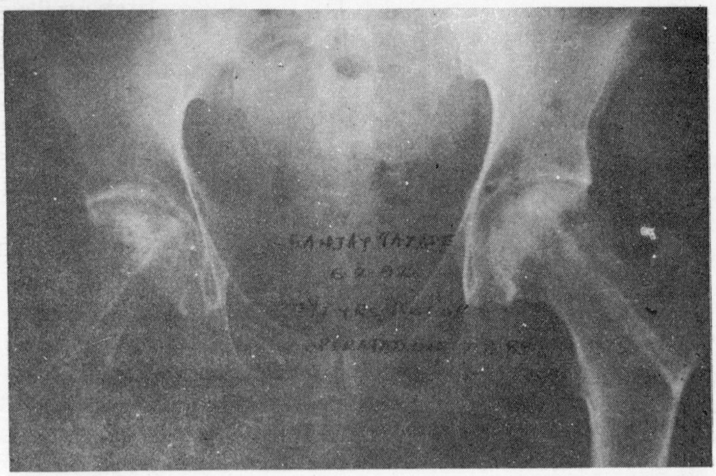

Fig. 6.20

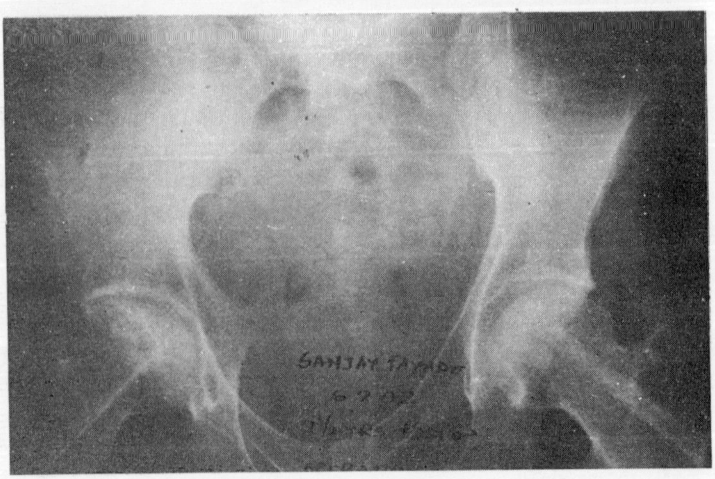

Fig. 6.19 and 6.20. X-ray pelvis of same patient (Fig.6.18) years after core decompression and Phemister bone grafting using long fibular graft. Contour of femoral head is well maintained even after 2.5 years.

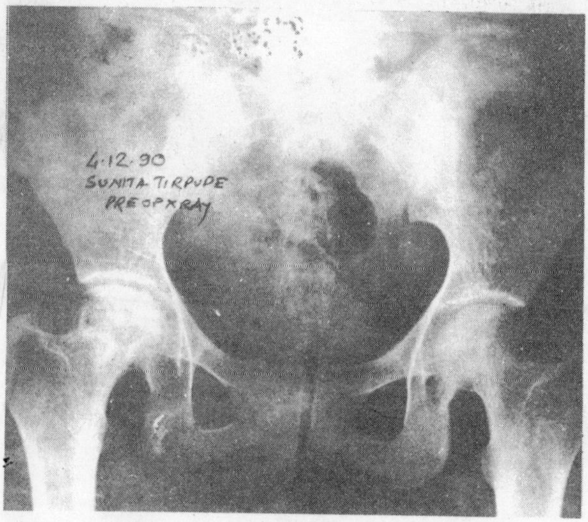

Fig. 6.21

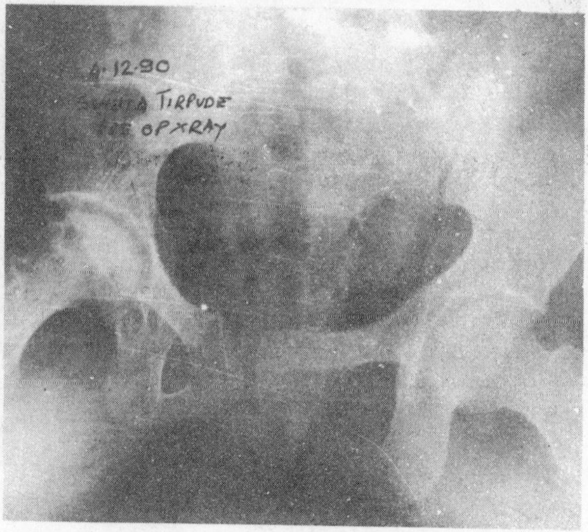

Fig. 6.22

Fig. 6.21 and 6.22. X-ray pelvis A.P. & Dunn's view in a young Sickle cell disease patient showing osteonecrosis of right femoral head.

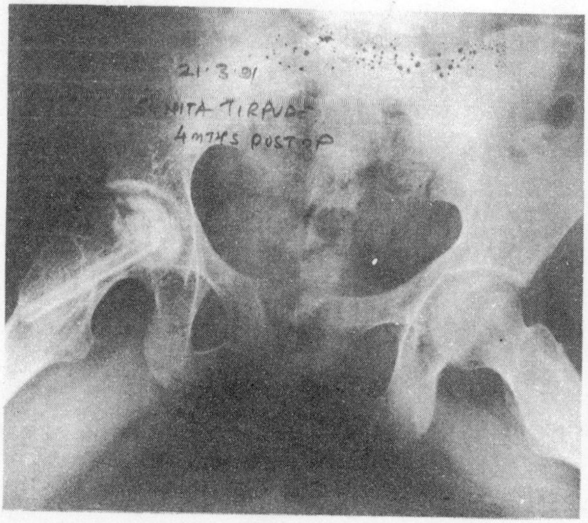

Fig. 6.23

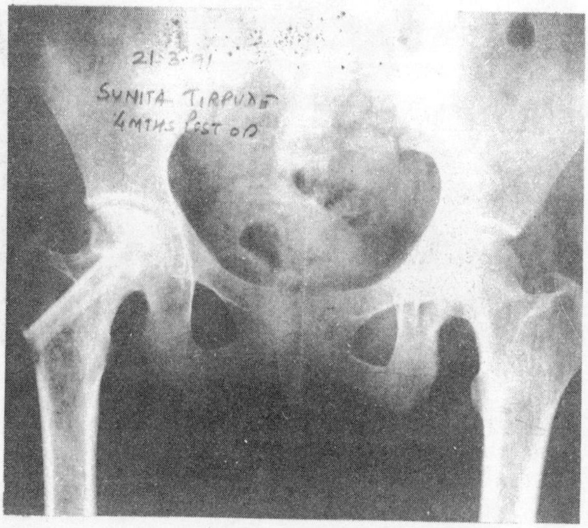

Fig. 6.24

Fig. 6.23 and 6.24. A.P. & Dunn's view same patient (Fig.6.21) postoperative X-ray four months after core decompression and Phemister bone grafting using long fibular graft.

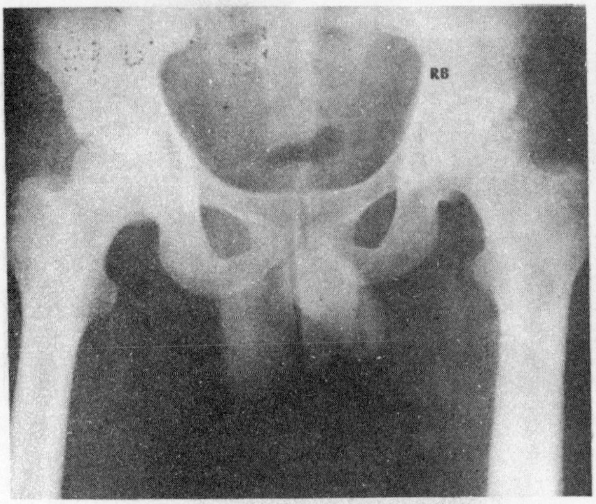

Fig. 6.25

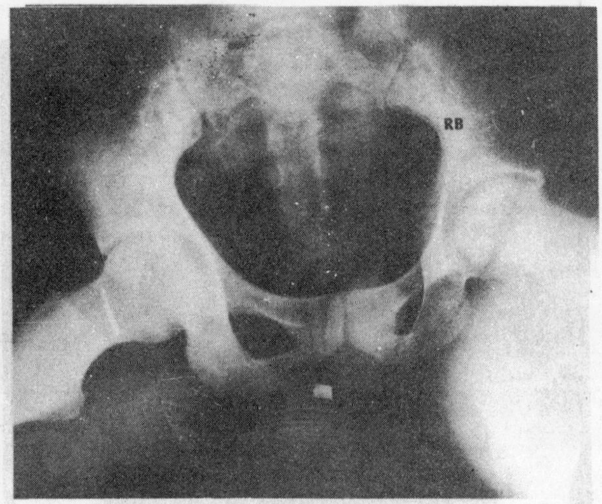

Fig. 6.26

Fig. 6.25 and 6.26. X-ray pelvis A.P. and Dunn's view of young Sickle cell patient with bilateral osteonecrosis with advanced changes on left side.

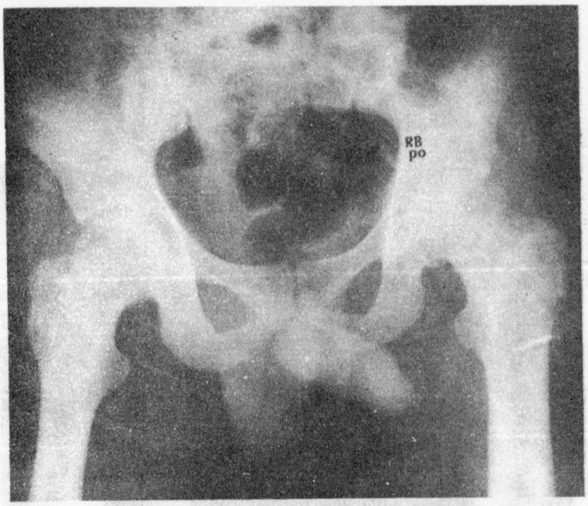

Fig. 6.27

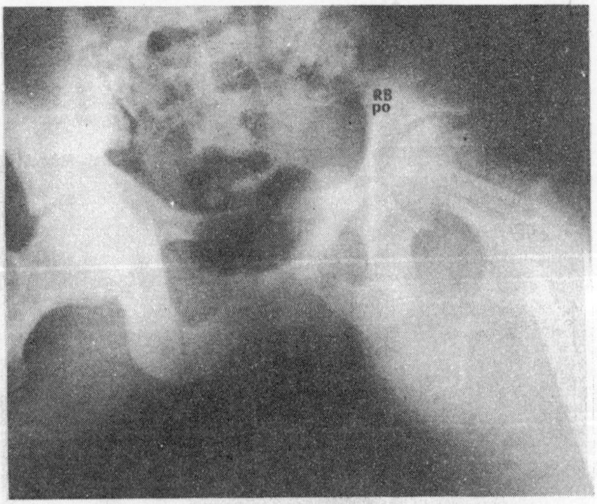

Fig. 6.28

Fig. 6.27 and 6.28. X-ray pelvis A.P. and Dunn's view postoperative after core decompression and fibular cortical graft.

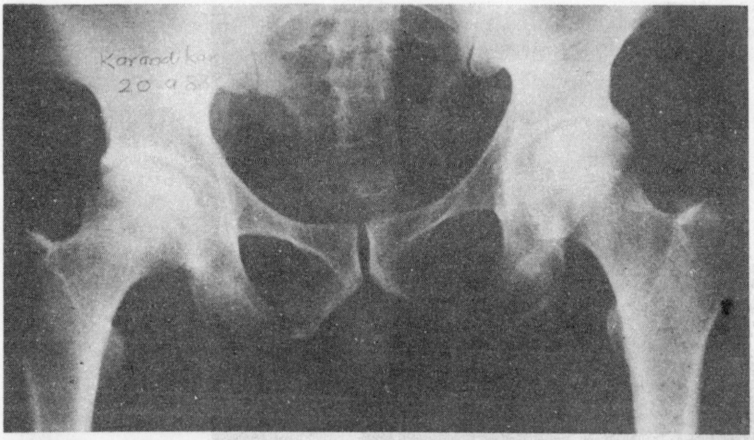

Fig. 6.29

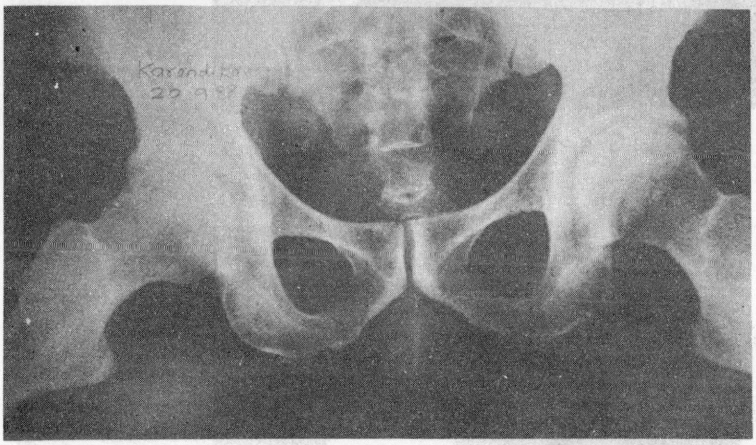

Fig. 6.30

Fig. 6.29 and 6.30. A.P. and Dunn's view of a young sickler in whom osteonecrosis was suspected but plain X-rays did not reveal any changes.

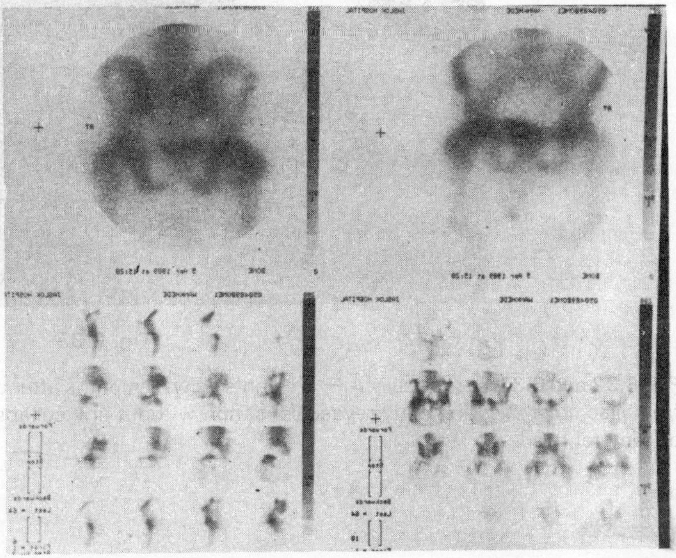

Fig. 6.31. Bone scan of young patient showing increased uptake in right femoral head suggestive of osteonecro-sis of femoral head in whom the plain X-rays were normal.

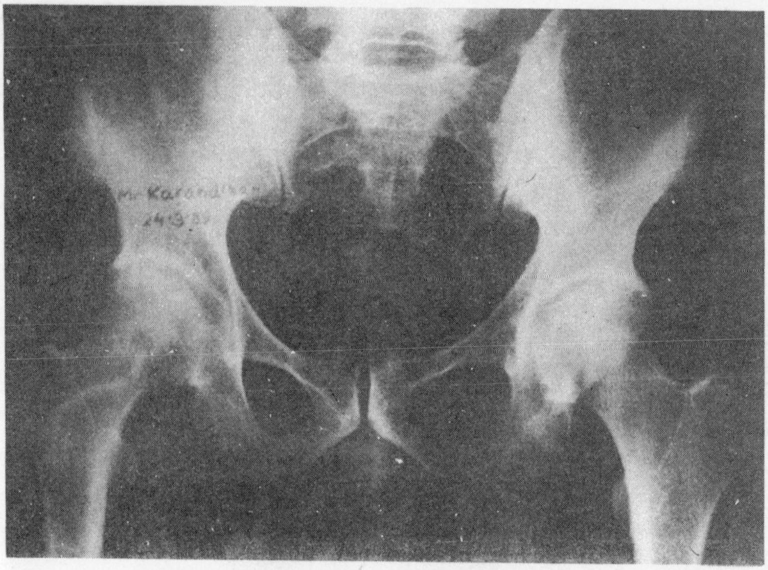

Fig. 6.32

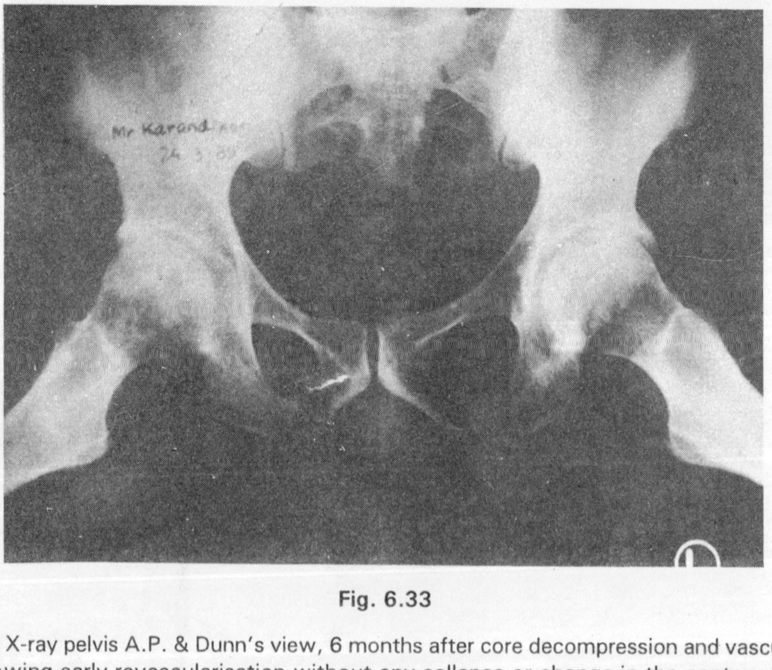

Fig. 6.33

Fig. 6.32 and 6.33. X-ray pelvis A.P. & Dunn's view, 6 months after core decompression and vascular pedicle grafting from iliac crest showing early revascularisation without any collapse or change in the contour of articular surface of femoral head.

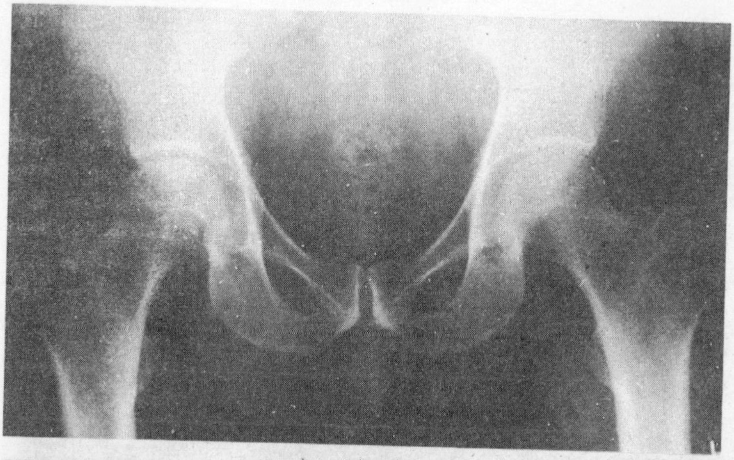

Fig. 6.34

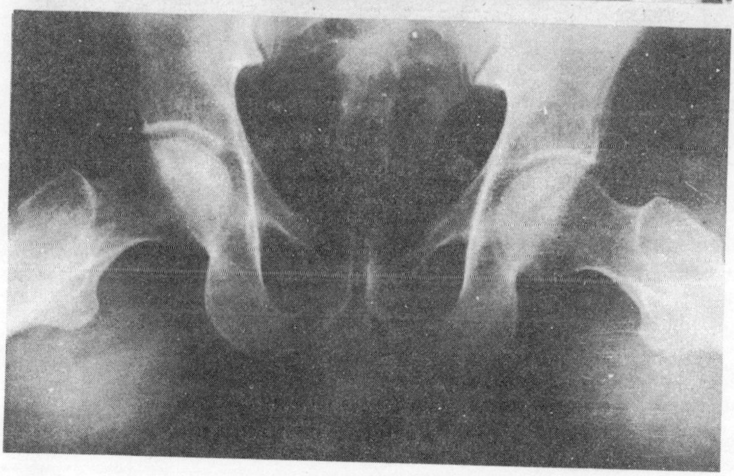

Fig. 6.35

Fig. 6.34 and 6.35. X-ray pelvis A.P. and Dunn's view of young lady 30 yrs. with S.S. pattern with osteonecrosis of right femoral head without any collapse.

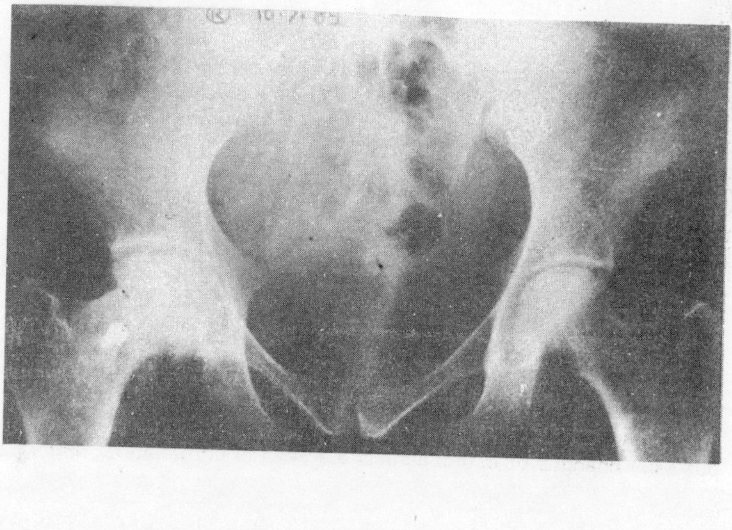

Fig. 6.36. X-ray pelvis A.P. same patient (Fig 6.34) two years after Meyer's procedure of Quadratus femoris muscle grafting showing minimal improvement. But there is no deterioration and no collapse. Contour of femoral head is well maintained with good hip joint space.

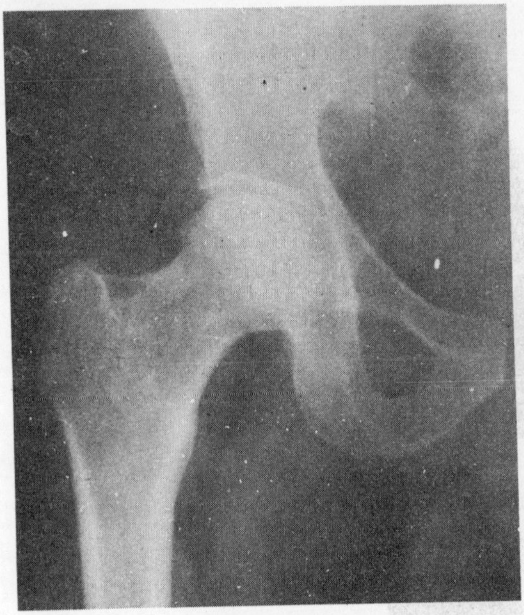

Fig. 6.37

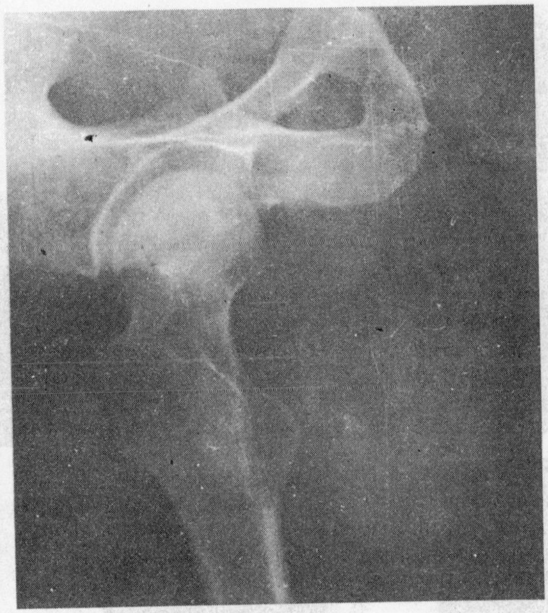

Fig. 6.38

Fig. 6.37 and 6.38. X-ray right hip A.P. and lateral view showing osteonecrosis of femoral head in young sickler of 36 yrs. but without any collapse of necrotic segment.

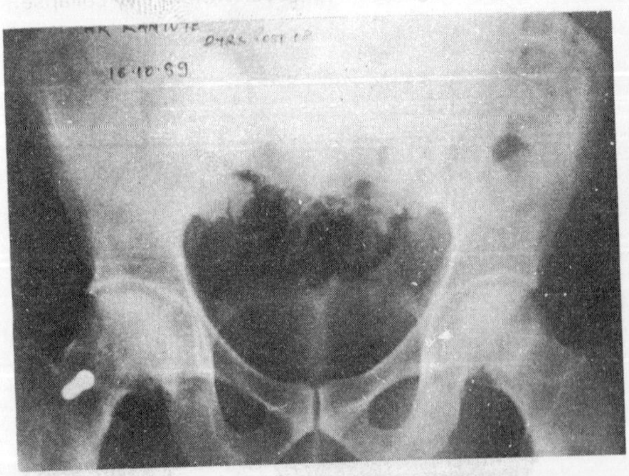

Fig. 6.39

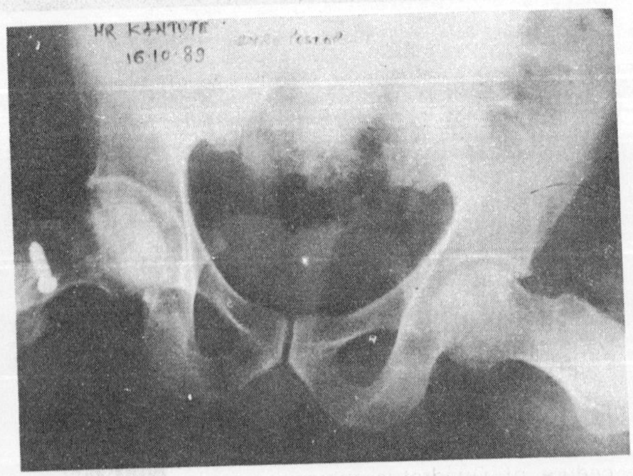

Fig. 6.40

Fig. 6.39 and 6.40. X-ray pelvis A.P. & Dunn's view of same patient (Figs.6.37 & 6.38) 2 years after Meyer's opera tion showing good vascularisation of right femoral head without any collapse. Good radiological improvement, but early changes of osteonecrosis are seen in contralateral femoral head.

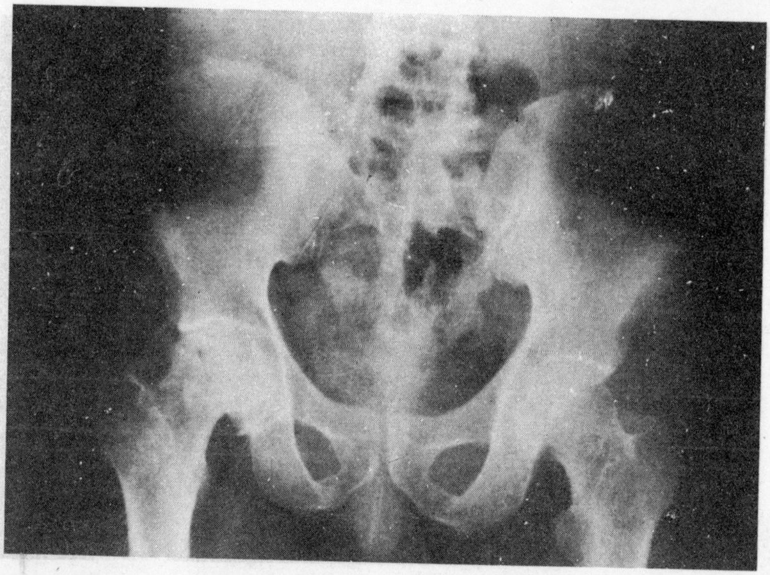

Fig. 6.41. X-ray pelvis A.P. showing advanced changes of osteonecrosis in right hip with fissuring and minimal collapse in a young 28 years sickle cell trait.

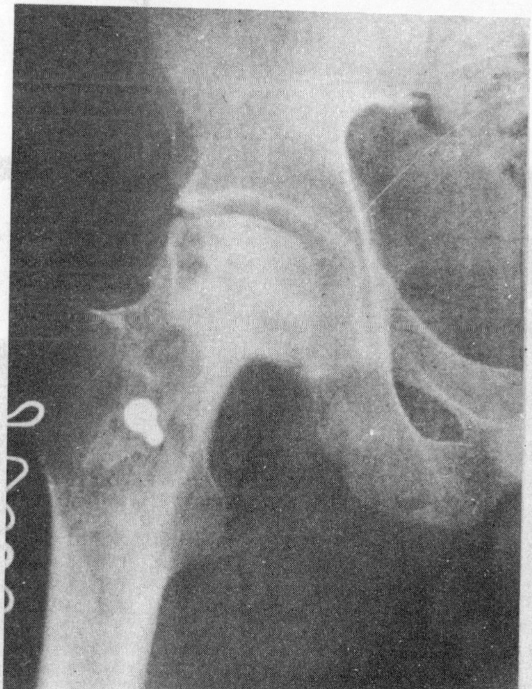

Fig. 6.42

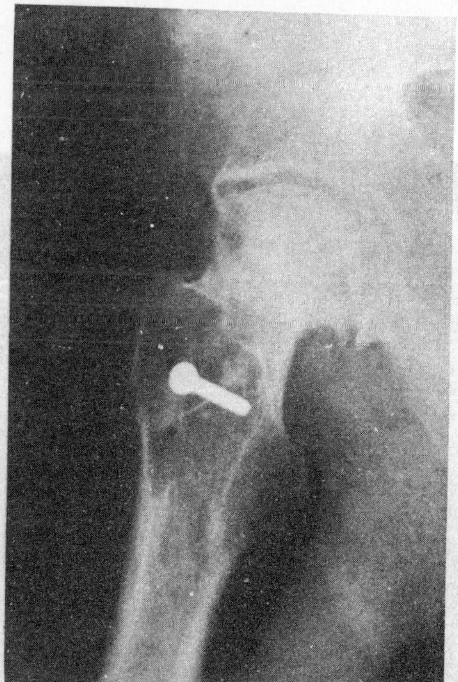

Fig. 6.43

Fig. 6.42 and 6.43. X-ray of same hip (fig.6.41) A.P. and lateral view 1.5 years after core decompression and Sartorius muscle pedicle grafting operation, showing revascularisation. No progression of osteonecrosis. Hip joint space is well maintained.

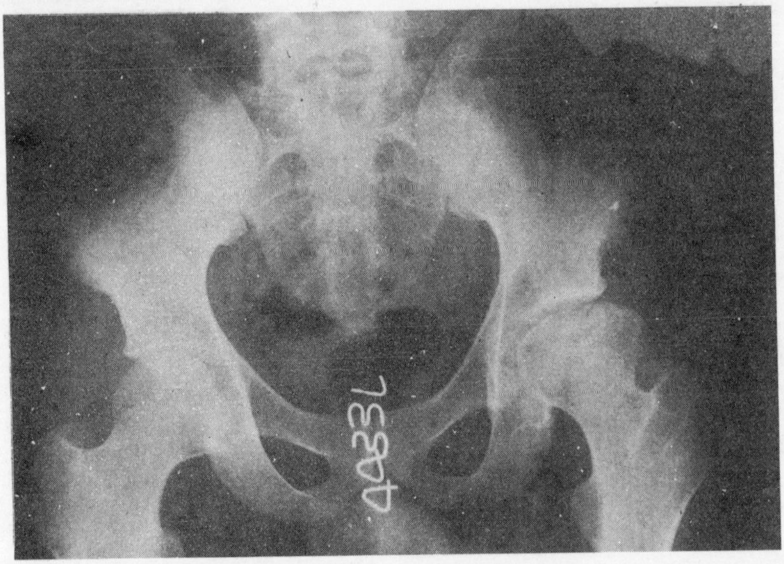

Fig. 6.44. X-ray pelvis A.P. showing osteonecrosis with collapse of small fragment in the centre of left femoral head in young 23 yrs. old sickler with S.S. pattern.

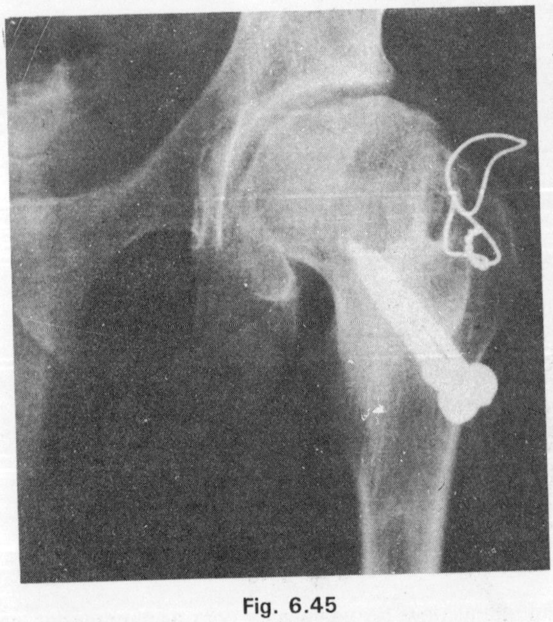

Fig. 6.45

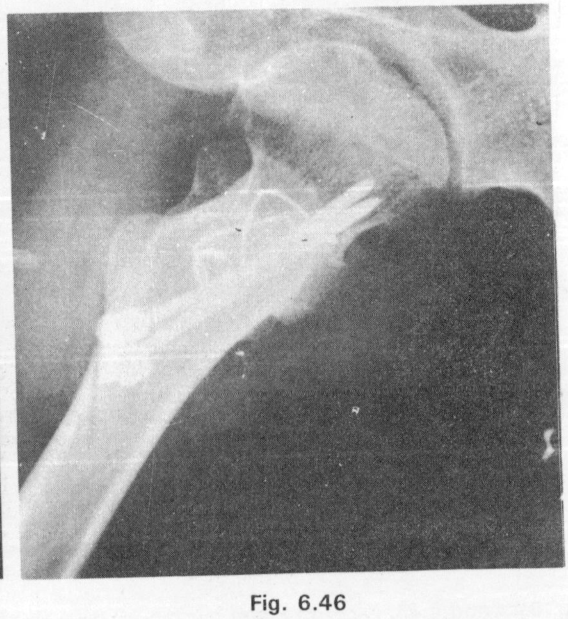

Fig. 6.46

Fig. 6.45 and 6.46. X-ray left hip A.P. and lateral view 2 years after ventral rotational osteotomy, showing good revascularisation of necrotic segment and smooth articular surface of weight bearing portion of femoral head.

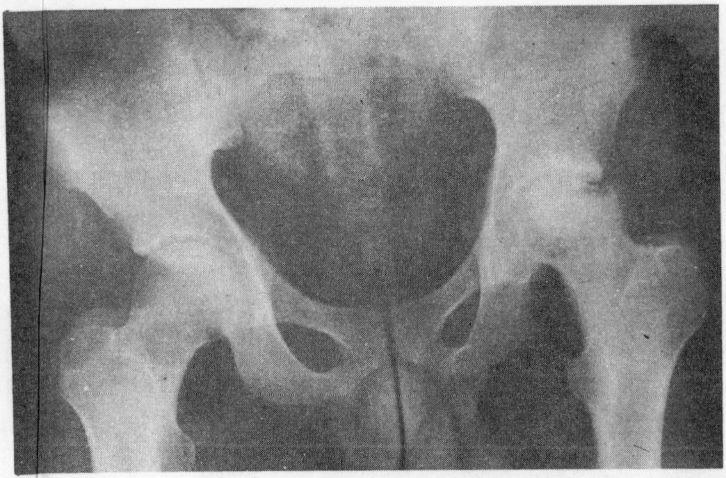

Fig. 6.47. X-ray pelvis A.P. showing osteonecrosis of left femoral head with collapse of necrotic segment in young sickler of 30 yrs.

Fig. 6.48

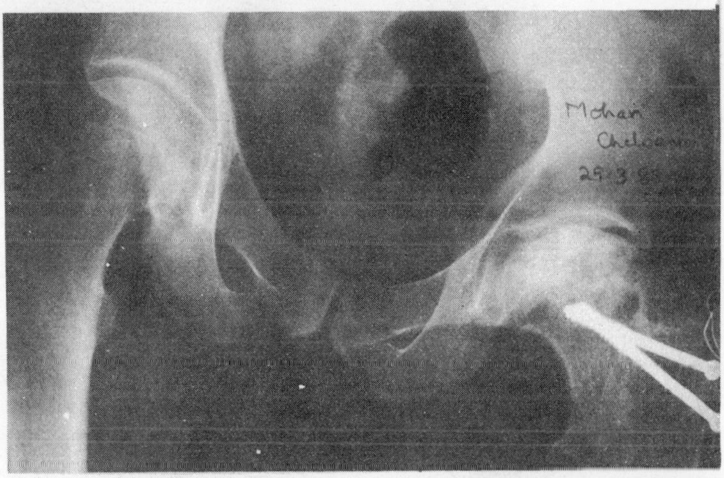

Fig. 6.49

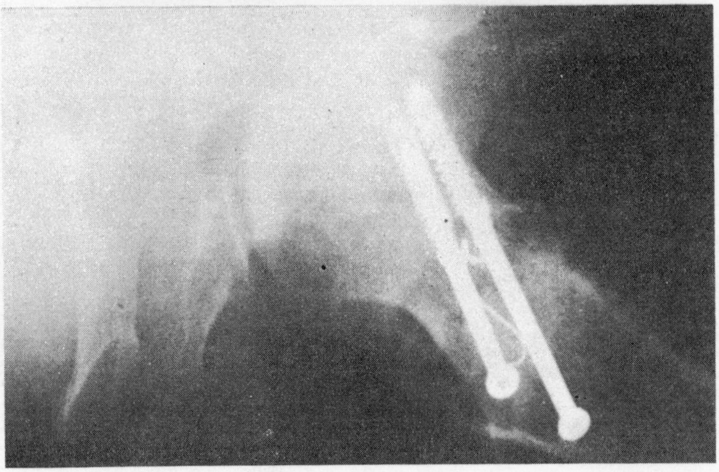

Fig. 6.48 and 6.49. X-ray pelvis (Fig. 6.47) A.P. and left hip lateral 14 months after ventral rotational osteotomy showing good revascularisation and smooth contour of articular surface.

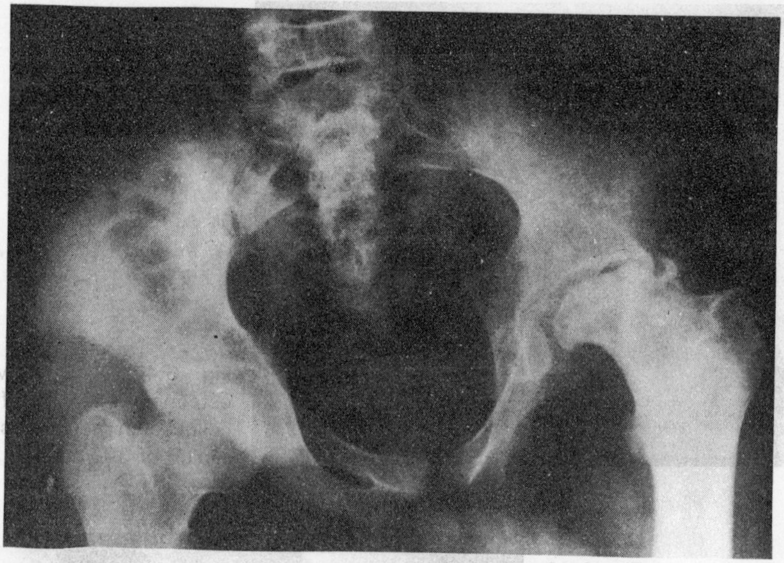

Fig. 6.50. X-ray pelvis A.P. showing advanced osteonecrosis in young patient of sickle cell haemoglobinopathy ith severe collapse of femoral head in young S.C. disease patient of 19 yrs.

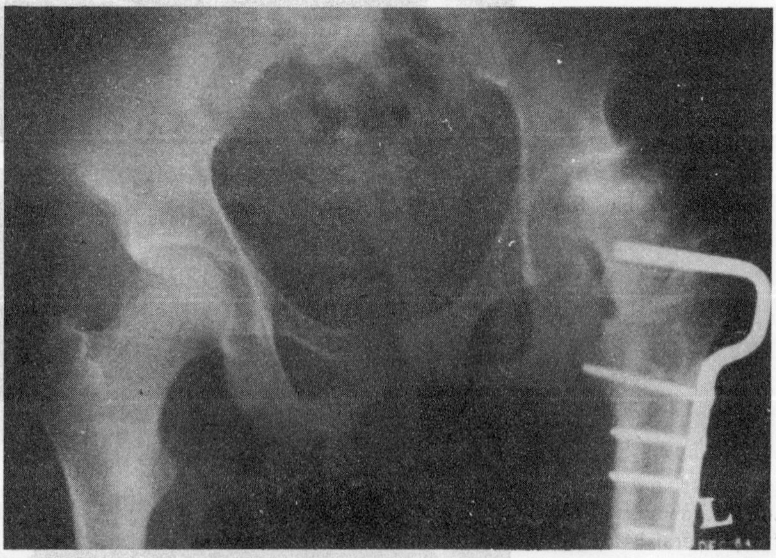

Fig. 6.51. X-ray pelvis of same patient (Fig. 6.50) one year after flexion rotational osteotomy showing improveme though minimal.

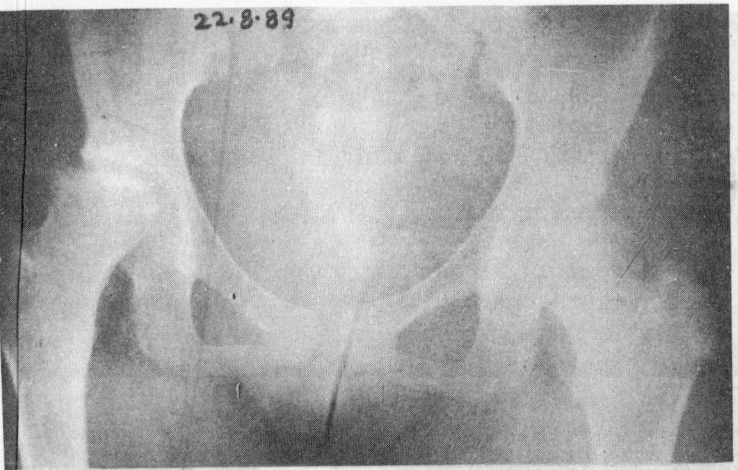

Fig. 6.52

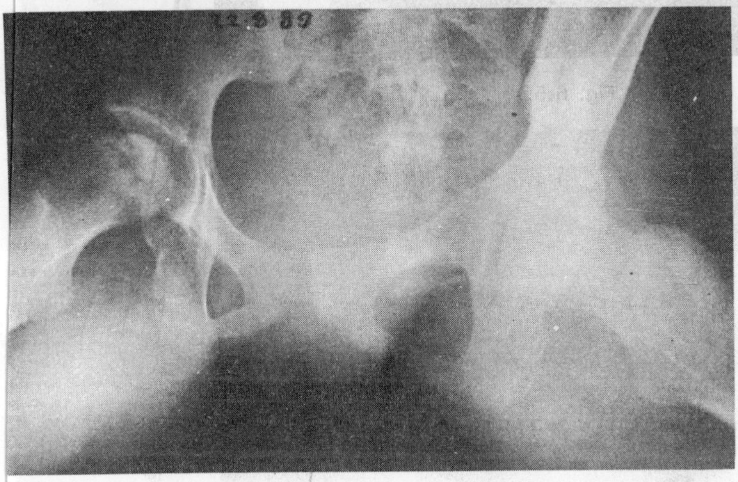

Fig. 6.53

Fig. 6.52 and 6.53. X-ray pelvis A.P. and Dunn's view showing osteonecrosis of right femoral head with collapse and lateral subluxation of femoral head in young girl of 20 years having S.S. pattern.

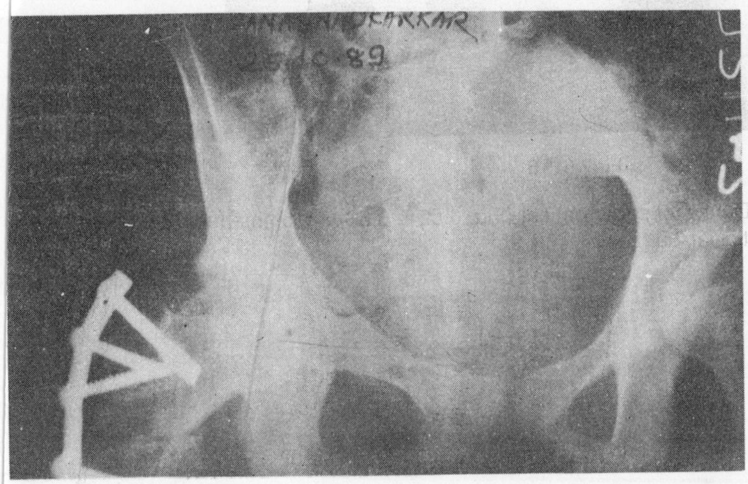

Fig. 6.54. X-ray pelvis of same patient of (Fig. 6.52 & 6.53) 2 months after varus osteotomy showing good containment and attempt towards revascularisation.

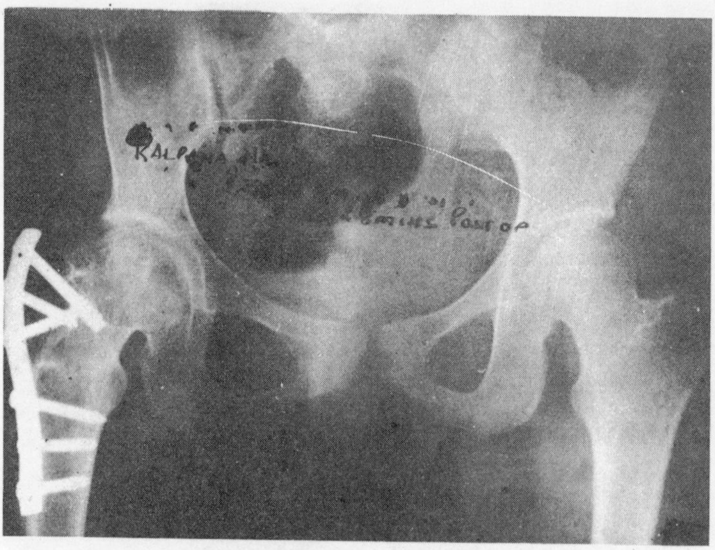

Fig. 6.55

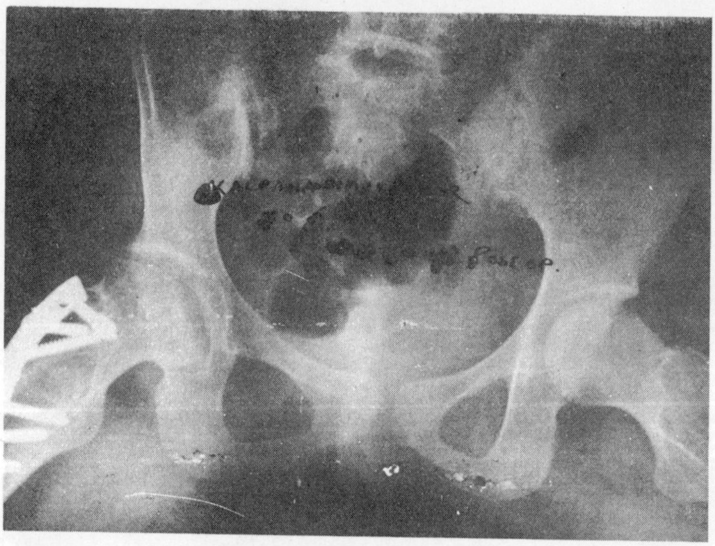

Fig. 6.56

Fig. 6.55 and 6.56. X-ray pelvis A.P. & Dunn's of same patient (Fig. 6.52 & 6.53) 8 months post-operative showir good containment and fairly smooth articular surface.

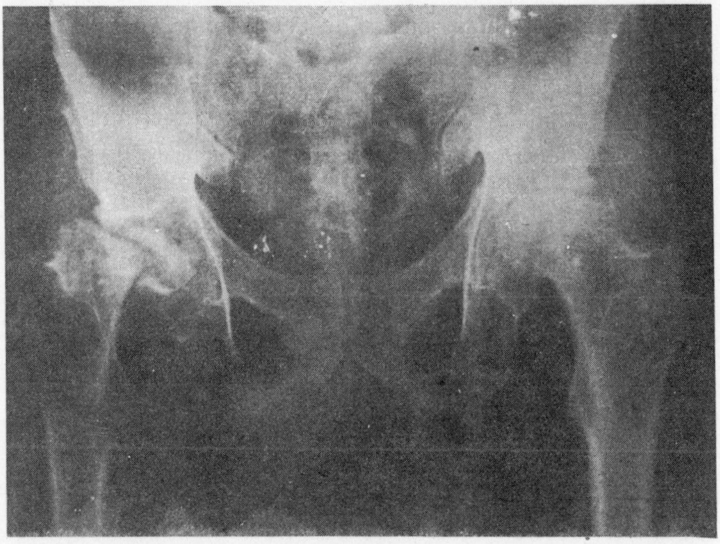

Fig. 6.57. X-ray pelvis showing gross collapse of femoral head on right side with fairly advanced changes on left side.

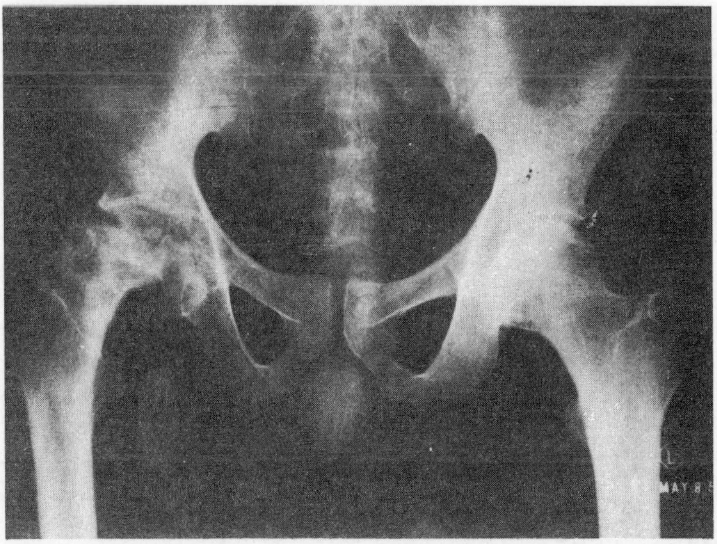

Fig. 6.58. X-ray showing collapse of femoral head, with subluxa- tion and arthritic changes.

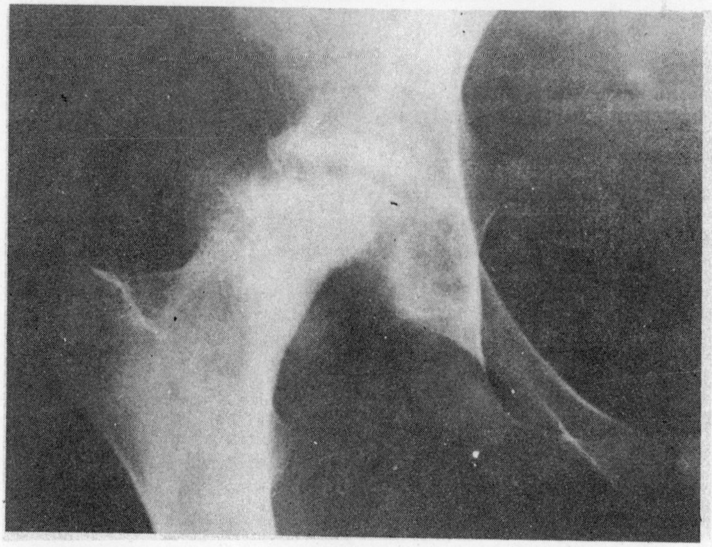

Fig. 6.59. X-ray of the hip showing advanced necrosis with subluxation.

Though in earlier days we had performed and promoted many patients for Girdlestone or arthrodesis, presently we encourage the patients more for replacement arthroplasty. Total Hip Replacement in these patients of Sickle cell haemoglobinopathy offers excellent quality of life. Since their life expectancy has improved because of better therapy and newer medical care. The patients of Sickle cell trait live almost normal life span as compared to other average patients of sickle cell disease.

In this duration in this series following surgeries were performed - 68 Hip Replacement surgeries, only 5 Girdlestone arthroplasty & 3 arthrodesis (Table 6.4 and 6.5). 68 total hip replacements were done in 60 patients who were suitable for surgery. These 60 patients form the part of this study, 34 hips were classified as Charnley Functional Class A (unilateral disease); 9 as Class B (Bilateral disease); 17 as Class C (Systemic disease affecting the ability to walk). Amongst these patients the younger 20 patients had Isoelastic Hip Replacement (Non-cemented femoral and acetabular components) and the physiologically older 38 patients had Charnley's type of hip replacement (Cemented Femoral & acetabular components). Amongst other replacement we did bipolar prosthesis on 9 occasions, A.M.P. on 3 occasions. We had no experience of osteochondral allograft (Meyer M. 1978) or spongioplasty or vascular bundle transplantation (Hori) or electrical stimulation (Steinberg et al. 1984, 1985). The patients were evaluated pre-operatively and post-operatively with the use of the system of **Merle d'Aubigne and Postel as modified by Charnley** for the assessment of pain and walking ability. Although the scores for pain and walking were prospectively evaluated for each patient each year, only the results of the most recent post-operative assessment were analysed for this study (Table 6.8). The scoring system awards 6 points each for pain and walking, with the maximum score being 12 points. A combined score of 11 or 12 points was considered to indicate an excellent result : 9 or 10 points, a good result : 8 points, Fair and 7 points or less a clinical failure. Any pain score of 3 points or less at the time of most recent evaluation was also considered to represent a failure. This clinical scoring system was used at yearly intervals for the first 5 years post-operatively and then at 2-year intervals.

PERIOPERATIVE MANAGEMENT

The management of a patient of Sickle cell disease, to undergo surgery demands a planned control of various factors which can precipitate sickling or aggravate the already existing anaemic state. The management aims at maintenance of a steady state of haemoglobin and avoidance of factors that are known to precipitate sickling like hypoxia, acidosis, hypotension, peripheral circulatory stasis, hypothermia, dehydration, respiratory depression.

Blood Transfusion

Preoperatively or during surgery, transfusion with packed red cells is sometimes necessary but is not without risk. The rationale for preoperative transfusion is to achieve reduction in the level of HbS by diluting with HbA blood. By their presence normal red cells limit the maximum increase in viscosity resulting from the condition of lower pH and decreased oxygen tension. This raises the Hb level to normal and thereby live sickle cells to be removed from circulation. Such a procedure simultaneously dilutes the sickle cells with normal cells and increases the blood volume and thus without producing circulatory overload.

Anaesthesia

Wherever possible, general anaesthesia should be avoided and spinal anaesthesia or epidural block should be used.

Hypoxia

Hypoxia can be prevented by taking following precautions during surgery and postoperatively.

* Before inducing a patient 100% oxygenation for 3 to 5 minutes.
* Intubation should be smooth without any episode of breath holding or laryngeal spasm.
* Maintenance with gas (N_20) or Halothane should be combined with proper oxygen concentration (30 to 50 percent) in the inspired air.
* Extubation should be preceded by 100% oxygenation.
* Postoperatively oxygen supplementation under supervision should be continued till full recovery of the patients from anaesthesia.

Acidosis

This can be prevented by pre operative oral soda bi-carb 0.5 to 1 g/kg/day. Intra-operatively administration of intravenous soda bi-carb 3.3 mEq/kg/hr over a period of 90 minutes is recommended. It should be continued after surgery for 24 to 48 hrs.

Hypotension, Peripheral Stasis and Dehydration

This can be avoided by encouraging oral intake preoperatively and proper intravenous fluid infusions intra operatively. Tourniquets should be avoided as far as possible. Their use should be kept limited to only those situations where their omission will jeopardise the surgical safety or success. Low molecular weight dextran to prevent hypotension is given intra-operatively.

Hypothermia

Hypothermia has two-fold effect :

1. Vasoconstriction leading to peripheral stasis and thus precipitating sickling.
2. Shivering leading to increased oxygen demand.

Measures to prevent hypothermia include:

* Prevention of excessive cooling of the theatre.
* Judicious use of halothane intra-operatively because halothane is known to cause post operative shivering.
* Infusing I.V. fluids of optimum temperature.

Drugs

1. Zinc orally preoperatively and post-operatively.
2. Folic acid orally.
3. Low molecular weight dextran intra-operatively to replace the fluid loss is recommended.
4. Sodium bicarbonate orally & I.V. preoperatively, during surgery and post-operatively.

COMPLICATIONS

Postoperative haematoma was commonly observed & was seen in 21 patients. Nine patients had deep-seated infection. In two patients head had to be excised, out of which total hip replacement was done in one patient after a year. Mechanical loosening was noticed in acetabular component in one patient of THR which required revision. Bacteraemia with generalised spread of infection occurred in these patients of Sickle cell disease. No other complications were noticed. Though Sickle cell crises was precipitated on 11 occasions, total complications were observed in 36 patients in this study of 169 patients treated surgically (Table 6.7).

Table 6.7. Postoperative complications.

Name of Complication	*No. of patients*	
	A *Head preserving group*	*B* *Head sacrificing group*
1. Haematoma	19	02
2. Infection	08	01
3. Mechanical loosening	—	02
4. Septic loosening	—	01
5. Bacteraemia	03	—
Total	30	06
6. Precipitation of haematological crisis	08	03
7. Post traumatic fracture of the tip of stem	—	—

FOLLOW-UP AND RESULTS

169 patients were followed who required surgery on 252 Hips. Amongst 164 head preserving surgeries on 88 occasions core decompression and various types of bone grafting were done. And on 76 occasions different types of intertrochanteric osteotomies were done to change the site of necrotic segment into non-weight bearing portion. Whereas in 75 patients surgery to preserve the integrity of femoral head was not possible and were subjected to Head sacrificing surgery. The patients were routinely followed every month and the results were analysed by Merle d' Au bigne & Postel modified by Charnley's system at the end of 12 months (Table 6.8).

In 60 patients 68 THR's were done, where as in 15 patients 20 surgeries of Girdlestone, Hemiarthroplasty, Bipolar & Arthrodesis were done.

DISCUSSION

Need to treat ischaemia of femoral head is becoming more common since many cases are detected in early stages in young patients. One must consider the possibility, of osteonecrosis if individual has pain in the vicinity of hip who has history of Sickle cell disease. Osteonecrosis of the femoral head is a common skeletal manifestation and complication observed in Sickle cell disease. Osteonecrosis affecting femoral head might be the first presentation of the Sickle cell disease. The symptomatology varies depending upon

Table 6.8. Analysis of results by Merle d'Aubigne & Postel modified by Charnley's system

Operative procedures	*No. of patients*	*Score points*		*Results*	
		Excellent 11-12	*Good 9-10*	*Fair 8*	*Poor 7 or <*
Core decompression and Bone Grafting	**88**				
Vascular Ped. Gft.	18	12	03	02	01
Phemister Fib. Gft.	26	12	05	05	04
Cancellous Iliac Gft.	14	04	03	04	03
Mayer's Mus.Ped.Gft.	30	15	04	07	04
Total		43	15	18	12
Osteotomy	**76**				
Ventral Rot.Ost'omy	42	18	10	08	06
Flexion Osteotomy	16	06	04	04	02
Valgus/Varus Ost'omy	13	05	03	03	02
McMurray's Osteotomy	05	00	01	01	03
Total		29	18	16	13
Total Hip R'cements	**68**	58	06	02	02

whether it is a trait or disease and the stage of the osteonecrosis . Once there is a collapse of articular surface by and large patients are likely to require replacement arthroplasty. Obviously if segmental collapse is minimal one could consider head preserving surgery but whereas collapse of articular surface is more & if weight bearing surface of more than 60% is involved replacement arthroplasty is the surgery of choice. Hypoxia, hypotension, circulating stasis, hypothermia, hypovolumia, respiratory depression, acidosis are all possible causes of Sickle cell crisis which can cause and lead to complications of anaesthesia and surgery which can predispose and precipitate sickling. Unless these patients are given plenty of parenteral fluids, (they cannot tolerate pre-operative oral fluid) restoration duc to renal concentrating defects is difficult and they become dehydrated leading to a vaso-occlusive crisis. Non-weight bearing conservative management of ischaemic necrosis has not been proved to be beneficial and hence various operative procedures are done depending upon the stage of necrosis of femoral head. Core decompression offers the opportunity to study histological changes of early bone ischaemia. It also achieves reduction in the symptoms of precollapse stage of ischaemic necrosis. With this study emphatically it is agreed that core decompression is the effective treatment in preradiological and pre-collapse stage of osteonecrosis of femoral head (Hungerford 1979; Ficat 1983, Camp J.1986) but it is necessary to add Cortical graft at the tract of core to avoid iatrogenic fracture. Certainly early diagnosis is the key to the success for head preserving operations. Once the crescent sign appears it is desirable to couple the bone grafting procedure in addition to the core decompression preferably vascular pedicle grafting. In patients with ischaemic necrotic segment without crescent sign, Phemister bone grafting is superior since it provides biomechanical and biological graft, where as once crescent sign appears without any collapse vascular or muscle pedicle graft is a good procedure. Once the collapse of ischaemic segment occurs all the procedures of core decompression and bone grafting are not expected to do any more good, and at this stage various osteotomies amongst head preserving operative groups are indicated (Sugioka Y.1978, Simonnet et al. 1984, Kempt I. et al. 1984). In such situations one must analyse the possible future development in osteonecrosis, so that failed osteotomy do not affect or worsen the situation for performing Total hip replacement. However this does not reduce the importance of effectiveness of osteotomies, since at this stage, this is the only group of operation in which relatively young patient does not undergo joint replacement and a benefit of 10-15 years can be easily drawn from osteotomy. Different types of intertrochanteric osteotomies are performed which preserve the joint as an important and efficient method to treat the cases of ischaemic necrosis of femoral head, which usually threatens the younger patients by its rampant destruction of joint which may result in severe disability. Basically in osteonecrosis of femoral head which is common in young age group a conservative approach is chosen (Kerboul et al. 1974) than a radical approach of reconstructive surgery. Essentially the results depend on the preoperative condition of the joint and the site of necrotic focus. If the ischaemic necrosis of femoral head is diagnosed early in stage 0 and I, core decompression by and large gives very good results. Head preserving operations certainly gives satisfactory results in Stage II, III and IV. The prognosis of Stage II and III is fairly good where as in Stage IV it is satisfactory, since about one third of this group are likely to progress further and may require joint surface or total hip joint replacement or resurfacing operations (Dutton R.O. & Amstutz H.C. et al. 1982). If there is a collapse of the articular surface, head preserving operation may be considered but with >60% articular surface involvement and degenerative changes total hip replacement is the treatment of choice. Replacement of the femoral head with a metal prosthesis may restore function and aid in rehabilitation of bed-ridden patients. This procedure has not been tried on a sufficient number of patients to appraise its work and its risk. The relatively short life of patients with Sickle cell anaemia and the inability of these patients to be gainfully employed should be taken into consideration in planning major elective operative procedures.

Joint replacement is being done on an increasing number of patients with the advent of general medical care of these sickler patients and advances in anesthetic agents and techniques. The relatively short life-span of these patients should be taken into consideration before planning such a major surgical procedure. Haddad (1967) presented several cases and recommended hemi-arthroplasty, and not arthrodesis, Girdlestone or total joint replacement. The clinical outcome of total joint replacement performed within the last twenty years has been excellent. The result have been disappointing in younger patients combined with the traditional older technique of cementing which has resulted into poorer results thus bringing non-cemented joint replacement in vogue. The theoretical advantage is biological ingrowth of bone thus leading to less likelihood for mechanical failure at implant bone interface. However two potential problems challenge this theory i.e. stress-shielding of proximal femur and osteolysis due to particulate debris.

Dorr et al. reviewed the results of 108 hip arthroplasties performed with cement in 81 patients who had been less than 45 years old. After four and one-half years follow up, they found a 19 percent of revision, a 29 percent of impending failure in hips that were not revised, and radiolucent lines at the bone-cement interface in 95% cases. In a more recent review of the same patients after nine years of follow-up, the rate of revision had almost tripled, to 33% of hips, the rate of impending had risen to 56% in the hips that had not been revised and radiolucent lines were present in all but one hip. Chandler et al. reviewed results of thirty-three total hip arthroplasties performed with cement in twenty-nine patients who were 30 years or less. After an average follow-up of 67 months, 21% of patients had a revision, 33% an impending failure, and 97% radiolucency at bone-cement interface.

In the present study of 68 hips in which cemented and non-cemented both varieties are used with satisfying results in either group, but it seems better to use non-cemented in the physiologically younger patients and to use cemented in physiologically older patients based on a better survivorship. The overall rate of revision compares quite favourably with the earlier reported series. With the modern cementation techniques the earlier known complications of cementation can be avoided on long term.

Gunderson reported results after joint replacement and enumerated the complications like heamatological crisis, infected haematoma, bacteraemia, post-traumatic fracture of the tip of the stem. Epps & Castro.1978; Sebes & Krous, 1993 reported the results of arthroplasty in Sickle cell disease. Sickle cell disease patients are at considerable risk of post-operative morbidity including infection, early mechanical and septic loosening. In this study the patients complicated with deep infections belonged to Charnley Class C. High rate of failure of joint replacement combined with high incidence of complications in patients of Sickle cell disease suggested that the risk to benefit ratio of this procedure should be assessed carefully for each patient.

Hanker, 1988, suggested peri operative care of patients of Sickle cell disease and these recommendations should be followed to minimise post operative complications.These patients must have adequate hydration and oxygenation to avoid acidosis, hyposthesia and vascular stasis. They may require pre operative transfusion to raise the haematocrits to more than 30% and to lower the level of haemoglobin S.

To improve the quality of life, to achieve painless mobile hip it is necessary to perform total hip replacement, even if the rate of complications is very high in these young patients of Sickle cell haemoglobinopathies once the collapse of femoral head has occurred.

CONCLUSION

After the study, observation and follow-up of these patients of osteonecrosis of femoral head the surgical treatment is streamlined. The stage wise treatment options for these patients of osteonecrosis is suggested (Table 6.9). However early diagnosis is the key to the success of head preserving operations in these sickler patients.

Presently we advocate following surgical procedures according to the stage of involvement in these patients of Sickle cell haemoglobinopathy.

Table 6.9.

Stage 0 & I	II	III	IV & V
Core decompression and bone grafting 1. Phemister fibular graft 2. Vascular pedicle graft	Core decompression and . bone grafting 1. Phemister fibular graft 2. Vascular ped. graft 3. Muscle pedicle grafting A. Quadratus femoris B. Sartorius C. TFL	1. Intertrochanteric osteotomy (Various types) 2. Vascular ped. graft 3. Muscle ped.	1. THR 2. Hemiarthroplasty A. AMP B. Bipolar 3. Girdlestone arthroplasty or arthrodesis

REFERENCES

1. Acurio M.T., Richard J. Friedman. Hip arthroplasty in patient with sickle cell Haemoglobinopathy. JBJS Vol. 74-B No 3 May 1992. 367-371.
2. Ballas S.K., Talacki C.A., Rao V.N., Steiner R.M. The prevalence of avascular necrosis in Sickle cell anaemia, haemoglobin 1989, 13(7-8);649-55.
3. Baumgard S.H., and Leach R.E. Avascular necrosis of the femoral head secondary to sickle cell disease. Case reports of the two Caucasian Sisters. Clin Orthop , 69 : 207-212, 1970.
4. Bishop A.R., Roberson J.R., Eckman J.R., Fleming L.L. Total hip arthroplasty in patients who have sickle cell haemoglobinopathy.:J.B.J.S (Am) 1988 July, 70(6); 853-5.
5. Blau S. and Hamerman D. Aseptic Necrosis of Femoral Head in sickle cell Anaemia. Arthitis Rheum. 10:397-402, 1967
6. Boettcher W.G. and Bonfiglio M., Smith K. : Nontraumatic necrosis of the femoral head. Part I. Relation of altered Haemostasis to etiology - J. Bone & Joint Surgery (Am.) 1970, 312-319.
7. Boettcher W.G. and Bonfiglio M., Smith K. : Non traumatic necrosis of the femoral head. Part II - experiences in treatment. J. Bone and Joint Surgery [Am.] 1970; 52A:322- 329.
8. Bomelberg D, Ehringhaus C, Zeigler R, von Lengerke H J, Timm C; Femur head necrosis in sickle cell anaemia;Monatsschr Kinderheilkd 1986 Apr. 134[4]; 212-5.
9. Brooks B.J. Jr. et al.: Erythropoietin therapy for sickle cell anaemia in Jehovah's witnesses (letter); South Med Jr. 1991 Nov, 84(11) 1416-7.

10. Camp J.F. and Colwell C.W. : Core decompression of the femoral head for osteonecrosis. J. Bone and Joint Surgery [Am.] 1986; 68-A 1313-1319.
11. Charache, Samuel, and Page, D.L. Infarction of bone marrow in the Sickle cell disorders.Ann.Intern.Med, 67:1195-1200, 1967.
12. Chung & Ralston: Necrosis of femoral head in Sickle cell disease. JBJS 51A, 33-58, 1969.
13. Clarke H.J., Jinnah R.H., Brooker A.F. Total replacement of hip for avascular necrosis in Sickle cell disease; J.B.J.S. [Br] 1989 May; 71[3]; 465-70.
14. Clark Gunderson, Robert D.D'Ambrosia, and Hiromu Shoji. Total hip replacement in patients with Sickle cell disease J.B.J.S. Vol. 59-A, No. 6 Sep 1977. Page 760-762.
15. Diggs L.W. Bone and joint lesions in Sickle cell disease Clinical orthopaedics and related reaserch No.52 May-June 1967. Page 119.
16. Diggs L.W. Sickle Cell Crisis, The American Journal of Clinical Pathology, Vol. 44, No. 1, July 1965, 1-19.
17. Donald G. Mitchell, Herbert Y., Kressel, Peter H. Arger, Murrey Dalinka, Charles E. Spritzer, Marvin E. Steinberg; Avascular necrosis of the femoral head ; Radiology 1986, Vol. 161, No.3; 739-742.
18. Donald G. Mitchell, Michael Fallon, Herbert Y. Kressel, Vijay M. Rao, Murray K. Dalinka, Charles E. Spritzer, Abbas Alavi & Marvin E. Steinberg; Femoral head avascular necrosis, coorelation of MRI, radiographic staging, radionuclide imaging and clinical findings, Radiology 1987, Vol 162, No.3.;709-715.
19. Edward O'Hara : Roentgenographic osseous manifestation of the anemias and the Leukemias, Clinical orthopaedics and related research No. 52, May-June 1967, Pg.63
20. Ebong W.W. Avascular necrosis of the femoral head associated with hemoglobinopathy. Tropical & Geographical Medicine, 29(1977) 19-23.
21. Ebong W.W., Kolawole T.M. Aseptic necrosis of the femoral head in Sickle disease; Br. J. Rheumatol 1986 Feb.; 25[1]; 34-9.
22. Elke R., Morscher E. Total prosthesis arthroplasty in femoral head necrosis, Orthopade. 1990 Aug., 19(4), 236-41.
23. Emilio. S. Musso, Sharon N Mitcheel, Marry Schink Ascani, C Andrew Barett; Results of conservative management of osteonecrosis of the femoral head. CORR 1986, Vol. 207, 209-205.
24. Epps, C.H., Jr and Castro.Oswaldo: Complications of the Total hip replacements in Sickle cell disease. Orthop trans. 2 : 236-237, 1978.
25. Ficat R.P. : Treatment of avascular necrosis of femoral head "The Hip". The Hip Society 1983, 279-295.
26. Ficat R.P. : Idiopathic bone necrosis of femoral head. Early diagnosis and treatment. J. Bone and Joint Surgery [Am.] 1985; 67-B, 3-9.
27. Genin P., Vouge M., Bloch P. Osteonecrosis of the femoral head caused by Sickle cell anaemia in benign epidemiologic and radiological aspect. Bull. Asso. Pathol. Exot. Filiales 1985; 78(2); 249-55.
28. Golding J.S.R. Conditions of the hip associated with hemoglobinopathies. Clinical orthopaedics and related reasearch. No. 90 Jan.-Feb. 1973, Page 22.
29. Golding J.S.R. Bone changes in Sickle cell anaemia Ann. Roy. Colle. Surg. England 19, 296-314, 1956.
30. Golding J.S.R., MacIver JE & Went LN The bone changes in Sickle cell anemia and it's genetic variant. JBJS 41B, 711- 718, 1959.
31. Gregory J. Hanker , Van Nuys, and Herlan C. Amstutz. Osteonecrosis of the hip in the Sickle cell disease.JBJS Vol.70- A, No.4, April 1988.Page 499-506.
32. Haddad R.J., Jr. Sickle cell disease involvement of the hip and its surgical treatment.Clin.orthop, 55:135-149, 1967.
33. Hawker H., Neilson H., Hayer R.J. and Sergaent, G.R. Haematological factors associated with avascular necrosis of the femoral head in homozygous Sickle cell disease. British J Haematal, 50:29-34, 1982.
34. Hanker G.J., Amstutz H.C. Osteonecrosis of the hip in the Sickle cell diseases. J.B.J.S. (Am); 1988 Apr; 70(A); 499-506.
35. Herold H.Z. Avascular necrosis of the femoral head in children under the age of 3; CORR 1977, No. 126, 193-195.
36. Hernigou P, F.Galacteros, D Bachir and D. Goutallier: Deformities in the hip in adults who have Sickle cell disease and had avascular necrosis in childhood JBJS (Am.) 1991 Jan., 73 (1), 81-92.
37. Hernigou P. Avascular necrosis of the femoral head in Sickle cell disease.Treatment of collapse by the injection of acrylic cement. JBJS (Br)1993 Nov, 75(6), 875-80.

38. Hernigou P, Bachir D, Galacteros F; Hip dysplasia, a complication of Sickle cell disease; Rev Rhum Ed Fr 1993 Jul-Sept;60[7-8];505-13.
39. Hernigou P, Galacteros F, Bachir D, Goutellier D; Natural history of hip necrosis in Sickle cell disease; Rev Chir Orthop 1989; 75[8]; 542-57.
40. Hungerford D.S. and Zizic T.M. : Pathogenesis of ischaemic necrosis of the femoral head. "The Hip": The Hip Society, 1983 : 249-262.
41. Hungerford D.S. and Dennis W. Lennox : The importance of increased intraosseous pressure in development of avascular necrosis of femoral head; Implication for treatment - Orthopaedic Clinics of North America, 1985 : 16:4635-668.
42. Hungerford D.S. : Bone marrow pressure, venography and core decompression in ischaemic necrosis of femoral head - Hip Society Meeting, proceedings, 1979, 218-237.
43. Iwegbu C.W., A.F. Fleming Avascular necrosis of the femoral head in Sickle cell disease. JBJS (Br.)67B, 1985 Page 29-32
44. Jones J.I.P. and Sakovich L. : Fat embolism of bone. J.Bone and Joint Surgery 1966, [Am.] 48-A, 149-163.
45. Jones J.I.P., Jamenson R.M., Engelman E.P. : Alcoholism, Fat embolism and avascular necrosis of femoral head. J. Bone and Joint Surgery, [Am.] 1968, 50A, 1065.
46. Jones J.I.P.: Fat embolism and osteonecrosis. Orthopaedic Clinics of North America - 1985 16:4:595-633.
47. Kanoley & Ahulum FID, Lancet, 999, 1970
48. Kauichi R. Ţanaka, George O. Clifford & Arnold R Axerold: Sickle Cell Anaemia (homozygous S) with Aseptic necrosis of Femoral Head; J.B.J.S. 1956, Blood - 11, 998-1007.
49. Kempt I., Karger C. and associates : Post rotational osteotomy of femoral head in avascular necrosis Rev. Chir. Ortho. 1984, 70:271-282.
50. Kenzora J.E., Steele r.E., Yosipovitch Z.H. et al. : Experimental osteonecrosis of femoral head in adult rabbits. Clinical orthopaedics and related research 1978, 130, 8-46.
51. Kenzora J.E. and Glimcher M.J. : Accumulative Cell Stress : The multificatorial etiology of idipathic osteonecrosis. Orthopaedic Clinics of North America, 1985; 16:4, 669-679.
52. Kenzora J.E. and Glimcher M.J. : Pathogenesis of idiopathic osteonecrosis. The ubiquitous crescent sign. Orthopaedic Clinics of North America 1985, 16:4 681-696.
53. Kenzora J.E. : Treatment of idiopathic necrosis : Orthopaedic Clinics of North America 1985, 16:4, 717-725.
54. Kerboul M., Thomine J. et al. : The conservative surgical treatment of idiopathic aseptic necrosis of femoral head. J. Bone and Joint Surgery [Br.] 1974, 56-B : 291-296.
55. Koren A : Avascular Necrosis of bones in children with Sickle cell anaemia ; Pediatr.Hematol. Oncol.;1993 Oct-Dec; 10(4) 385-7.
56. Khermosh O & S L Weissman; Coxavara, avascular necrosis and osteochondritis dessicans complicating solitary bone cysts of the proximal femur. CORR 1977, No. 126; 143-146.
57. Lifeso RM Total Joint replacement in Sickle cell disease. Orthop trans, 9:453, 1985.
58. Lee R E J, J.S.R. Golding & G.R. Serjeant The radiological features of avascular necrosis of the femoral head in homozygous Sickle cell disease., Clinical radiology (1981)32, 205-214
59. Marle D'Aubingne R., Postel M., Mazabraud A., et al. : Idiopathic necrosis of femoral head in adults. J. Bone and Joint Surgery [Br.] 1965, 47-B, 612-633.
60. Meyer's M.H. : The treatment of osteonecrosis of hip with fresh osteochondral allografts and with the muscle pedicle graft technique. Clinical orthopaedics and related research, 1978 : 130, 202-209.
61. Mijiyawa M , Pfudie S, Pitche V, N'Dakena K, Amedegnato MD, Doury P, ; Coxofemoral pathology in Rheumatology; Med Trop (March) 1994, 54(1), 38-42.
62. Milner P F, Kraus A P, Sebes J I, Sleeper L A, Dukes K A, Emry S H, Bellebue R, Koshy M, Moohr J W, Smith J; Sickle cell disease as a cause of osteonecrosis of femoral head, N. Engl. J. Med. Nov. 1991, 325(21), 1476-81.
63. Moseley J E, & Manly J B.Aseptic Necrosis of Bone in Sickle Cell Disease, Radiology/Roentgenology- 60, 656, 1953.
64. Moran M C, Huo, Garvin, Pellicci, Salvati; Total hip arthroplasty in Sickle cell haemoglobinopathy.; Clin Orthop' 1993 Sept; [294];140-8.
65. Matthew D Mitchell, Harold L Kundel, Marvin E Steinberg, Herbert Y Kressel, Abass Alavi, Leon Axel, : Avascular necrosis of the Hip; AJR 1986; 147; 67-71.

66. Mitchell DG, Kressel HY, Arger PH, et al.. Avascular necrosis of the femoral head: morphologic assesment by MR imaging, with CT correlation. Radiology 1986; 161:739-42.

67. Mitchell DG, Rao VM, Dalinka MK, et al..Femoral head avascular necrosis:correlation of MR imaging, radiographic staging, radionuclide imaging, and clinical finding. Radiology 1987; 162 : 709-15.

68. Musso ES, Mitchell SN, Schink-Ascani M, Basset CAL. Result of conservative management of osteonecrosis of the femoral head:a retrospective review. Clin. Orthop 1986; 207 : 209-15.

69. Ndugwa C M; Aseptic necrosis of the head of femur among Sickle anaemia patients in Uganda.; East African Medical Jr. Oct. 1992, 69(10), 572-6.

70. Omojala M F, Annobil S, Adzaku F, Addae S K, Mohammad S; Bone changes in sickle cell anaemia: East African Med. Jr. 1993 March 70 (3) 184-88.

71. Phemister D.B. : Treatment of necrotic head of femur in adults. J. Bone and Joint Surgery [Am.] 1949, 31-A, 55-56.

72. Pierce R.O., Jr. Aseptic necrosis of the hip in Sickle cell disease. J. Nat. Med. Assan, 71 : 45-48, 1979.

73. Rand C et al.: Avascular Necrosis of Femoral Head in Sickle Cell Syndromes: A Report of 5 cases; Acta Hematol, 1987, 78(2-3), 186-92

74. Rijke A M, Pope T L Jr., Kent T E ; Bilateral protrusio acetabuli in Sickle cell anaemia, South Med. Jr. March 1990, 83(3), 328-9.

75. Roesingh G.E. and James J. : Early phase of avascular necrosis of femoral head in rabbits. J. Bone and Joint Surgery [Br.] 1969:51 B 165-176.

76. Russel J. : An essay on necrosis - "The Classic" Clinical Orthopaedics and related research 1978, 130:5-7.

77. Rand C, Pearson T C, Heatley F W, Avascular necrosis of femoral head in sickle cell syndrome, Acta Haematol, 1987; 78(2-3), 186-92.

78. Reich RS & Rosenberg NJ: Aseptic necrosis of bone in caucasians with Sickle cell anemia JBJS 35A, No.4, 894-904, 1953.

79. Rutt A, Kusswetter W; Sickle cell anaemia and it's skeletal and joint changes as an orthopaedic problem; Z Orthop 1986 Mar- Apr; 124[2]; 140-3.

80. Sadat M. Ali Avascular necrosis of the femoral head in Sickle cell disease. An integrated classification Clin.Orthop 1993 May, (290), 200-05.

81. Sennara H & F Gorry : Orthopaedics aspects of Sickle cell anaemia & haemoglobinopathies, CORR 1978, No.130, 154-157.

82. Sebes J I, Diagnostic imaging of bone and joint abnormalities associated with Sickle cell haemoglobino-pathies.; AJR Am J Roentgenol 1989 Jun; 152[6]; 1153-9.

83. Smith E W & Conley CL Clinical features of genetic variants of Sickle cell disease. Bull. John hopkins Hosp. - 94, 289- 1954.

84. Sebes Jeno I: Diagnostic imaging of bone in joint abnormalities associated with Sickle cell haemoglobinopathies, AJR Am. J Roentgenol 1989 June, 152(6), 1153-9.

85. Sebes Jeno I, Alfred P.Kraus: Avascular necrosis of the hip in the Sickle cell hemoglobinopathies. Journal of the Canadian Association of radiologist Vol.34, June 1993, 136.

86. Sherman Mary; Pathogenesis of disintegration of the hip in Sickle cell anaemia, Soth Med. Jr. 1959, Vol. 52, 632-396.

87. Sheldon Blau & David Hamerman: Aseptic necrosis of the femoral heads in sickle-A Haemoglobin disease. Arthritis and rheumatism, Vol.10, No.4 (Aug 1967) 397- 400.

88. Simonnet J.H., Aubaniac J.M. : The results of intertrochanteric flexion osteotomy in idiopathic avascular necrosis of femoral head - 52 cases - Rev. Chir. Ortho. 1984, 70:219-229.

89. Soloman L, Mechanism of idiopathic osteonecrosis; Orthop. Clinic. North Am. 1985, Oct 16(4);655-67.

90. Stanley M.K., Chung & Edgar L. Ralston; Necrosis of the femoral head asociated with Sickle cell anaemia and its genetic variants, J.B.J.S. 1969, 51A(1), 33-58.

91. Stanley M.K. Chung, , Abass Alavi And Marie O.Russell Management of osteonecrosis in Sickle cell anemia and it's genetic variants. Cl.Orthop NO.130 Jan-Feb 1978, 158.

92. Stanley M.K.Chung, and Edgar L. Ralston Necrosis of the femoral head associated with sickle cell anemia and it's genetic variants. JBJS Vol.51-A, No.1 Jan 1969, 33-58.

93. Steinberg M.E. and Brighton C.I. and others : Treatment of avascular necrosis of the femoral head by combination of bone grafting, decompression and electrical stimulation. Clinical Orthopaedics and related research 1984, 186:137-153.

94. Sugioka Y. : Transtrochanteric anterior rotational osteotomy of the femoral head in treatment of osteonecrosis affecting the hip. Clinical Orthopaedics and related research, 1978, 130:191-201.

95. Sugioka Y. : Transtrochanteric rotational osteotomy of femoral head - Proceeding of Hip Society, 1980, 3-23.

96. Sugioka Y. : Transtrochanteric rotational osteotomy in treatment of idiopathic femoral head necrosis, Perthes disease, osteoarthritis, Clinical Orthopaedics and related research, 1984, 184 : 12-23.

97. Taylor P W, Thorpe W P, Trueblood M C; Osteonecrosis in Sickle cell trait; J Rheumatol 1986 Jun; 13[3]; 643-6.

98. Tanaka K R., George O. Clifford & Arnold R. Axelrod: Sickle cell anemia (Homozygous S) with aseptic necrosis of Femoral head. Blood 1956, 11;998-1008

99. Theis JC, Owen R. Skeletal complications in Sickle cell disease in the UK. J R Coll Surg Edinb 1988;33:306-10.

100. Totty WG, Murphy WA, Ganz WI, et al.. Magnetic resonance imaging of the normal and ischaemic femoral head. AJR 1984; 143 : 1273-80.

101. Wang C.J., Seet D.E., Roger S.I., Thomson E.C. : Fat cell changes as a mechanism of avascular necrosis of the femoral head in cortisone treated rabbits. J. Bone and Joint Surgery [Am.] 1977, 59A, 729-735.

102. Wang C.J. and Dughman S.S. et al. : The effect of core decompression of femoral head blood flow in steroid induced avascular necrosis of femoral head. J. Bone and Joint Surg. [Am.] 1985 : 67-A, 121-124.

103. Ware H.E., Brooks A.P., Toye R., Berney S.I. Sickle cell disease and silent avascular necrosis of the Hip; J.B.J.S.(Br.) Nov. 1991, 73(6), 947-9

104. Washington E R, Root L, Conservative treatment of Sickle cell avascular necrosis of the femoral head, J. Paediatr. Orthop. 1985 Mar-Apr, 5(2), 192-4.

105. Wayne Alen S, Steven B Zelicof, Clement B Saldge, Total hip arthroplasty in Beta Thallassemia; CORR 1993, 294, 149-54.

7

Osteonecrosis of the Humeral Head in Sickle Cell Haemoglobinopathy

In Central India this multisystem disease may manifest in various forms. Skeletal changes are seen in a large number of patients and may be the first manifestation of the disease.

Osteonecrosis of the bone is one of the skeletal manifestation of Sickle cell haemoglobinopathy. The sites commonly involved in the decreasing frequency are the femoral head, the humeral head and rarely the lunate, talus, tarsal navicular and the vertebral end plates.

Osteonecrosis of the humeral head though rare, was commonly observed in this series. Inspite of the fact that most of the patients are asymptomatic in the early stages of the disease and the condition may not be detected, large number of patients were detected and followed in this study.

REVIEW OF LITERATURE

The first case of avascular necrosis was described by Bauer and Fischer in 1943 (Taylor 1985).

The prevalence of osteonecrosis of the femoral head in Sickle cell disease is well described (Diggs, Pulliam & King 1937, Ehrenpreis & Schwinger 1952, Smith & Conley 1954, Tanaka, Clifford & Axelrod 1956, Barton & Cockshott 1962, Becker 1962, Moseley 1963, Reynolds 1965, Diggs 1967, Lee, Golding & Serjeant 1981, Milner et al 1993).

Involvement of the humeral head is well recognised though very few studies have been done in details (Ehrenpreis & Schwinger 1952, Smith & Conley 1954, Tanaka, Clifford & Axelrod 1956, Cockshott 1958, Golding, MacIver & Went 1958, Reynolds 1965, Chung and Ralston 1971, Theis & Owen 1988, Milner et al 1993, David et al 1993).

PATHOPHYSIOLOGY

Blood containing long, multipointed, curved and rigid sickled cells are more viscid and flows less readily through terminal vessels. Utilisation of oxygen by living blood cells and by endothelial and tissue cells favours an exaggeration of sickling. Chronic stasis of blood in capillaries and defective oxygenation leads to infarction in various tissues. Sickle cells are mechanically more fragile, are phagocytosed more readily and are subject to haemolysis in the circulating blood. The imbalance between blood destruction and formation leads to chronic haemolytic anaemia, the degree of anaemia depending on the type of disease.

Osteonecrosis of humeral head though rare was commonly seen in this study. It is a common belief that humeral head has abundant blood supply compared to the femoral head. Our observation on dissecting 50 cadaveric shoulders in the Anatomy Department were different (Fig. 7.1, 7.2).

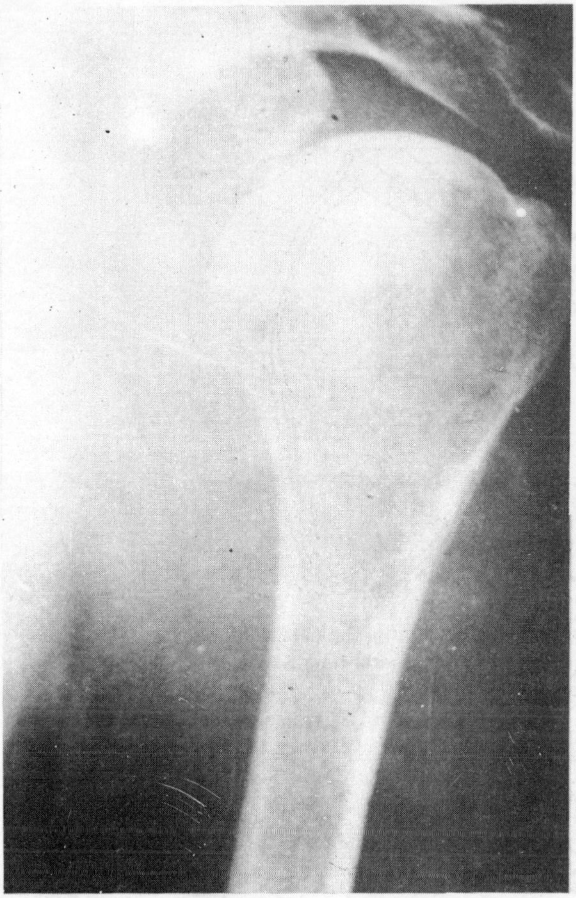

Fig. 7.1

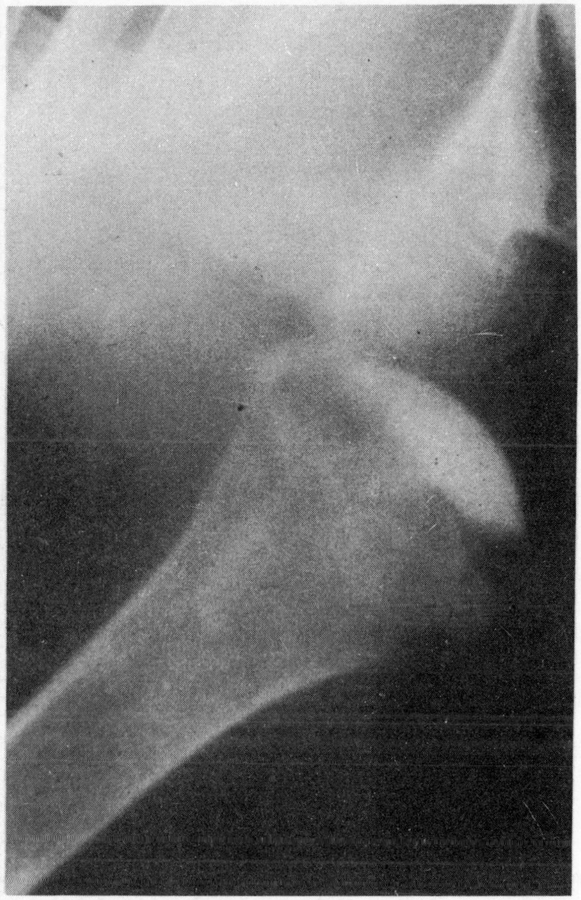

Fig. 7.2

Fig. 7.1 and 7.2. Osteonecrosis of the humeral head. Segmental sclerosis is seen involving about 90% of the articular surface with relative porosis in the metaphysis.

The observations were consistent in over 70% of shoulders dissected. About 80% of the size of humeral head has vascular supply from the ascending branch of the anterior circumflex humeral artery. This relatively large vessel supplies the supero-medial, supero-lateral and inferomedial quadrants. The infero-lateral quadrant is supplied by a branch from posterior circumflex humeral artery which pierces the humerus after traversing the quadrangular space along with the articular branch of axillary nerve (Fig. 7.3-7.5). It is observed that in patients with Sickle cell haemoglobinopathy the vaso-occlusive changes of osteonecrosis of humeral head mainly involve the quadrants supplied by anterior circumflex humeral artery and the infero-lateral quadrant is usually spared. Another explanation for peculiar affection is the longer course of this artery and the susceptibility for impingement underneath the subscapularis during abduction and rotation of shoulders as against the lax posterior circumflex artery which lies mainly postero-inferiorly. These findings appear similar to the changes of osteonecrosis of the femoral head secondary to vaso-occlusive changes in the ascending branch of lateral femoral circumflex artery seen frequently in Sickle cell disease.

Changes of osteonecrosis were seen in 258 humeral heads in 178 patients. Eighty patients had bilateral affection of the shoulder joints.

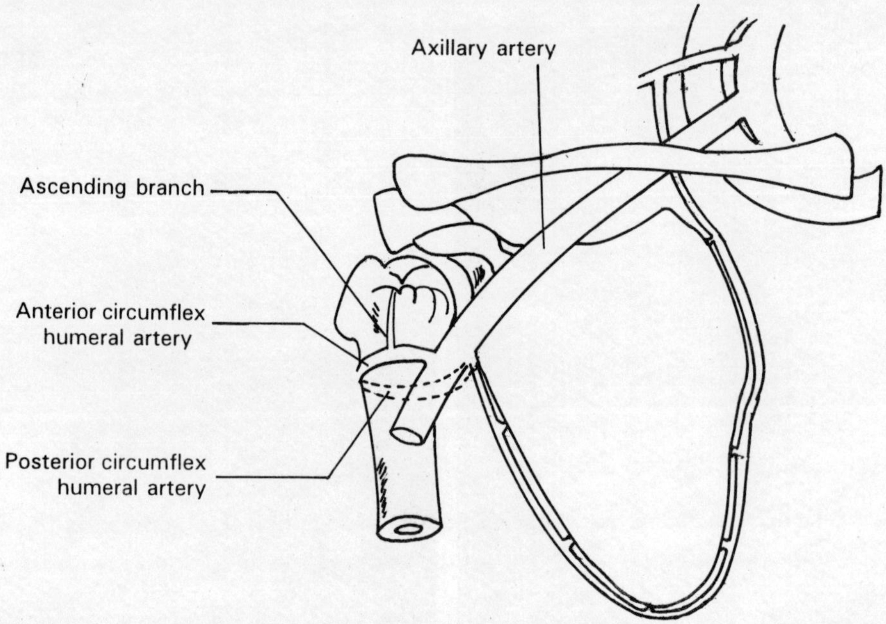

Fig. 7.3. Diagrammatic representation of anterior view of shoulder showing consistent presence of ascending branch of anterior circumflex humeral artery (Vascular supply of the humeral head).

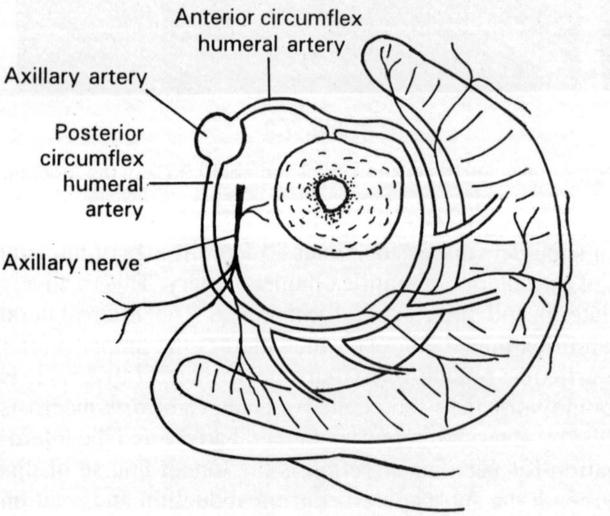

Fig. 7.4. Cross-section at upper end of humerus showing vascular supply of proximal humerus.

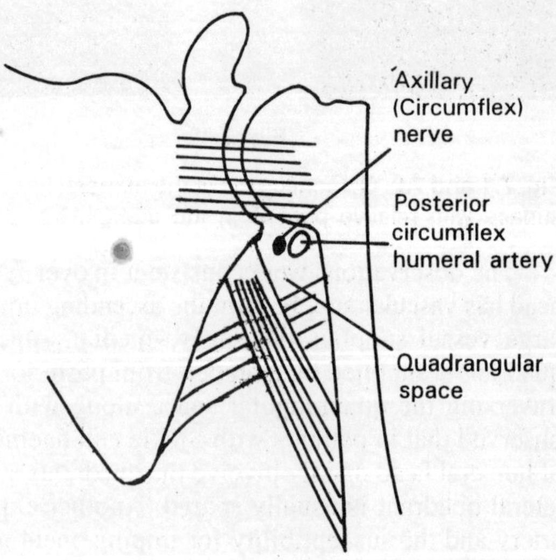

Fig. 7.5. Posterior view of shoulder showing quadrangular space with a branch from posterior circumflex humeral artery traversing to the humeral head along with articular branch of axillary nerve.

RADIOGRAPHIC CHANGES

Routine radiography is used for assessment of these patients. Advanced investigation like CT Scan & MRI were not used due to cost restraints and non-availability in many sickle cell centres. A new classification is proposed according to the changes seen in the humeral head in this study. The MRC classification (McCallum et al 1966) does not give details of pathological stages in the progression of osteonecrosis even in A type. The B Type of lesions are essentially different stages of infarcts and osteomyelitic changes rather than changes of osteonecrosis of the humeral head.

CLASSIFICATION

To know the severity of affection of the humeral head, we have classified osteonecrosis of the humeral head in different stages. One of the important observations of this study was predominant involvement of 3/4 th of the humeral head and the sparing of infero-lateral quadrant in osteonecrosis.

The patients were classified into various stages according to the radiological changes observed at the first presentation. Significant number of patients had progression of the disease on follow up. This gives us clear picture at a glance for better assessment.

Table 7.1. Radiological staging and number of patients

Stage	*Features*	*No.*	*Figs.*
I	Area of spotty irregularities & densities in the subchondral region	92	**7.7, 7.8**
II	Rim like area of increased density in juxta-articular portion of the humeral head. At times larger dense shadows in humeral head without any separation	40	**7.9, 7.10, 7.11, 7.12**
III	Crescent sign with incresed density as in Stage II with clear cleavage	15	**7.13, 7.14**
IV	Increased density with fragmentation without change in the contour of the humeral head.	47	**7.15, 7.16**
V	Mild collapse of humeral head with reduction of vertical height and width with irregularity of articular surface.	53	**7.17**
VI	Severe Collapse of humeral head with hypertrophic arthritic changes	11	**7.18, 7.19**

OBSERVATIONS

Age and Sex Distribution

There were 104 Males and 74 Females. The maximum number of patients were between 15 to 25 years of age. There were 4 patients under the age of 10 years.

Table 7.2. Age and sex distribution

Age (Years)	*Total*	*Male*	*Female*
0-5	1	1	0
6-10	9	8	1
11-15	12	7	5
16-20	62	38	24
21-25	57	31	26
26-30	29	13	16
Over 30	8	6	2
Total	178	104	74

CLINICAL FEATURES

Maximum number of patients (153) were diagnosed cases of Sickle cell haemoglobinopathy under regular follow up. In 12 cases the shoulder affection was detected when the patients were admitted in Sickle cell crisis. The changes were seen as early as four years of age in one patient (Fig. 7.6).

The commonest presenting complaint was vague pain in the shoulder. The restriction of movements was related to the stage of the disease. Wasting of the deltoid was a constant feature.

Table 7.3. Stagewise clinical features

Stage	*No. of Shoulders*	*No. Symptomatic*
I	92	10
II	40	19
III	15	-
IV	47	22
V	53	27
VI	11	10

Table 7.4. Electrophoresis pattern

Pattern	*Total*	*Males*	*Females*
AS	106	67	39
SS	43	22	21
ASF	29	15	14
Total	178	104	74

HAEMATOLOGY

The test for sickling was positive in all the cases. The electrophoretic pattern observed is as follows:

RADIOGRAPHIC FINDINGS

The changes of osteonecrosis and collapse of the humeral head usually occurs in the superomedial quadrant, where maximum pressure occurs with shoulder in abduction.

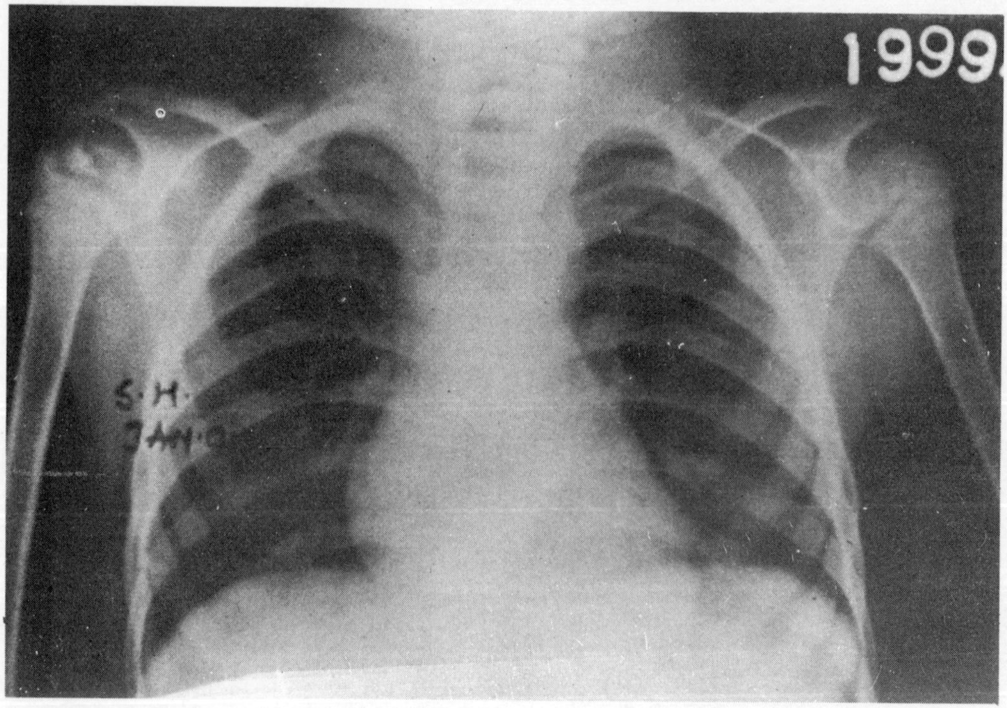

Fig. 7.6. Radiograph of a four years old child showing classical changes of osteonecrosis of the humeral head with fragmentation.

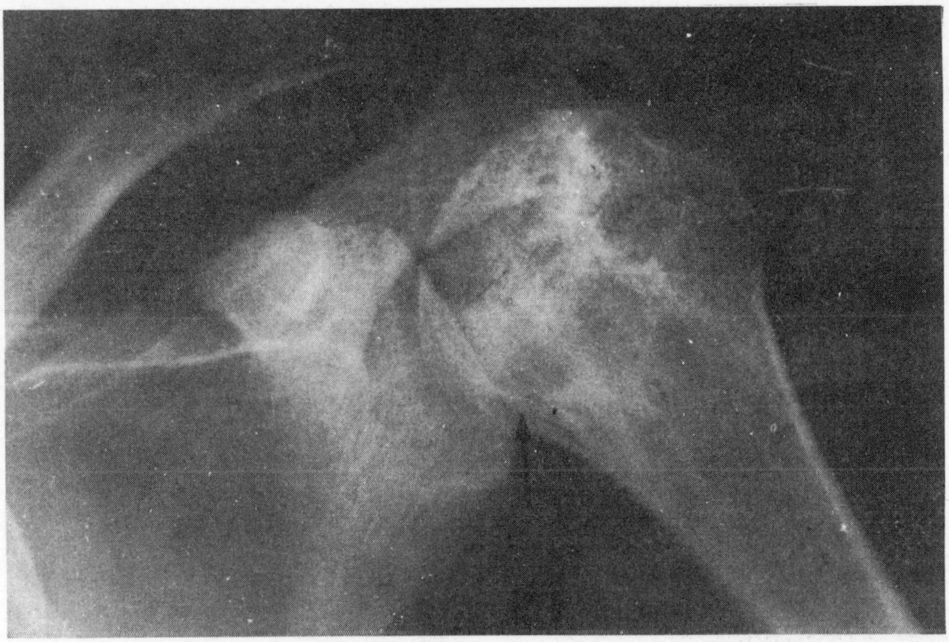

Fig. 7.7

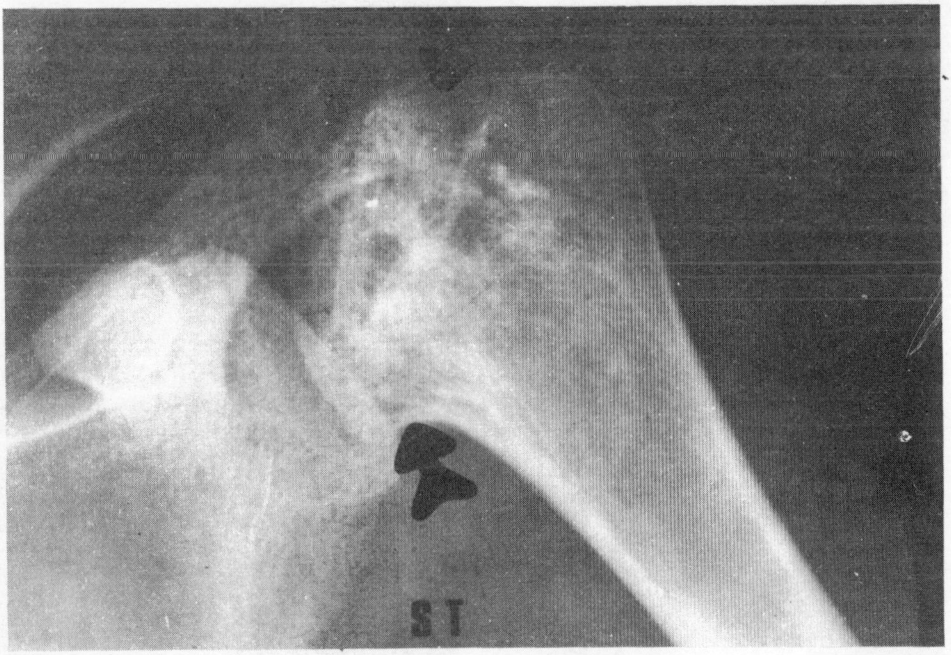

Fig. 7. 8

Fig. 7.7 and 7.8. 'Stage I' : Radiograph showing multiple dense sclerotic spots in the humeral head, at places fused to each other, deiineating the possible segmental involvement in osteonecrosis.

The radiographic findings were staged according to the initial assessment. In a few patients progression of the disease was observed at followup. Large number of patients had regression of the changes. Of the 178 patients, 80 had bilateral involvement. The findings are presented as seen in 258 humeral heads.

BILATERAL AFFECTION

This was seen in 80 patients maximum of which were between 20-25 years of age.

Table 7.5. Radiological staging at first presentation

Stage	*Number of Humeral Heads*
I	92
II	40
III	15
IV	47
V	53
VI	11
Total	258

Table 7.6. Age and sex-wise bilateral affection

Age (Years)	*Total*	*Male*	*Female*
0-5	0	0	0
6-10	1	1	0
11-15	11	7	4
16-20	13	7	6
21-25	32	21	11
26-30	14	10	4
Over 30	9	6	3
Total	80	52	28

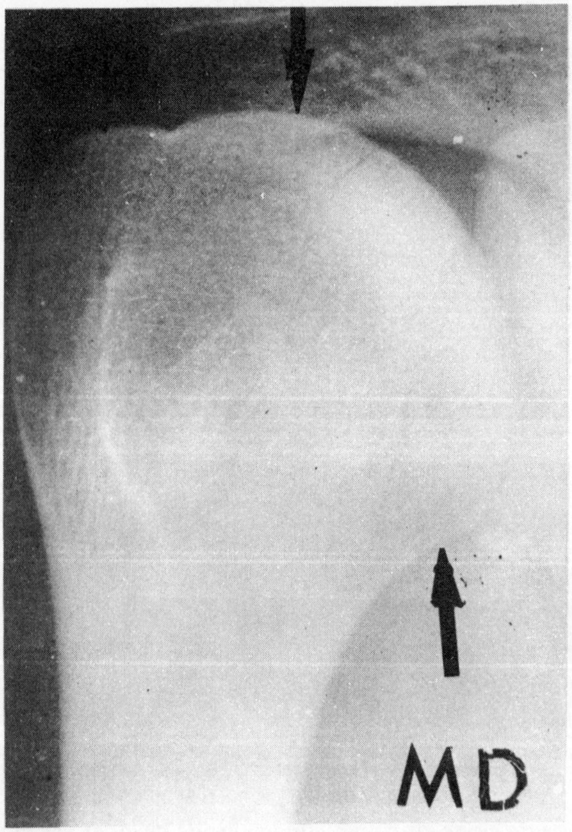

Fig. 7.9

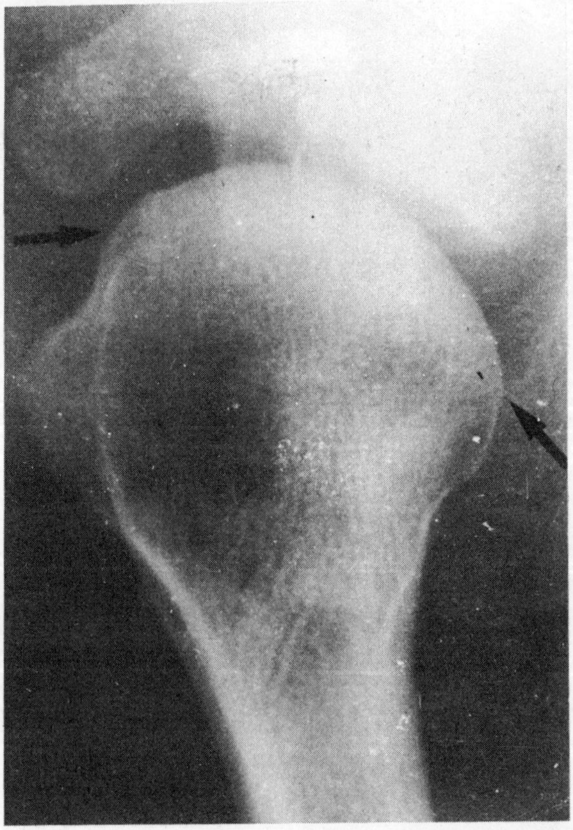

Fig. 7.10

Fig. 7.9 & 7.10. 'Stage II': Radiograph showing the juxtaarticular dense band of sclerosis seen in A.P. & lateral views. There is no cleavage or separation.

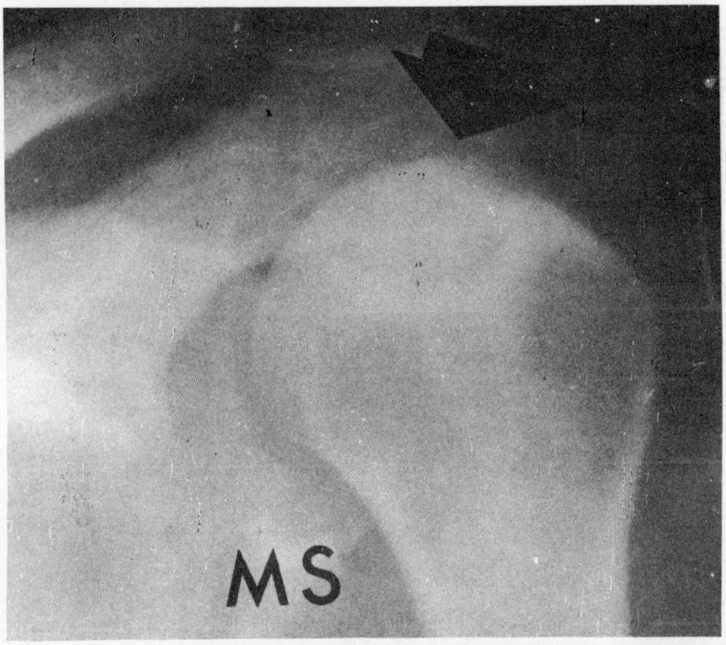

Fig. 7.11.

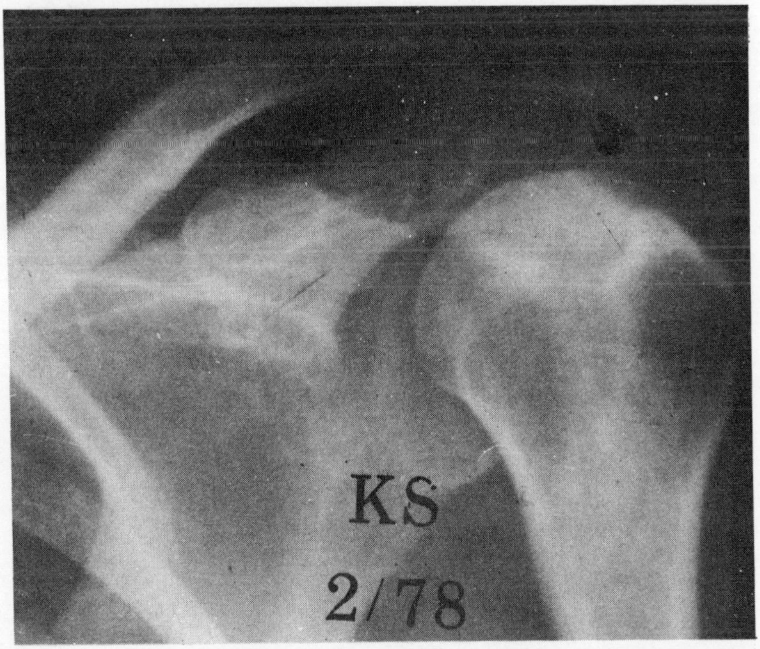

Fig. 7.12.

Fig. 7.11 and 7.12. 'Stage II': Radiograph showing segmental involvement of the humeral head in osteonecrosis without separation, with relative osteoporosis.

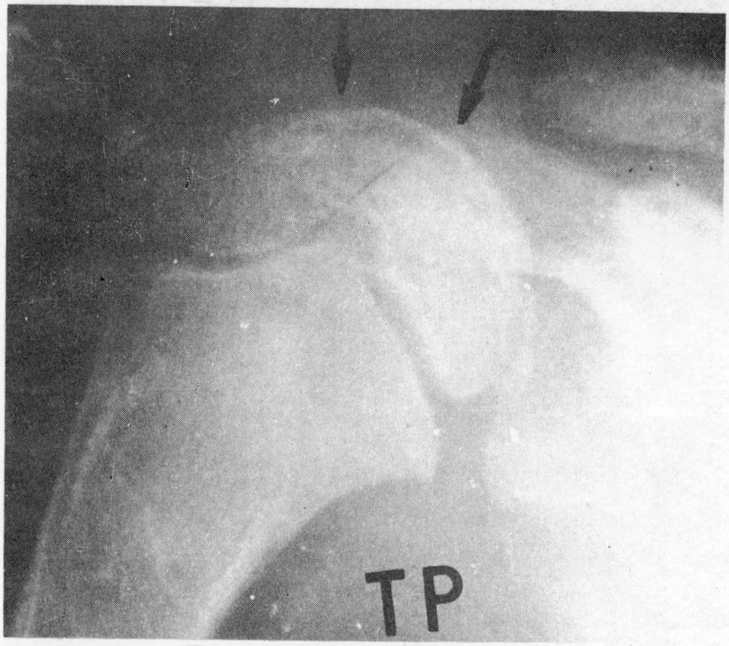

Fig. 7.13

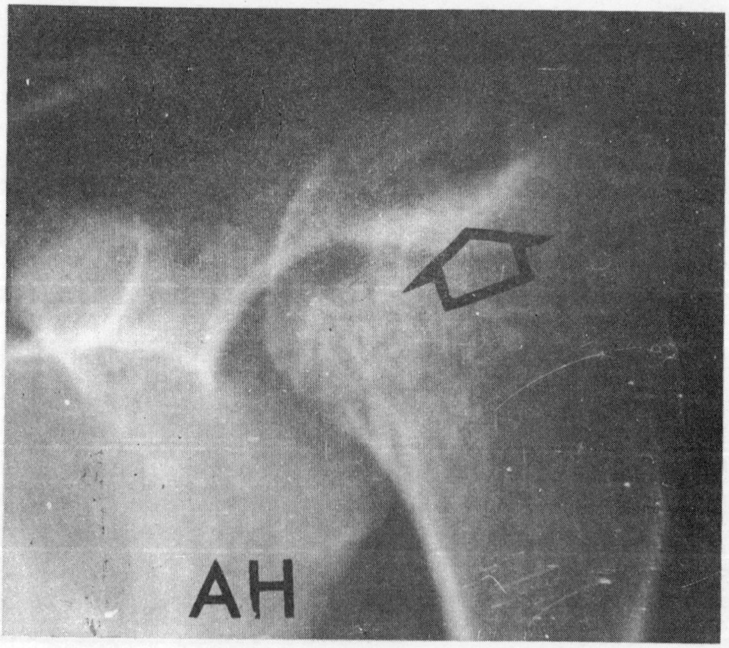

Fig. 7.14

Fig. 7.13 and 7.14. 'Stage III': Radiograph of shoulder showing clear separation of subchondral segment without deformation of the humeral head.

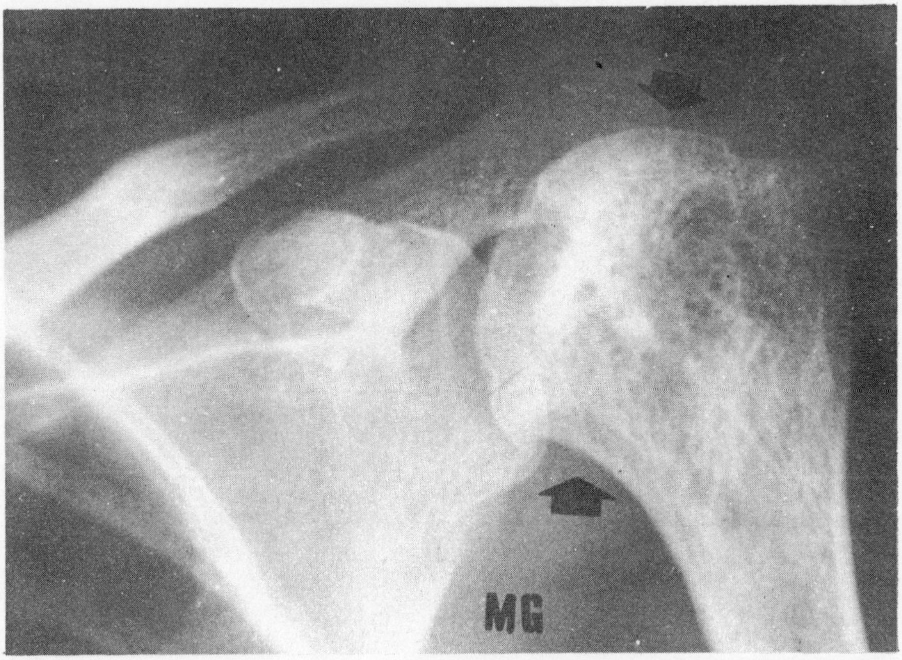

Fig. 7.15

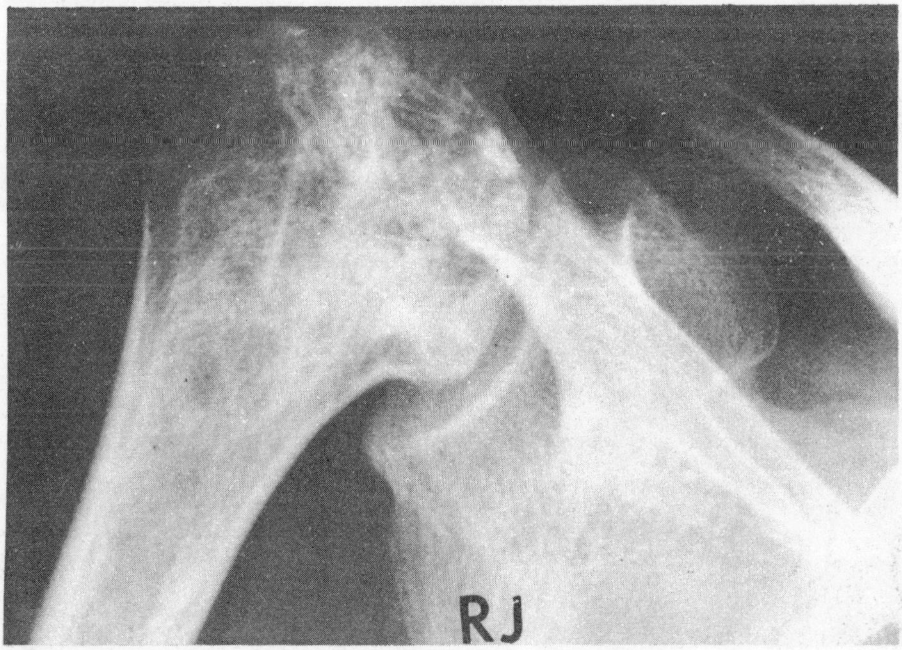

Fig. 7.16

Fig. 7.15 and 7.16. 'Stage IV': Radiograph of shoulder showing multiple dense areas with fragmentation of the humeral head without change in the contour.

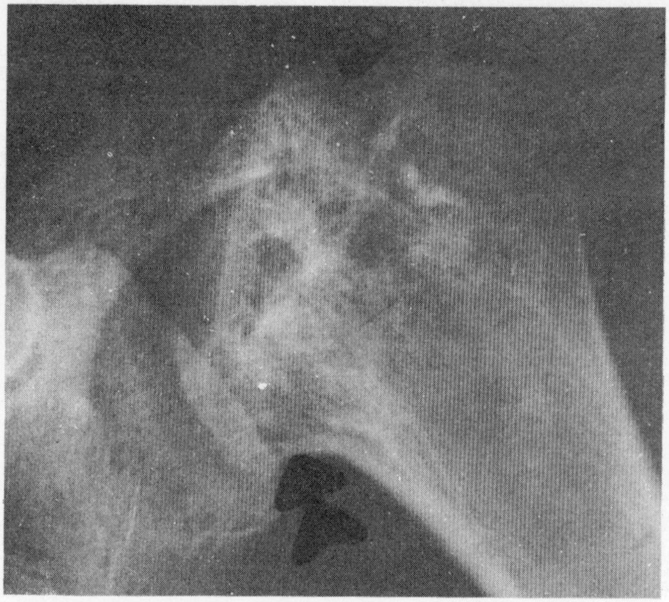

Fig. 7.17

Fig. 7.17. 'Stage V': Advanced changes of Osteonecrosis with partial collapse of the humeral head causing deformation and reduction in the vertical height of the humeral head.

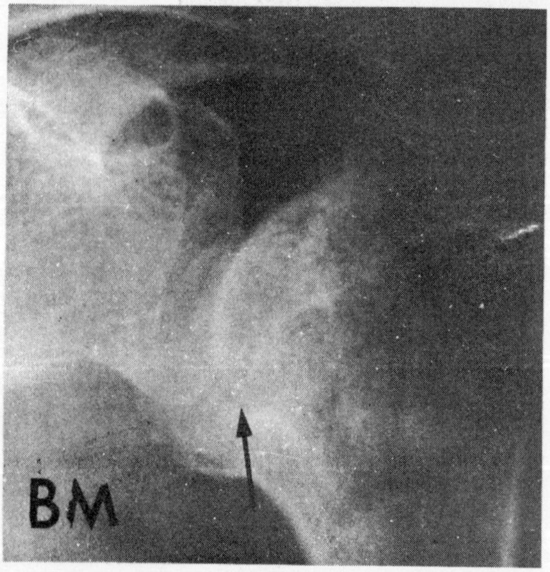

Fig. 7.18

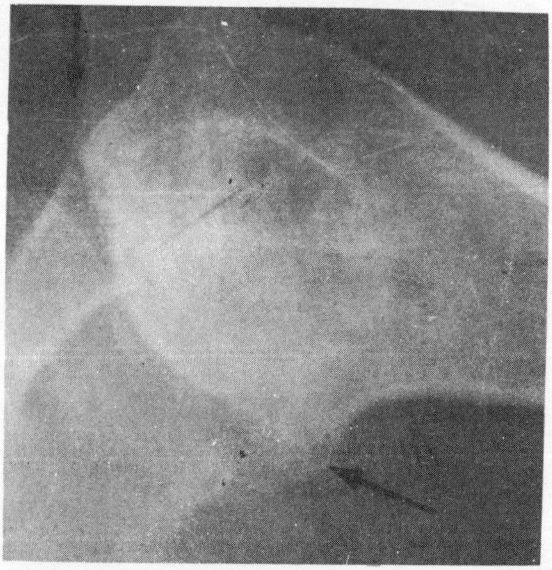

Fig. 7.19

Fig. 7.18 and 7.19. 'Stage VI': Residual changes of Osteonecrosis with collapse of the humeral head causing irregularity of the articular surface and secondary hypertrophic arthritic changes.

MANAGEMENT

Most of the patients with osteonecrosis of the humeral head were managed by conservative treatment. During the painful episode, the shoulder was rested in a sling till the pain subsided. Patients presenting during Sickle cell crisis were managed by similar means in addition to the specific treatment for crisis.

Core decompression was done in 12 humeral heads without bone grafting. Core decompression & free iliac bone grafting (Fig. 7.20-22) was done twice. Arthroplasty was indicated in only 6 patients but not done due to the morbid condition of the patient.

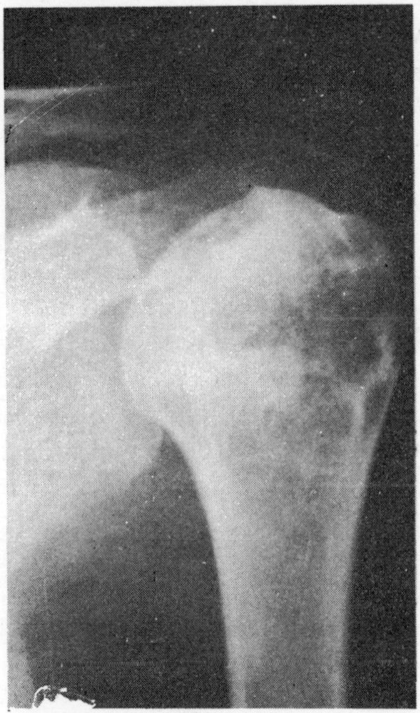

Fig. 7.20

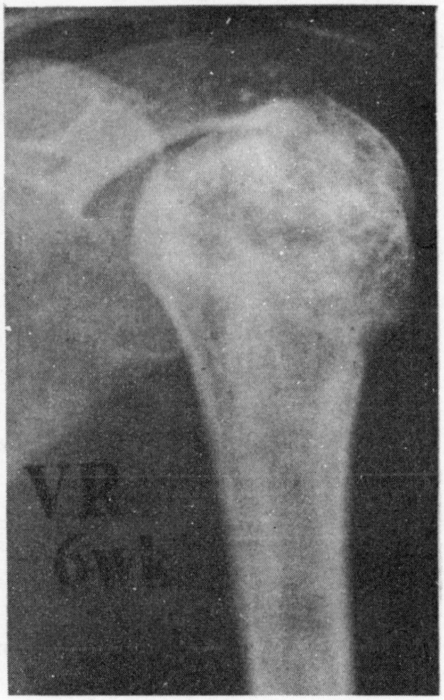

Fig. 7.21

Fig. 7.20 & 7.21. X-ray showing stage III-IV type of osteonecrosis of humeral head treated by core decompression.

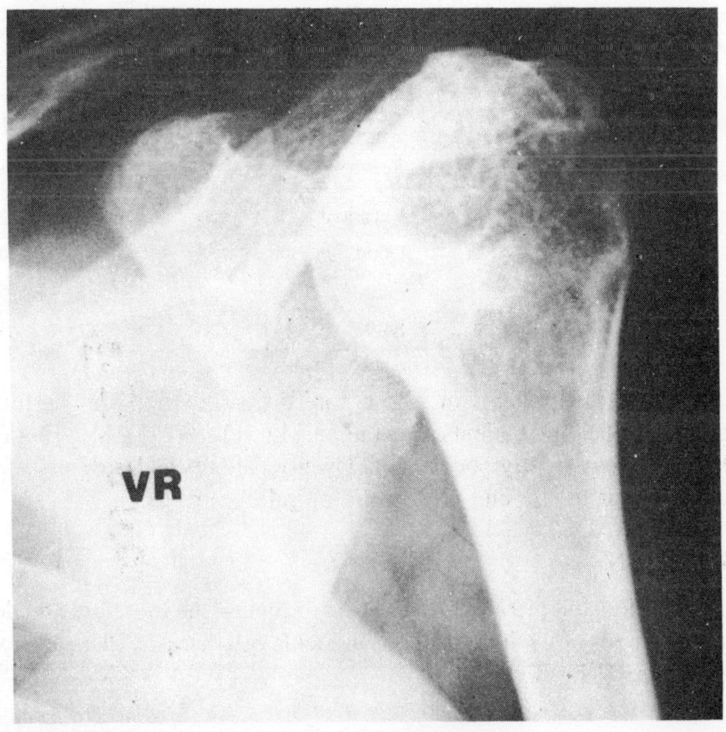

Fig. 7.22. X-ray of same patient (Fig. 7.21) 1 year postoperatively after core decompression showing good attempt towards revascularisation.

EVALUATION AND RESULTS

Clinical evaluation was done by the UCLA Shoulder Rating System (Kay & Amstutz, 1988). Ten points were assigned in each of the three categories, Pain, Function and Active movements. The maximum score possible was 30 points. An excellent result scored 27 points or more, a good result 24 to 26, a fair result 21 to 23 and a poor result scored less than 21.

Table 7.7. UCLA Shoulder Rating

Criterion	*Score*	*Findings*
Pain	1	Constant, unbearable, strong medications frequently
	2	Constant but bearable,strong medications occasionally
	4	None or little at rest, occurs with light activity, salicylates frequently.
	5	With heavy or particular activities only salicylates occasionally.
	8	Occasional and slight
	10	No Pain
Function	1	Unable to use arm
	2	Very light activities only
	4	Light house work or most daily living activities
	5	Most house work, washing hair, putting on brassiere, shopping, driving.
	8	Slight restriction only, able to work above shoulder level
	10	Normal activities.
Muscle power and motion	1	Ankylosis with deformity.
	2	Ankylosis with good functional position.
	4	Muscle power poor to fair, elevation less than 60°, internal rotation less than 45°.
	5	Muscle power fair to good, elevation 90° internal rotation 90°.
	8	Muscle power good or normal, elevation 140°, external rotation 20°.
	10	Normal muscle power, motion near normal.

Table 7.8. Results of osteonecrosis

Result	*No. of shoulders*
Excellent	125
Good	46
Fair	53
Poor	34

A total of 10 patients in whom core decompression was performed in Stage I or II had excellent to good result. Four patients had fair results (Fig. 7.20,7.21). Humeral heads with changes of stage V and VI had consistently poor result. Twenty patients had progress of lesion during the follow up and the result was fair at the end of 2 years of follow up.

DISCUSSION

Chung and Ralston (1971) were the first to review the literature and describe the orthopaedic implications of osteonecrosis of the humeral head in Sickle cell disease. There are a very few reports on the osteonecrosis of the humeral head.

The incidence of osteonecrosis of humeral head in this study was 3.5%. The reported incidence of humeral head involvement ranges from 0% (Becker 1962) to 31.5% (Golding et al 1959). Milner et al (1993) reported an incidence of 5.6% and David et al (1993) found humeral head involvement in 28.3% patients (Table 7.9).

Table 7.9. Review of literature

Author	*Hb*	*No. of patients*	*Humeral head No.*	*AVN %*
Ehrenpreis & Schwinger (1952)	-	72	1	1.4
Smith & Conley (1954).	SC	16	1	6.2
Tanaka et al (1956)	SS	38	1	2.6
Cockshott (1958)	SC	20	3	15.0
Golding et al (1959)	SS	51	5	9.8
	SC	19	6	31.5
Barton & Cockshott (1962)	SC	117	4	3.4
Becker (1962)	SC	12	0	0
Reynolds (1965)	SS	63	10	15.9
	SC	34	7	20.6
Chung & Ralston (1971)	SS	40	2	5

Early reports from Smith & Conley (1954) suggested that only patients with Sickle cell trait were affected by osteonecrosis. It has now been shown that it occurs in all types of Sickle cell haemoglobinopathy with the same frequency, giving a distribution proportional to that of the types of haemoglobin electrophoretic pattern in any given population or geographical area (Tanaka et al 1956, Golding et al 1959, Chung & Ralston 1969, Nachamie & Dorfman 1974, Ebong 1977).

As reported earlier, I found a higher incidence of osteonecrosis of humeral head in patients with heterozygous SC disease than in those with homozygous SS disease (Smith & Conley 1954, Tanaka et al 1956, Cockshott 1958, Barton & Cockshott 1962, Chung & Ralston 1969, David et al 1993). Milner et al (1993) found a higher incidence in patients with Hb SS.

Osteonecrosis of the humeral head has not been reported in a child below 5 years of age (David et al 1993). There was no patient under the age of ten years in their study. Milner et al (1993) reported 6 patients under the age of 10 years. In this study, there were 4 cases under the age of 10 years and one of them had radiological changes at the age of 4 years (Fig. 7.6). The age distribution otherwise is comparable to other studies (David et al 1993, Milner et al 1993).

There were 80 patients (45%) with bilateral involvement in this study. Chung and Ralston (1971) reported six cases with bilateral involvement out of 10. The reported incidence of bilateral disease in the study of Milner et al (1993) and David et al (1993) was 67.2% and 28% respectively.

It is generally agreed that the patients with osteonecrosis of the humeral head are not as disabled as those with involvement of the femoral head (Chung and Ralston 1971). In the study of Milner et al (1993), 79% patients were asymptomatic at the time of diagnosis. Only 22% patients reported pain and limitation of movement. In the present study, 34% patients were symptomatic at the initial assessment. In contrast to the above reports, Haddad (1967) found significant pain and disability in a similar group of patients.

Diggs (1967) opined that since the humerus does not bear weight, the cartilage is usually spared, hypertrophic changes are minimal and the glenoid fossa is normal. Only in rare instances, deformity and secondary hypertrophic arthritic changes are seen.

Changes of osteonecrosis of the humeral head are also reported with other disorders (Jones J.I.P. et al. 1965, Hunder G.G. et al. 1968, Fischer D.E et al. 1971, Solomon L. 1973, Hungerford D. S. 1983) and I have seen such changes in two patients of Gaucher's disease, six patients of corticosteroid consumption and five cases of alcohol abuse. I did not observe similar changes of osteonecrosis of humeral head in any other disease known to cause osteonecrosis like hyperuricaemia, alkaptonuria or following renal transplantation.

Various classifications have been proposed for the osteonecrosis of the humeral head (Mc Callum and Walder 1966, Ficat & Arlet 1980). David et al (1993) have used the Medical Research Council Decompression Panel Classification proposed by McCallum & Walder (1966).

A conservative treatment comprising of heat, massage, range of motion exercises and protection from undue stresses has been recommended in the early stages of the disease (Chung & Ralston 1971). A large number of patients in this study were satisfactorily managed by conservative means.

Chung and Ralston (1971) reported decompression and bone grafting for patients of osteonecrosis of the humeral head who did not respond to conservative treatment with good results. In this study a similar procedure without grafting was done in 12 shoulders and twice with bone grafting. In 10, the results were good to excellent and 4 patients had fair results. It was thus possible to arrest the progression of the disease. The results of this procedure are comparable to those obtained by Mont et al (1993) in patients with osteonecrosis of the humeral head due to causes other than Sickle cell disease.

Replacement arthroplasty using the Neer's prosthesis has been advocated in patients with intractable pain and secondary osteoarthritic changes (Chung & Ralston 1971, Milner et al 1993, David et al 1993). Infection and prosthetic loosening are common following this procedure in sicklers (David et al 1993). No patient in this study was subjected to replacement arthroplasty though it was indicated in 6 cases.

SUMMARY

Osteonecrosis of the humeral head is common than is usually recognised since a large number of patients are asymptomatic. It is less common than osteonecrosis of the femoral head. Pain and disability in these cases is mild and the progression of the disease is slow and most of them are managed conservatively with good results. Patients with Sickle cell disease and trait are equally affected with osteonecrosis of the humeral head. Early detection is important to prevent progression of the disease as the results of replacement arthroplasty are not satisfactory. Core decompression with or without grafting yields good results and helps in arresting the progress of the disease.

REFERENCES

1. Barton C.J., Cockshott W.P. : Bone changes in Haemoglobin SC Disease. Am. J. Roentgenol 1962; 88 : 523-32.
2. Becker J.A. : Haemoglobin SC Disease. Am. J. Roentgenol 1962; 88 : 503-11.
3. Chung S.K.M., Ralston E.L. : Necrosis of the femoral head asociated with Sickle cell anaemia and its genetic variants. J. Bone Joint Surg. [Am] 1969; 51-A: 33-58.
4. Chung S.K.M., Ralston E.L. : Necrosis of the humeral head associated with Sickle cell anaemia and its genetic variants. Clin. Orthop. 1971; 80 : 105-17.
5. Cockshott W.P. : Haemoglobin SC Disease. J. Fac. Radiologists 1958; 9 : 211-6.
6. David H.G., Bridgman S.C., Davies S.C., Hine, A.L., Emery R.J.H. : The Shoulder in Sickle cell disease. J.B.J.S. [Br] 1993; 75-B : 538-45.
7. Diggs L.W., Pulliam H.N., King J.C. : The bone changes in Sickle cell anaemia. Southern Med Jr. 1937; 30: 249-59.
8. Daland G.A., Castle W.B. : A simple and Rapid method of demonstrating sickling of red blood cells, the use of reducing agents. J. Lab. Clin. Med. 1948; 33 : 1082.
9. Ebong W.W. : Avascular necrosis of the femoral head associated with haemoglobinopathy. Tropical & Geographical Medicine 1977 : 29 : 19-23.

10. Ehrenpreis B., Schwinger H.N. : Sickle Cell Anaemia. Am. J. Roentgenol 1952; 68 : 28-36.
11. Golding J.S.R., MacIver J.E., Went L.H. : The bone changes in Sickle cell anaemia and its genetic variants. J. Bone Joint Surg. (Br. 59; 41-B : 71-8.
12. Herrick J.B. : Peculiar elongated and sickle shaped red blood corpuscles in a case of anaemia. Arch. Int. Med. (Chicago) 1910; 6 : 517.
13. Kay S.P., Amstutz H.C. : Shoulder Hemiarthroplasty at UCLA. Clin. Orthop 1988; 288 : 42-8.
14. Lee R.E.J., Golding J.S.R., Sergeant G.R. : The radiological features of avascular necrosis of the femoral head in homozygous Sickle cell disease. Clin. Radiol. 1981; 32: 205.
15. McCallum R.I., Walder D.N. : Bone lesions in compressed air workers with special reference to men who worked on the Clyde tunnels 1958 to 1963. J. Bone & Joint Surg [Br.] 1966: 48-B; 207-35.
16. Milner P.F., Kraus A.P., Sebes J.I., Sleeper L.A., Dukes K.A., Embury S.H., Bellevue R., Koshy M., Moohr J.W., Smith J. : Osteonecrosis of the humeral head in Sickle Cell Disease. Clin. Orthop. 1993 ; 289 : 136-143.
17. Mont M.A., Marr D.C., Urquhart M.W., Lennox D., Hungerford D.S. : Avascular necrosis of the humeral head treated by core decompression. J. Bone Joint Surg. [Br.] 1993; 75-B ; 785-788.
18. Moseley J.E. : Bone changes in haematologic disorders. New, Grune and Stratton, 1963.
19. Nachamie B.A., Dorfman H.D. : Ischaemic necrosis of bone in Sickle cell trait. Mt. Sinai J. Med. NY 1974; 41 : 527-36.
20. Nixon J.E. : Avascular necrosis of bone : A review. J. of the Royal Soc. Med. 1983 : 76 : 681-692.
21. Reynolds J. The roentgenological features of Sickle cell disease and related haemoglobinopathies. Springfield, Ill : Charles C. Thomas, 1965.
22. Smith E.W., Conley Cl. : Clinical features of the genetic variants of Sickle cell disease. Bull John Hopkins Hosp. 1954 : 94 : 289-318.
23. Tanaka K.R., Clifford G.O., Axelrod A.R. : Sickle cell anaemia (homozygous S) with aseptic necrosis of the femoral head. Blood 1956 : 11 : 988-1008.
24. Taylor L. : Sickle cell disease in Britain : A review. Jacksonian Prize Essay, 1985.
25. Theis J.C., Owen R. : Skeletal Complications in Sickle cell disease in the UK. J.R. Coll. Surg. Edinb. 1988; 33 : 306-10.

8

Osteomyelitis in Patients with Sickle Cell Haemoglobinopathy

Osteomyelitis is an frequent presentation of Sickle cell haemoglobinopathy resulting secondary to bone marrow hyperplasia and vascular insufficiency. A study of 192 patients amongst sicklers is presented with osteomyelitic changes in various bones affecting 378 bones. *E. coli* was found to be the commonest organism as against the Salmonella which was frequently observed in western studies. The various changes of osteomyelitis occurring clinically as well as radiologically in long bones have been presented in detail. Multifocal Sickle cell osteomyelitis was observed in 18% patients of osteomyelitis. Ischaemia, infarction, impaired immunity with decreased phagocytosis, defective opsonin and bile froth formation and hypoxia play a major role in causation of infection by bacteria in Sickle cell osteomyelitis.

All these patients mainly reported for the pain in bones and joints, swelling over the bones and frequent recurrent infections. A few had difficulty in walking and painful limp. All these patients were thoroughly examined and investigated in detail. Total 192 patients of osteomyelitis, affecting 378 bones were detected and studied with an average follow up of 8 years, there were 120 males and 72 females, ranging from 4 years to 45 years. The following table shows the age and sex distribution of osteomyelitis in 192 patients.

Table 8.1. Age and Sex distribution

Age Group	*Males*	*Females*	*Total*
04-10	19	08	27
11-20	30	20	50
21-30	28	15	43
31-40	31	18	49
41-45	12	11	23
Total	120	72	192

CLINICAL MANIFESTATIONS

Most of the patients reported with history of fever, malaise, cough with expectoration, severe joint and bone pains with either localised or generalised tenderness of 3 - 10 days history. Range of the movement of the neighbouring joint was restricted and painful. One patient of 4 years and 2 months old presented with irritability, fever with swelling of the right foot and leg and refused to walk. Mother and elder sibling of this patient were known sicklers of SS pattern. Jaundice was noticed in 28 patients. six patients presented with ulcer over lower end of leg and subsequently were diagnosed as secondary to Sickle cell anemia. Splenomegaly was not found in any of the patients in our study. More than 30% patients were admitted into the hospital during the stage of crisis.

INVESTIGATIONS

All the patients were subjected to routine blood chemistry which revealed leukocytosis, raised erythrocyte sedimentation rate. Haemoglobin levels found to be below 7-8 gm% and reticulocyte count raised over 8-10%. Sickling test (Daland & Castle 1948) and haemoglobin electrophoresis were done in all the patients. Sickling was positive and the various electrophoretic patterns observed in these 192 patients with osteomyelitis are as follows:

Table 8.2. Electrophoresis pattern

Electrophoresis pattern	*No. of patients*
SS	61
AS	78
SF	34
ASF	19

Sickle cell trait (AS) formed the major group i.e., 50%. Radiographs in acute osteomyelitis of the affected parts showed no obvious bony changes in early stages or showed only soft tissue swelling but later on, after 10-15 days revealed bone destruction with periosteal reaction. Mottled radiolucent areas were found in entire shaft of tibia in 2 patients. Upper end of tibia was involved more when compared with the lower end of the tibia. All these findings were correlated clinically to differentiate osteomyelitis from bone infarction. Radionuclide scan studies may be useful to differentiate the bone infarction from osteomyelitis. But because of non availability of the scan in our Institute and since most studies showed no firm establishment to confirm the diagnosis with scans either of technetium 99 or gallium, we have not subjected any patient to this costly investigation. Positive pus and blood cultures helped to clinch the diagnosis of osteomyelitis and to differentiate from bone infarction. Based on physical and clinical findings the preliminary diagnosis of osteomyelitis was done and confirmed with pus and blood culture reports.

ETIOPATHOLOGY OF SKELETAL CHANGES

Skeletal changes occur mainly due to severe bone marrow hyperplasia and vascular insufficiency resulting in thrombosis and infarction (Barton C.J. et al 1962, Edward O'Hara A. 1967, Givner L.B. et al 1981, Keeley et al 1982, Koren A. et al 1984). Vascular insufficiency is triggered off by crowding of sickle cells, anoxia, reflex vasospasm, increased viscosity, capillary stasis and resultant ischaemic necrosis.

Associated bone infection is quite common, leading to osteomyelitis and sequestration (Johnston R.B. 1974, Launder W.J. 1979, Onwubalili J.K. 1983, Mallouh et al. 1985). In our study osteoporosis, infarction and sequestration resulted in pathological fractures in 12 patients of osteomyelitis.

OBSERVATIONS

Generalised osseous changes take place as microvascular circulation of bones is a favourite site of sickle cell to harbour. Out of 944 patients of osseous involvement, osteomyelitis was observed in 192 patients.

Table 8.3. Affection of various bones in Osteomyelitis of 192 patients involving 378 bones

Affected Bone	*No. of Bones*
1. Tibia	138
2. Fibula	84
3. Femur	63
4. Humerus	33
5. Radius Ulna	51
6. Lumbar spine	03
7. Iliac bone	03
8. Calcaneum	03

Changes were seen in multiple sites involving more than one bone in 36 patients making the total of 378 bones in 192 patients with the 18% incidence of multifocal osteomyelitis. The highest incidence being observed in tibia (138).

RADIOGRAPHIC CHANGES

Long bones in the patients of Sickle cell haemoglobinopathies usually reveal widening of medullary cavity, fine trabeculations, cortical thinning and osteoporosis. Infarcts of the marrow in the ends of long bones causing necrosis, lysis, fibrosis and sclerosis were observed in our study similar to the findings reported by Almklov J.R. et al 1950, Barton C.J. 1962, Reynolds J. 1965 and Aksoy M. et al 1966 (Fig. 7.20, 8.1). Patients of Sickle cell haemoglobinopathy are peculiarly susceptible to bacterial infections of bone. It is thought that ischaemia and necrosis of bone furnish a formidable nidus for the growth of bacteria. The infection usually starts in the medullary cavity of long and tubular bone but can occur in any bone. The infection from bone rarely spreads to the joint. Necrosis of the bone, periosteal inflammatory reaction and sinus formation are frequent and at times the pathological fractures are seen. Larger areas of necrosis which also include the cortex are characterised by severe pain and swelling clinically due to periosteal reaction. Occasionally there is separation of periosteum. The periosteum appears as a thin line of opacity parallel with the shaft. This defect is due to infarction of large segment of cortical bone followed by periosteal inflammatory reaction and sub-periosteal new bone formation. This gives a typical appearance called as "cortex within the cortex" (Figs. 8.3, 8.4). There is cortical fissuring, bone sclerosis and laminated bone formation on the inner surface of cortex as also reported by Wigh R. et al. 1950, Hewett B.V. et al. 1964, Reynolds J. 1965, Rao et al. 1985. Chalky density is seen in marrow cavity because of bone infarcts. At times there is formation of concentric thin cylinders in the medullary cavity parallel with the shaft and separated from the cortex and from each other by marrow spaces and trabecular bridges. This peculiar pattern which was observed in this series is also called as "Bone within bone" appearance and is supposed to be because of recurrent episodes of medullary infarction and periosteal separation (Fig. 8.5). In a few of the patients there was a lot of new bone formation giving " Overflowing bone around bone " appearance (Luxuriant, exuberant, abundant, copious, profuse) meaning there by addition of new bone on the top of the cortex, because of periosteal reaction secondary to infection (Figs. 8.6-8.10). According to my observation many layers of such new bone formation were seen which resulted in increase in the width of bone and at times widening of cavity. There is a clearcut demarcation between original cortex, and this new bone giving a classical appearance. This is mainly because of infarction resulting in to profuse, abundant, swarming, polluting, new bone formation which at times looks like candle grease appearance of Melorrheostosis (Figs. 8.9 and 8.10).

Radiographic changes varies from mild to severe form but massive destruction is usually seen. The periosteum is elevated, irregularly thickened, cortex within cortex, bone within bone and bone around bone appearance, cortical fissuring, lysis, fragmentation of necrotic cortex, sclerosis, bone abscesses and large sequestrae have been observed (Carroll D.S. et al 1949, Barton C.J. et al 1962, Hewett B.V. et al 1964, Edward O'Hara A. 1967, Gardner R.V. 1985, Ebong W.W. 1987, Ben Dridi et al 1987) as seen in Fig. 8.11-8.13 which may spread to the adjoining joint.

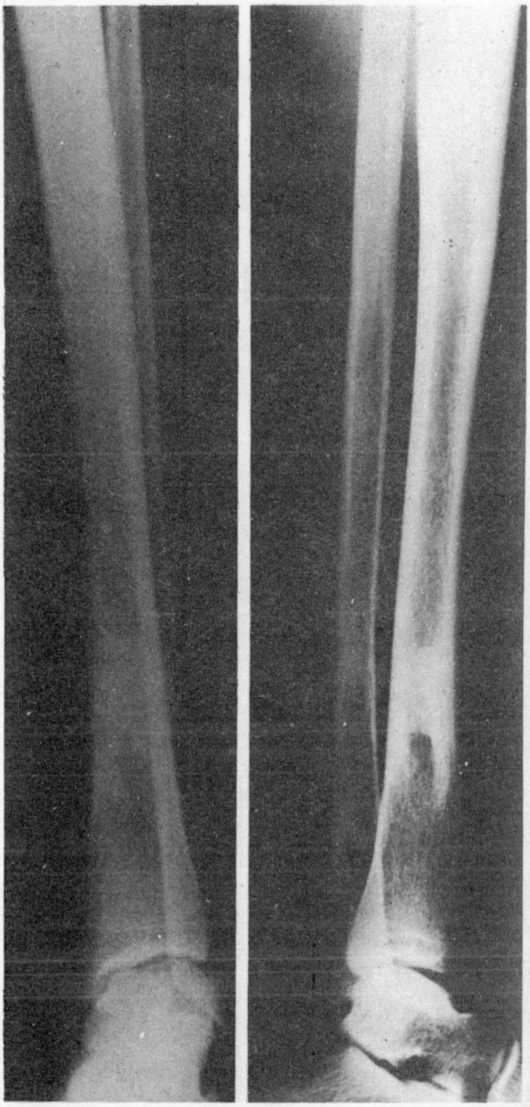

Fig. 8.1. X-ray of tibia showing bone infarct in tibia lower end.

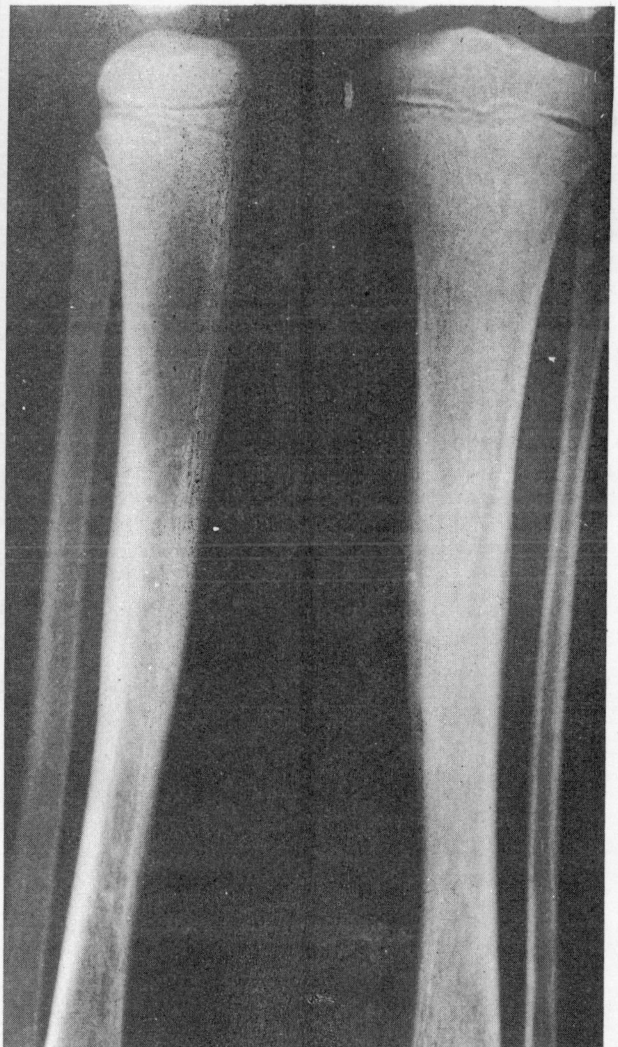

Fig. 8.2. Patient presented with acute symptoms mimicking suppurative osteomyelitis which subsided in 3-4 days treatment by analgesics only.

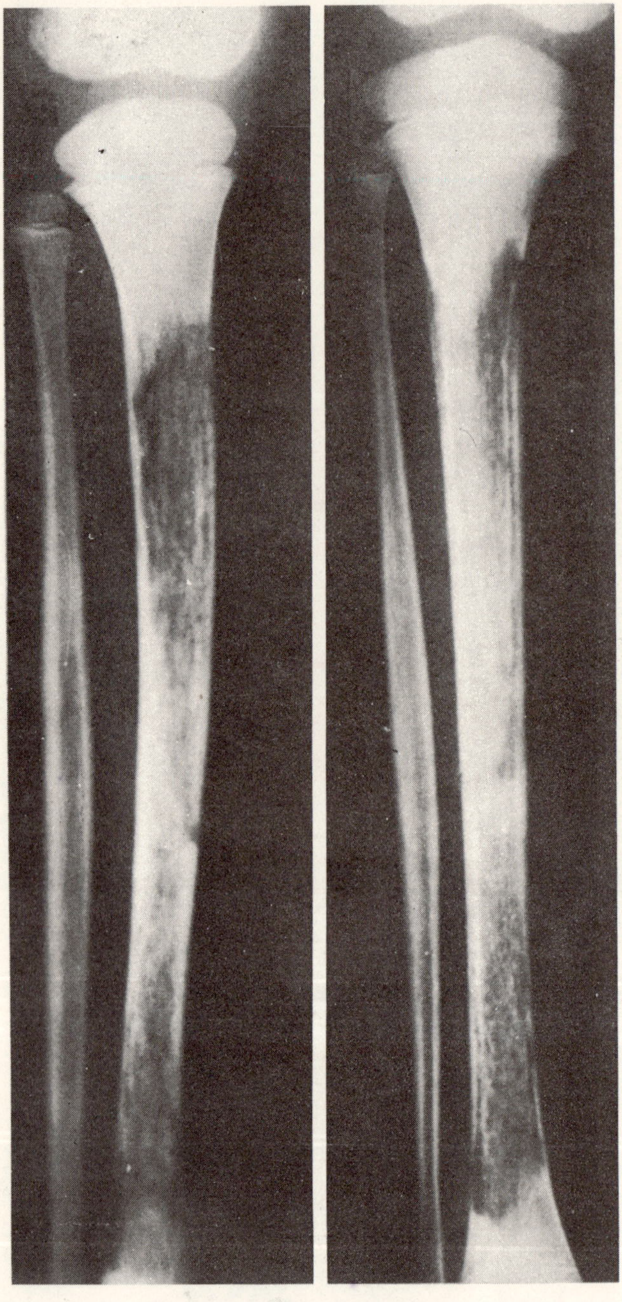

Fig. 8.3

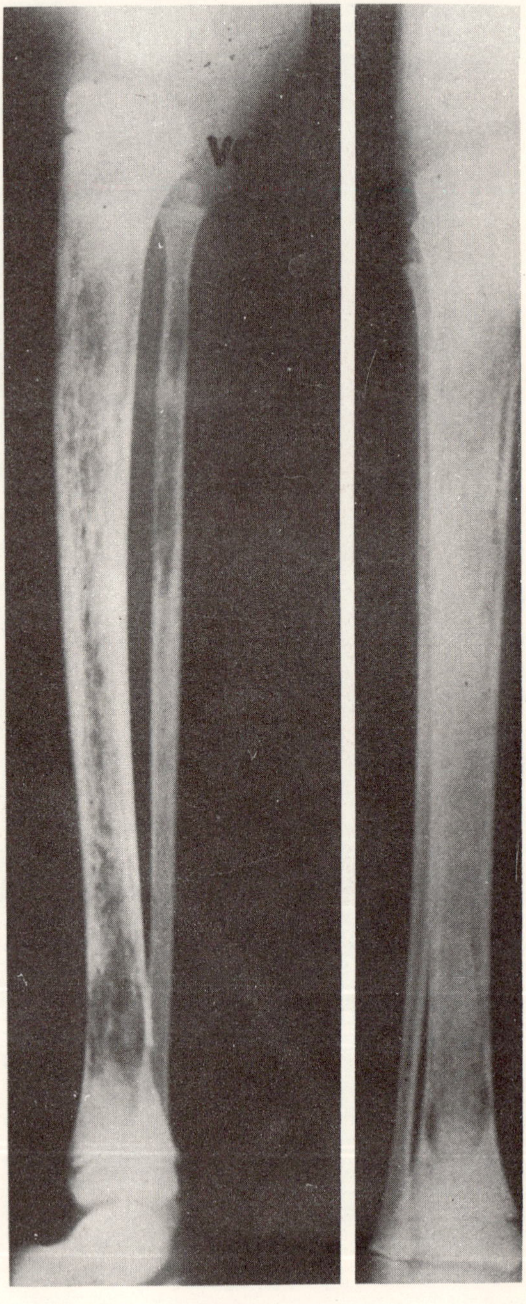

Fig. 8.4

Fig. 8.3 & 8.4. Typical X-ray appearance of " Cortex within Cortex " of both the tibia of the same patient. There is cortical fissuring and new bone formation beneath the periosteum.

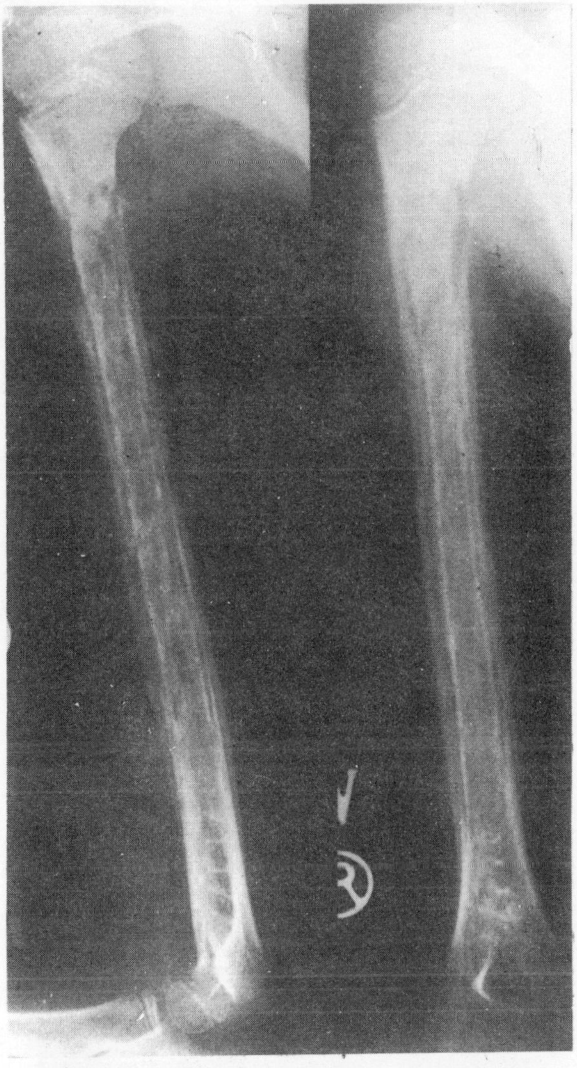

Fig. 8.5. X-ray humerus showing "Bone within Bone" appearance. There is formation of concentric layers of new bone parallel with the shaft and separated from cortex with marrow spaces.

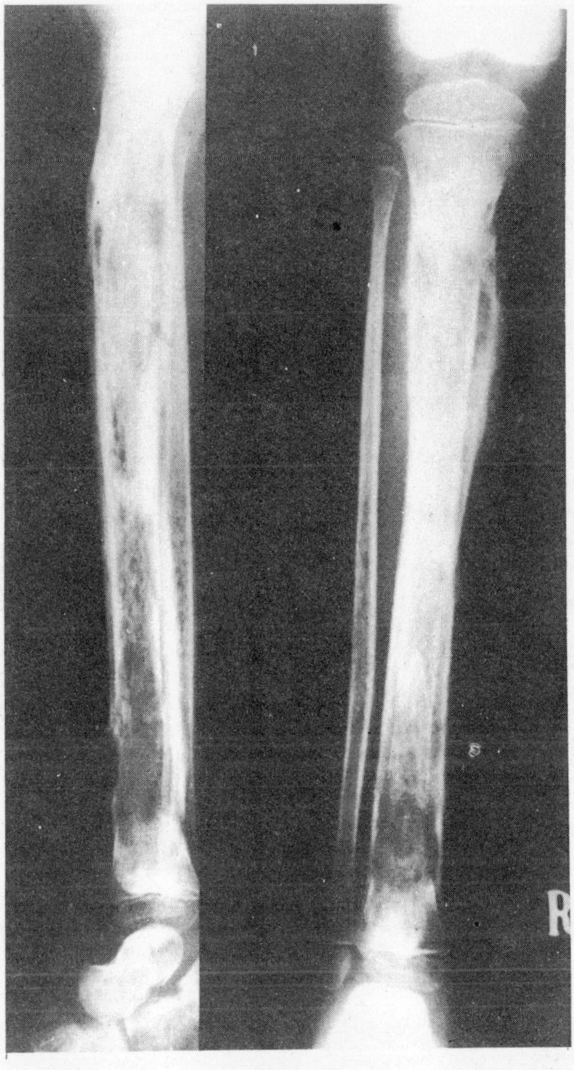

Fig. 8.6. X-ray of tibia and radius ulna showing "Overflowing.

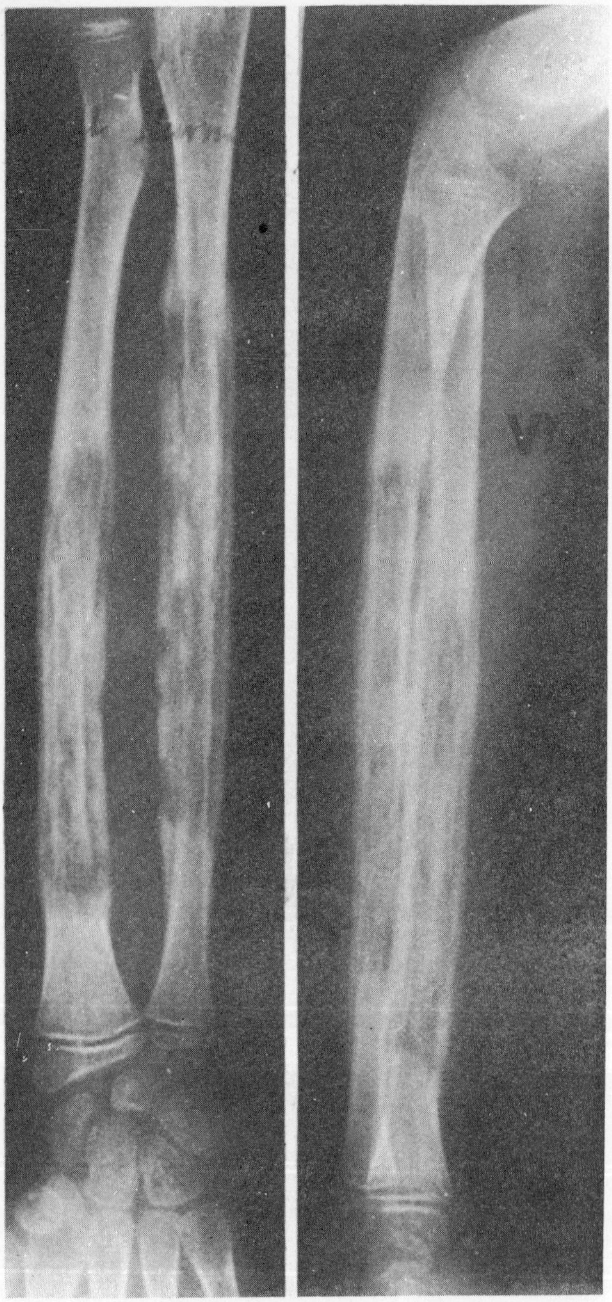

Fig. 8.7

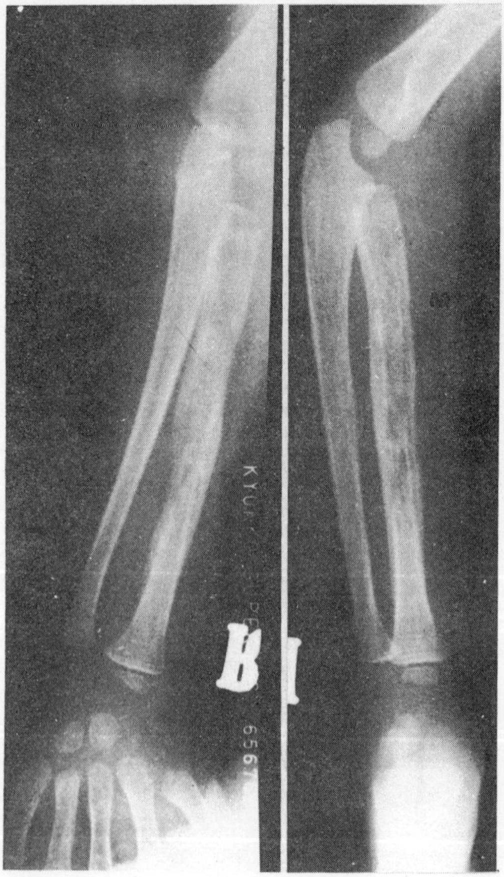

Fig. 8.8

Fig. 8.7 & 8.8. Bone around bone "appearance" showing profuse new bone formation on the top of the cortex with increase in the width of bone.

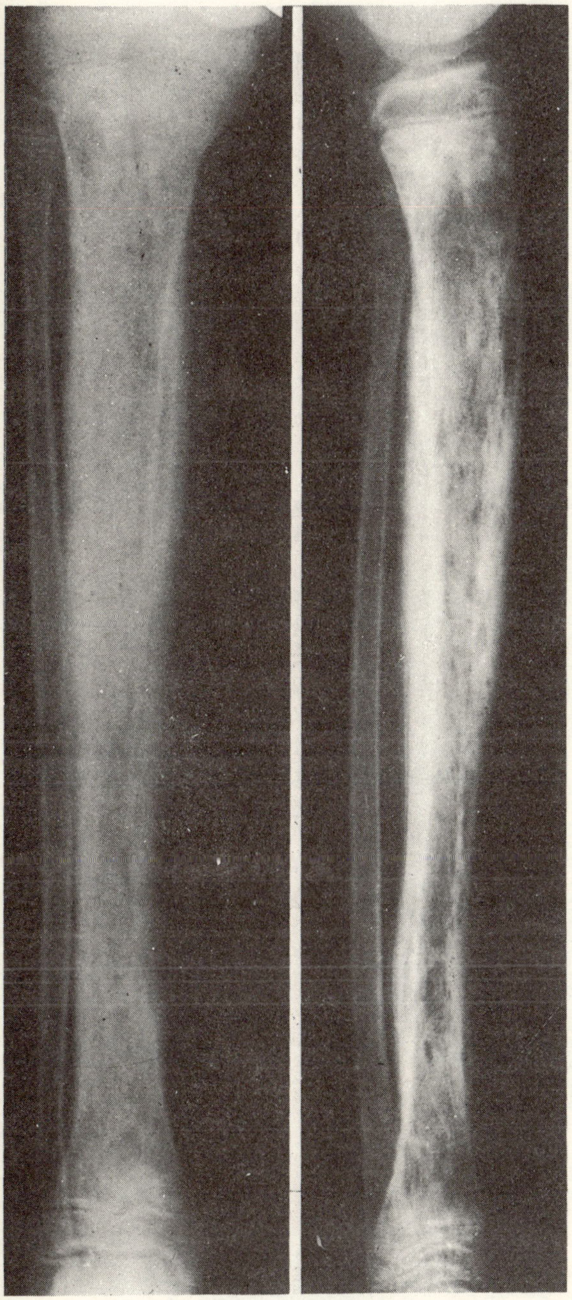

Fig. 8.9

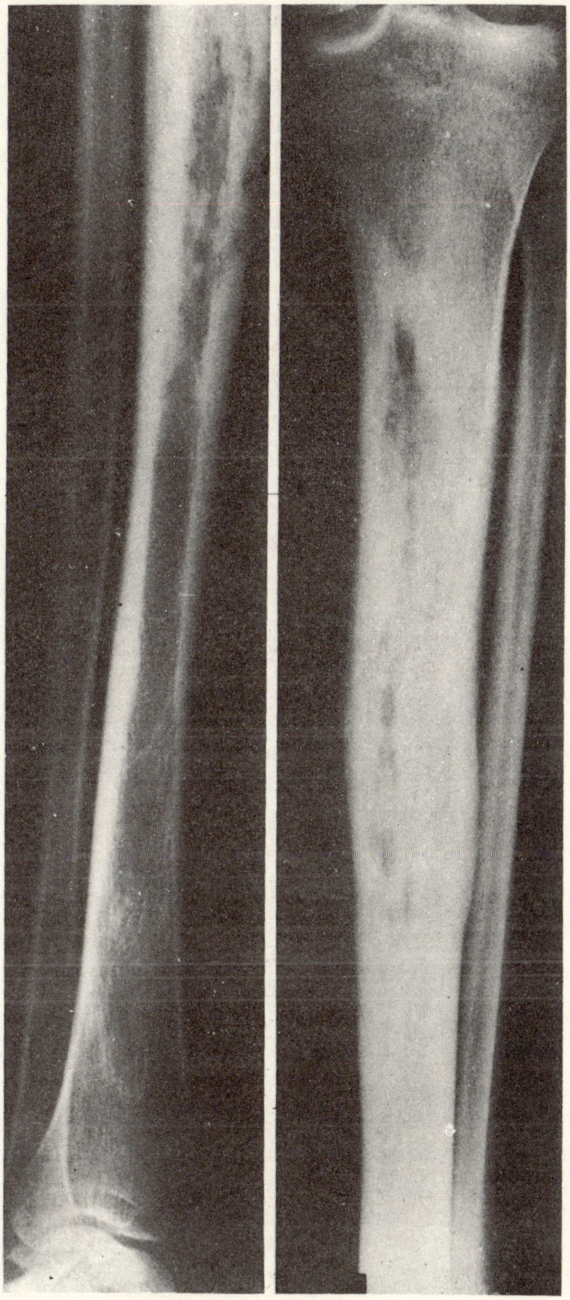

Fig. 8.10

Fig. 8.9 & 8.10. X-ray of tibia showing "Overflowing bone around bone" appearance with irregular exuberant copious new bone formation looking like candle grease appearance of Melorrheostasis.

MICROBIOLOGICAL CONFIRMATION

In all these patients the diagnosis was confirmed by aspiration of pus which was sent along with the blood for culture sensitivity. This has definite importance to differentiate from bone infarction in acute stage where as in chronic cases usually there is sinus formation with discharge of pus. In our series organisms were isolated in 36 cases who were operated in acute stage (100%) and in 15 patients of chronic cases who required sequestrectomy and saucerisation (31%). Only those patients of chronic discharging sinuses for more than 6 months with radiological signs and who failed to respond to conservative treatment for more than 10-16 weeks were subjected for surgery (saucerisation and sequestrectomy). Whereas all cases of acute osteomyelitis if confirmed by pus aspiration were subjected for drainage and corticotomy. The organisms were isolated either from pus in acute stage or from granulomatous tissue in chronic stage obtained during the surgery.

Table 8.4. Causative organisms of osteomyelitis in sickle cell disease

Organisms	*Number isolated*
E. coli	23
Staphylococcus	17
Salmonella species	8
Pseudomonas	3

The infecting organism was *E. coli* in majority of occasions instead of *Salmonella* which was highest in the studies reported by western literature (Ellenbogen et al 1955, Hughes J.G. et al 1957, Robert A.R. et al 1958 Hendrickse R.G. 1960, Greenberg L.W. et al 1970, Specht E.E.1971, Adeyokunnu A. et al 1980, Al-Awamy B. et al 1982, Noonan W.J. 1982, Gardner R.V. 1985, Greene W.B.et al 1987, Epps H.C. et al 1991).

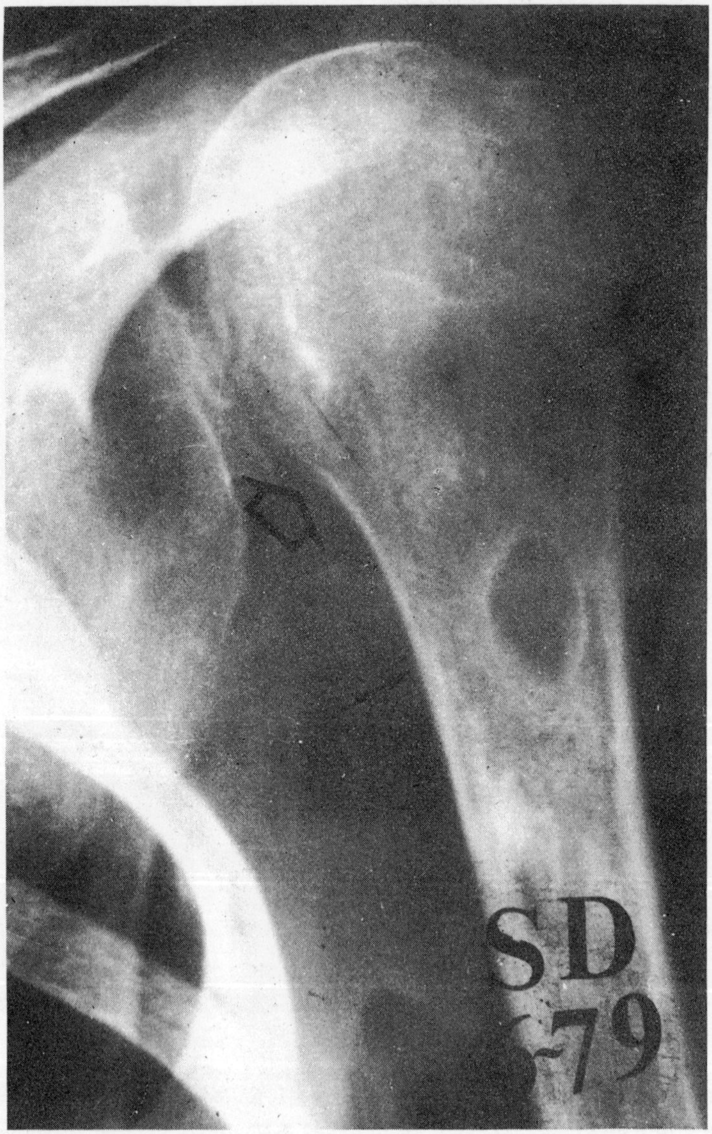

Fig. 8.11. X-ray showing chronic osteomyelitis of upper end of humerus.

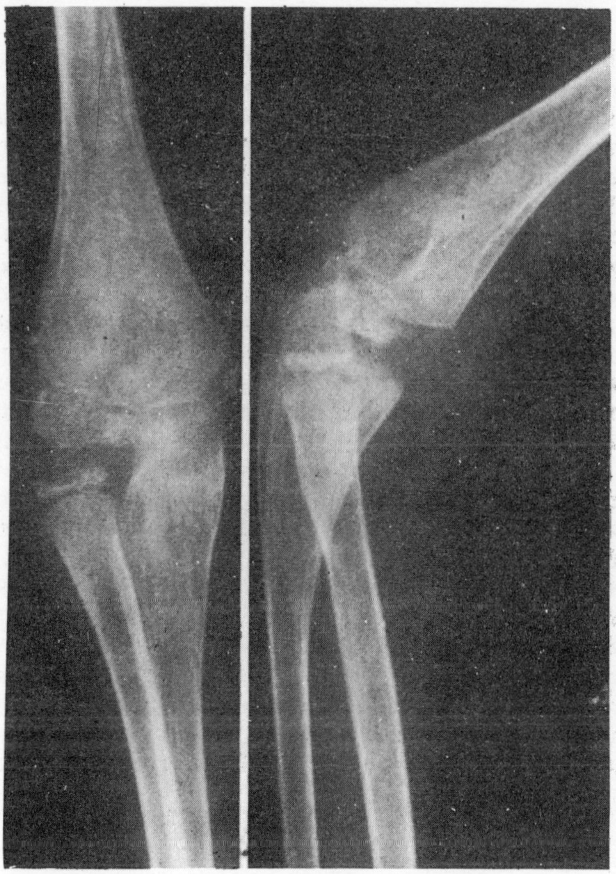

Fig. 8.12. X-ray of elbow showing osteomyelitis of distal Humerus and proximal ulna.

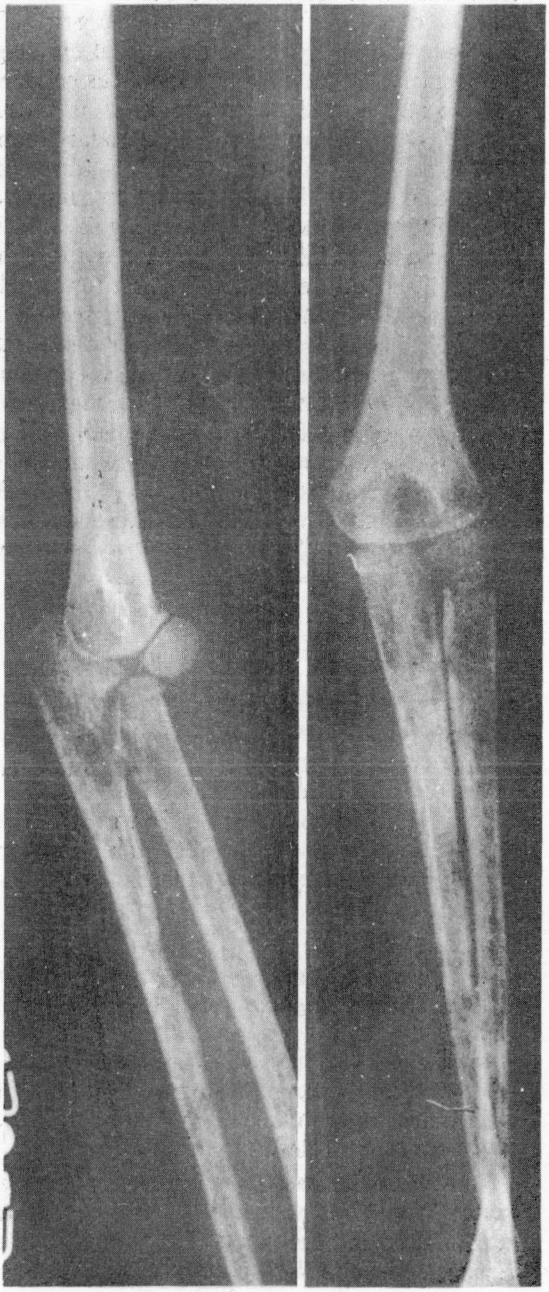

Fig. 8.13. X-ray forearm showing changes of osteomyelitis of radius and ulna with extension into elbow joint.

MANAGEMENT

Whenever there are specific changes of osteomyelitis, it requires specific treatment for that part. Antibiotics were given according to the pus culture or rarely of blood culture sensitivity report. The parts were immobilised either by splintage, traction or at times protected by plaster (Engh C.A. et al. 1971, Sadat Ali et al. 1985). Patients who were subjected to surgical decompression, pre-operatively required adequate maintenance of fluid balance and at times blood transfusion, preferably packed cells to bring up the haemoglobin level to minimum of 10 gms%. The rationale for preoperative transfusion is reduction of the level of HbS by dilution or partial exchange with HbA blood. This raises the haemoglobin level to the requirement and thereby suppresses endogenous erythropoiesis and allows time for short-lived sickle cells to be removed from the circulation. Adequate hydration is necessary with I.V. fluids to minimise sickling of RBCs which is seen secondary to increased viscosity and vascular stasis. Anaesthetist should take extra care by using safe techniques with adequate oxygenation, ventilation, maintenance of the circulating volume. Premedication with atropine and promethazine was used, avoiding respiratory depressant drugs. Preventive measures of sickling like alkalinisation with soda bicarbonate regimens, prophylactic folic acid and zinc, magnesium sulphate and low molecular weight dextran were taken (Oduntan S.A. et al. 1971, Oduro K.A. et al. 1972, Homi John et al. 1979). Arterial blood gas analysis should be performed intra as well as postoperatively and correct the acidosis accordingly. Adequate oxygenation, maintenance of fluid volume, monitoring cardiopulmonary status, acid-base levels are mandatory during and after surgical procedure. Anoxia and unphysiological conditions were avoided (Gilbertson A.A. 1965, Oduro K.A. 1972, Searle J.F. 1973). In acute stage drainage of pus and corticotomy was frequently required once the pus was aspirated and diagnosis confirmed. Whereas in chronic cases the operation of sequestrectomy and saucerisation was performed in those patients who did not respond to conservative treatment of at least 4 to 6 months and continued to have chronic discharging sinuses. Out of these 192 patients, 68 patients in chronic stage were subjected to sequestrectomy and saucerisation and 42 patients in acute stage to drainage and corticotomy. 48 patients of chronic osteomyelitis were managed by conservative treatment only. Antibiotics sensitive to either gram positive or gram negative organisms as per culture report were given for 6-8 weeks parenterally.

COMPLICATIONS

In addition to the pathological fractures in 12 patients, periarthritis of shoulder in 25 patients, stiffness of elbow was observed in 25 patients, and pericapsulitis of ankle in 7 patients. Septic arthritis of hip joint was found in 3 patients, (Figs. 8.14, 8.15) knee joint on 2 occasions and of elbow joint in 2 patients (Figs. 8.18). Associated changes of osteonecrosis were observed in 16 femoral heads and 11 humeral heads. Residual findings were seen in 36 patients in the form of shortening because of growth arrest, deformity secondary to infective epiphyseal damage and bending deformity due to malunion, osteoporosis, pathological fracture and deformity and stiffness because of spread of infection into the joint.

DISCUSSION

Sickle cell osteomyelitis was one of the commonest osseous manifestations observed in this study. Patients of Sickle cell disease are prone to bone infarction and infection. Almost all the long bones showed the radiological changes, in which there was fine and prominent trabeculation, marked cortical thinning and osteoporosis. Also there was widening of medullary cavity and increase in the width of diaphysis. Multiple infarctions in the bone causing necrosis, lysis, fibrosis and sclerosis were seen. Larger areas of necrosis were characterised clinically by severe pain, swelling due to periosteal inflammatory reaction and mild to severe form of destruction radiologically.

There was a classical appearance of "Cortex within cortex" and "Bone around bone". "Cortex within cortex" means, there is a new bone formation on the inner sides, due to vascular insult. There is no real increase in bone width, but reduction in the medullary cavity. There is a cortical fissuring which separates medulla from cortex and gives this classical appearance. The infected bone apart from above changes many times resulted in fragmentation, lysis or sclerosis and formation of bony abscesses and sequestras.

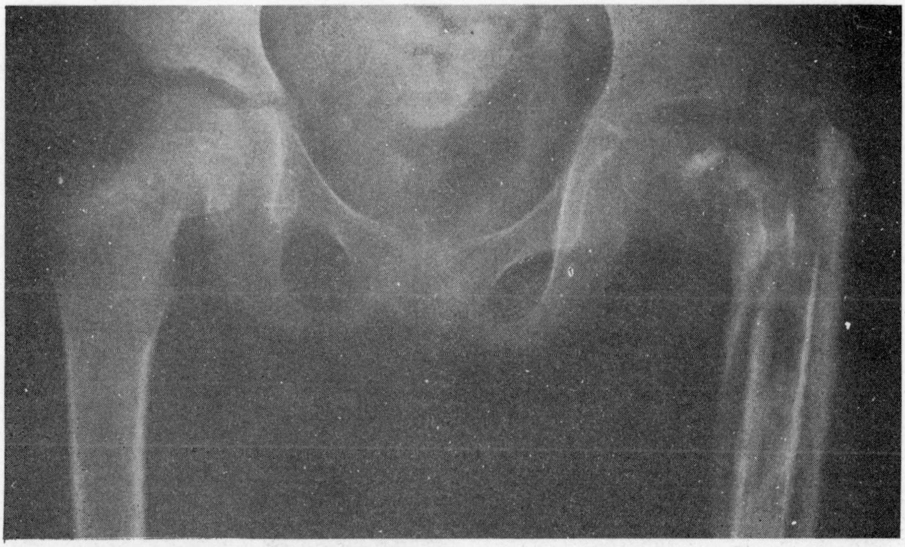

Fig. 8.14. Chronic osteomyelitis Femur (with sequestration) and spread of infection into the hip joint.

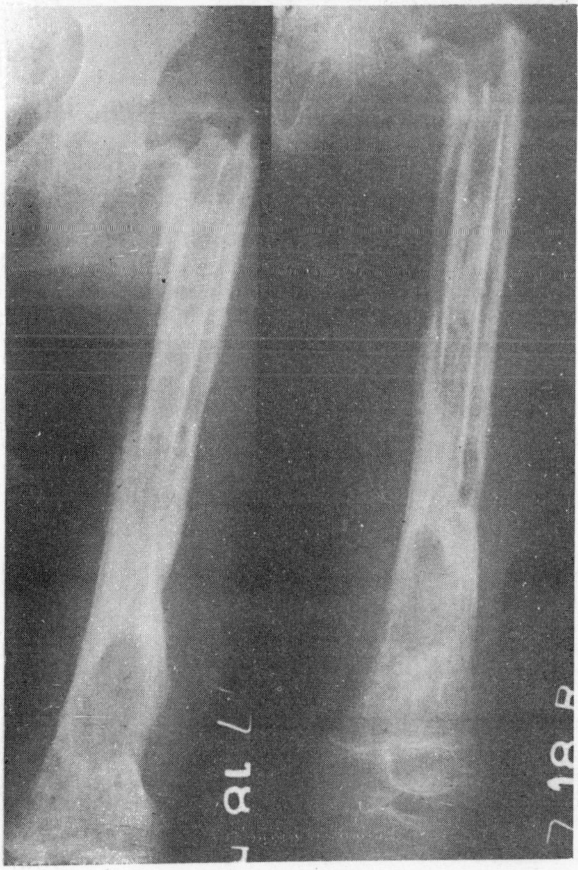

Fig. 8.15. Chronic osteomyelitis of Femur with extension into hip joint and pathological fracture.

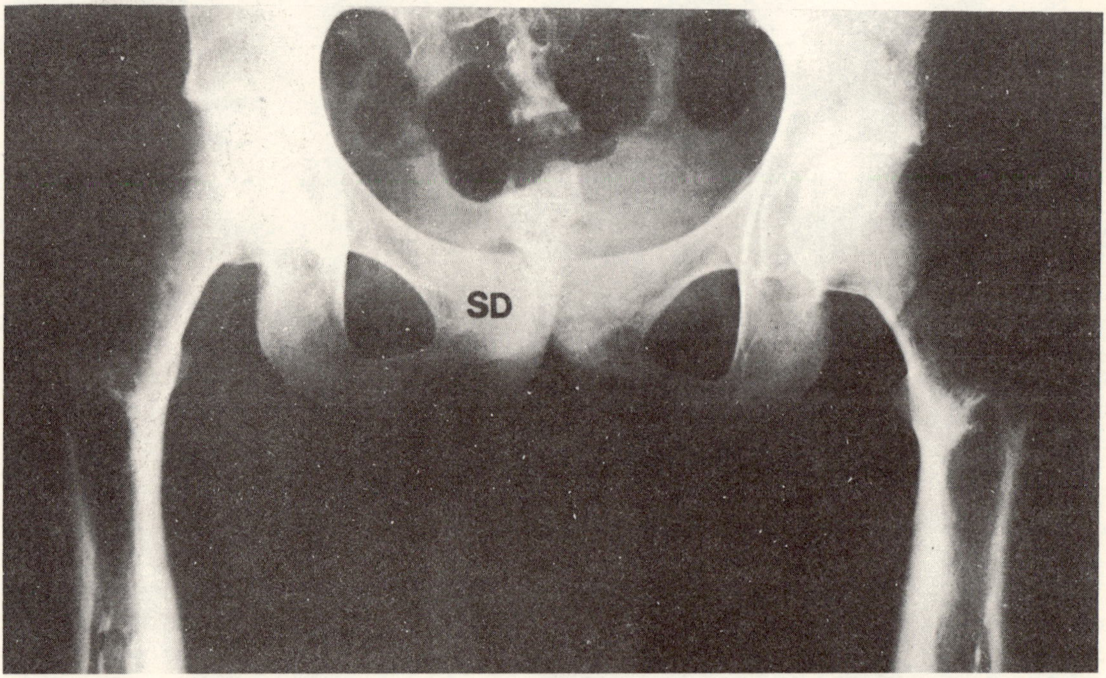

Fig. 8.16. X-ray pelvis showing changes of chronic osteomyelitis of both upper femora.

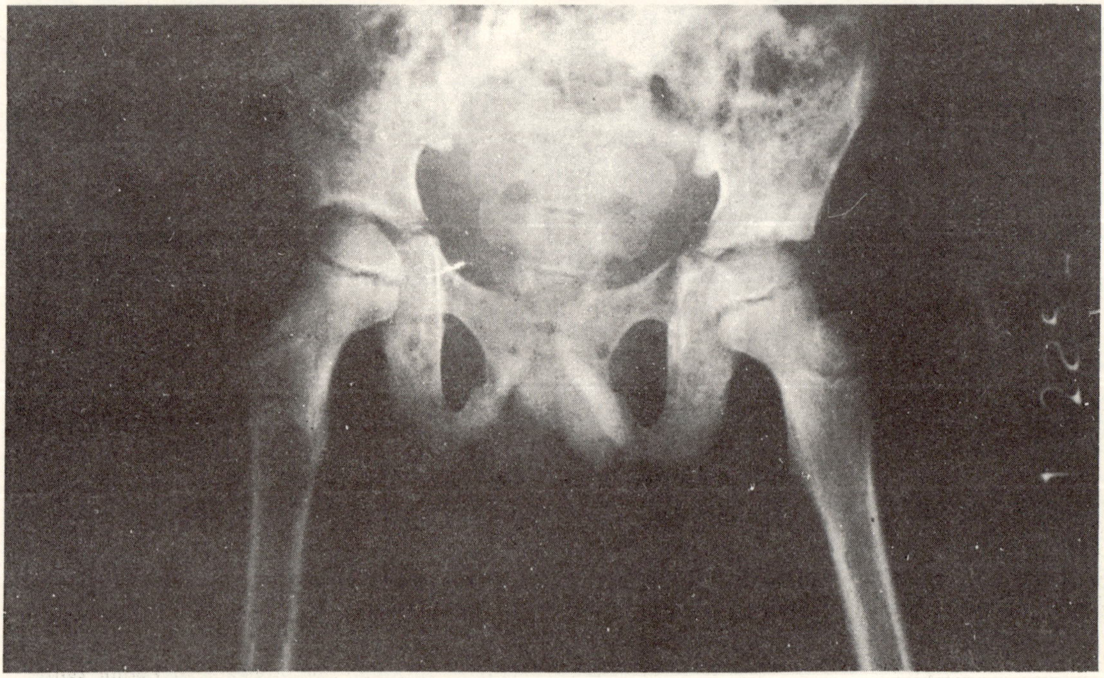

Fig. 8.17. X-ray femur showing changes of chronic osteomyelitis in the diaphysis of right femur with cavitation.

"Overflowing bone around bone" appearance (Luxuriant, exuberant, abundant, copious, profuse) means, there is addition of new bone on the top of the cortex, because of periosteal reaction secondary to infection. Many layers of such new bone formation results in increase in the width of bone and at times widening of cavity. There is a clear cut demarcation between original cortex and the formed new bone giving a classical appearance. This is mainly because of infarction resulting in to profuse, abundant, swarming, polluting, subperiosteal new bone formation as the haversian system in bones of sicklers is wide open.

Varied presentation of osteomyelitis from small to big sequestration (feathery to diaphyseal, tubular) was also observed (Figs. 8.15-8.17). Infrequently pathological fractures (Bohrer S.P. 1971, Ebong W.W. 1986) were seen and was noticed in 12 patients. The earliest radiological sign is nonspecific swelling of soft tissues and obliteration of fat planes in cases of acute osteomyelitis. The radiological demonstration of destruction of bone at the site of infection requires approximately 30 to 50 percent demineralisation before the lytic process can be appreciated and is noticed after 2-3 weeks. This lytic process is the earliest change in bone followed by classical changes as observed above.

The infecting organism was commonly *E. coli* as against the *Salmonella* infection which was commonly observed in the western studies. The second commonest organism was found to be *Staphylococci*.

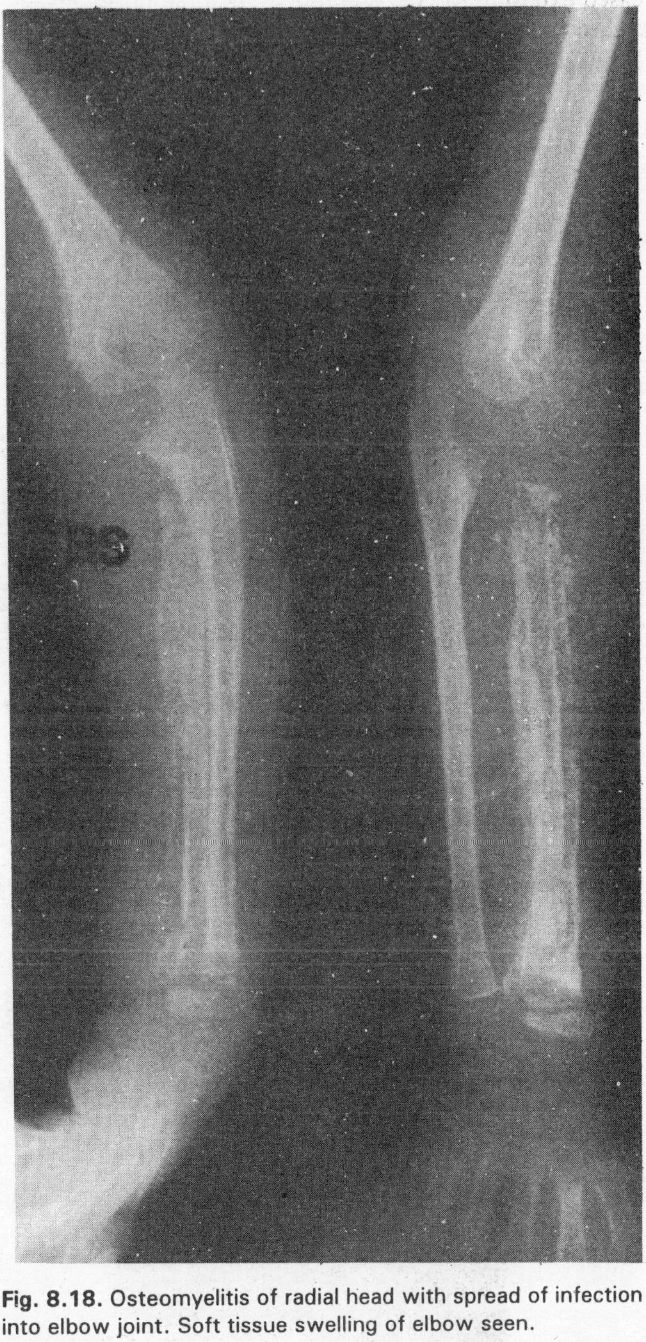

Fig. 8.18. Osteomyelitis of radial head with spread of infection into elbow joint. Soft tissue swelling of elbow seen.

There are various factors which make the patients of Sickle cell haemoglobinopathy prone to develop infection. The factors includes tissue injury from vascular insufficiency and infarction, impaired phagocytosis at low oxygen tension, increased haemolysis with stasis of sickled erythrocytes in sinusoidal bed of liver and spleen which overburdens and inhibits normal phagocytic function of macrophages in reticuloendothelial system, decreased splenic function due to fibrosis (Autosplenectomy), defective opsonin formation and abnormalities of compliments. There are more additional factors like peripheral bile froth formation, elevated serum levels of iron following haemolysis due to sickling (This potentiates the infection by bacteria which requires iron for growth), impaired bactericidal capacity of leucocytes in areas of focal hypoxia which develops during Sickle cell crisis where anaerobic bacteria still can grow, which increases the incidence of infection.

Increased exposure to infection due to multiple hospitalisations and recurrent episodes of infection with generalised debility predisposes to osteomyelitis.

In all these cases aspiration of pus, blood and pus culture was attempted. In this series organisms were isolated in 36 cases (100%) who were operated in acute stages (since they did not respond to

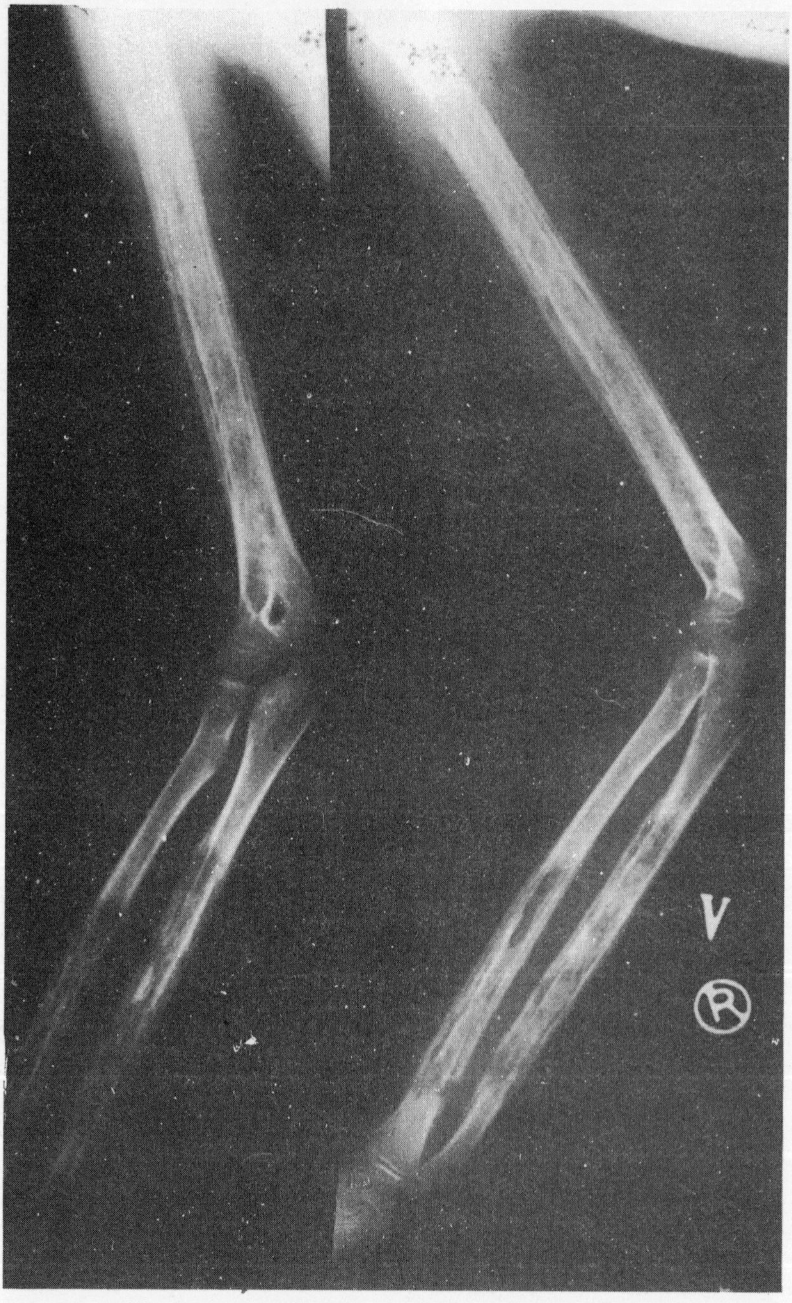

Fig.8.19. X-ray of multiple bones of a patient-Humerus , Radius, Ulna showing multi focal changes of Osteomyelitis.

conservative treatment) and in 15 patients of chronic cases (31%) who required sequestrectomy and saucerisation.

Very high percentage of the patients of osteomyelitis results into residual permanent disabilities like shortening, deformity and stiffness which was observed in about 20% of patients. Multifocal osteomyelitic changes were observed in about 18% of cases (Pande & Babhulkar, 1995) in this study (Fig. 8.19).

CONCLUSION

Sickle cell disease being a multisystem genetic hereditary familial chronic disease, early detection and awareness of its sequelae is necessary.

In acute stage drainage of pus and corticotomy was frequently required once the pus was aspirated and diagnosis confirmed. Whereas in chronic cases the operation of sequestrectomy and saucerisation was required in those patients who did not respond to conservative treatment for at least 4 to 6 months and continued to have chronic discharging sinuses.

Patients require protection and antibiotic cover on most of the occasions especially to prevent pathological fractures and other complications which might result in permanent disability. Basic effort and treatment is directed towards avoidance of unphysiological condition and hypoxia so that patients do not go into the crisis and thus hyperplasia of marrow is minimal. Usual treatment of chronic osteomyelitis is conservative but at times surgery is necessary. A genetic and marriage counselling alone would help in dilution of the disease (Headings V. et al 1974, Jackie Myrie 1983).

REFERENCES

1. Adeyokunnu A. and Hendrickse R.G. : Salmonella osteomyelitis in childhood Arch. Dis. Child., 1980, 55 : 175-84.
2. Almklov, J.R., Hansen, A.E., and Schneider, M. : Long bone involvement in Sickle cell anemia. Pediatrics 1950; 5 : 204 - 209.
3. Aksoy, M., Camli, N., and Erdem, S. : Roentgenographic bone changes in chronic iron deficiency anemia. Blood 1966; 27 : 677 - 686.
4. Al-Awamy B., Wilson W.A., Esmail S.M. and Abu-Nawarig M.: Sickle cell haemoglobinopathy and Salmonella osteomyelitis in Eastern Province of Saudi Arabia. Trop. and Geogr. Med 1982, 34 : 51-54.
5. Barton C.J., and Cockshott W.P. : Bone changes in hemoglobin S-C disease. Amer. J. Roentgenol, Rad. Therapy and Nuclear Med. 1962 ; 88 : 523-32.
6. Ben Dridi, M.F., Oumaya A., Gastli H., Doggaz, C., Bousnina S., Fattoum S., Ben Osman R., Gharbi H.A. Abnormalities of the skeleton in patients with Sickle cell anemia. A study of 222 cases in Tunisia. Pediat. Radiol., 1987, 17:293-302.
7. Bohrer, S.P. Fracture complicating bone infarcts and/or Osteomyelitis in Sickle-cell disease. Clin. Radiol., 1971, 22:83-88.
8. Carroll DS, Evans JW : Roentgen findings in Sickle cell anemia. Radiology 1949; 53 : 834-844.
9. Daland G.A. and Castle W.B. : A simple and rapid method for demonstrating the sickling of red blood cells; the use of reducing agents. J. Lab. Clin. Med. 1948, 33 : 1082-1088.
10. Ebong, W.W.: Pathological fracture complicating long bone osteomyelitis in patients with Sickle cell disease. J. Pediat. Orthop., 1986, 6 : 177-81.
11. Ebong, W.W.: Septic arthritis in patients with Sickle cell disease. British J. Rheumatol. 1987, 26: 99-102.
12. Ellenbogen, N.C., Raim, J., and Grossman, L. : Salmonella osteomyelitis. Amer. J. Dis. Children 1955 ; 90 : 275-79.
13. Engh C.A., Hughes J.L., Abrams R.C., Bowerman J.W. : Osteomyelitis in the patient with Sickle cell disease. Diagnosis and Management. J. Bone and Joint Surg., 1971, 53-A : 1-15.
14. Epps H. C., Bryant D'O.D., Coles M.J.M., Oswaldo C., and Washington D.C. : Osteomyelitis in patients who have Sickle cell disease. J Bone Joint Surg 1991, 73A : 1281 - 1294.

15. Gardner, R.V.: Salmonella vertebral osteomyelitis and epidural abscess in a child with Sickle cell anemia. Pediat. Emerg. Care, 1985, 1 : 87-9.
16. Givner L.B., Luddy R.E., Schwartz A.D. : Etiology of osteomyelitis in patient with major Sickle cell hemoglobinopathies. J. Pediat., 1981, 99: 411-13.
17. Gilbertson A.A. : Anaesthesia in West African patients with Sickle Cell Anaemia, Haemoglobin SC disease and Sickle Cell Trait. Br J Anaesth 1965, 37 : 614.
18. Greenberg L.W., Haynes R.E.: Escherichia coli osteomyelitis in an infant with Sickle cell disease. Clin. Pediat., 1970, 9: 436-38.
19. Greene W.B., Mcmillan C.W.: Salmonella osteomyelitis and hand foot syndrome in a child with Sickle cell anemia. J. Pediat. Orthop. 1987, 7: 716-18.
20. Headings V., Fielding J. : Guidelines for counselling young adults with Sickle cell trait. Am. J. Publ. Health 1974, 64 : 799.
21. Hendrickse, R.G. and Collard, P. : Salmonella osteitis in Nigerian children. Lancet 1960 ; 1 : 80 - 82.
22. Hewett, B.V., and Nice, C.M. : Radiographic manifestation of Sickle cell anemia. Rad. Clinics N.A. 1954 ; 2 : 249-59.
23. Homi John, Jennifer. Reynolds, Alison skinner, Wadia H., Graham serjeant : General anaesthesia in Sickle cell disease British Medical Journal 1979,
24. Hughes J.G., Carroll D.S. : Salmonella osteomyelitis complicating Sickle cell disease. Pediatrics 1957, 19 : 184-90.
25. Jackie Myrie : Complications of Sickle cell disease - Family planning and genetic counselling. Nursing Clinics of North America 1983, 18: 177-83.
26. Johnston, R.B. Jr.: Increased susceptibility to infection in Sickle cell disease. Review of its occurrence and possible causes. Southern Med. J. 1974, 67:1342-48.
27. Keeley Katherine and Buchanan, G.R.: Acute infarction of long bones in childern with Sickle cell anemia. J. Pediat.1982, 101: 170-75.
28. Koren A., Garty I., Katzuni E. : Bone infarction in childern with Sickle cell disease. Early diagnosis and differentiation from osteomyelitis. European J. Pediat.1984, 142: 93-97.
29. Launder W.J.: Musculoskeletal manifestations of the hemoglobinopathies. Orthop. Rev., 1979, 8(9): 111-18.
30. Mallouh Ahmad, Talab Younis.: Bone and Joint infection in patients with Sickle cell disease. J. Pediat. Orthop.1985, 5: 158-62.
31. Noonan W.J.: Salmonella osteomyelitis presenting as "Hand Foot Syndrome" in Sickle cell disease. British Med. J.1982, 284: 1464-65.
32. Oduro K.A., Searle J.F. : Anaesthesia in Sickle cell states : A plea for simplicity, British Medical Journal 1972, 4 : 596-98.
33. Oduntan S.A., Isaacs W.A. : Anaesthesia in patients with abnormal haemoglobin syndromes-a preliminary report. Br. J. Anaesth 1971, 43 : 1159.
34. O'Hara A.E. Roentgenographic osseous manifestations of the anemias and the leukemias. Clin Orth and Related Research 1967, 52 : 63-82.
35. Onwubalili J.K.: Sickle cell disease and infection. J. Infect.1983, 7: 2-20.
36. Pande Ketan C, Babhulkar Sushrut S, K Prasad S R S; Multifocal Osteomyelitis in a Case of Sickle Cell Disease, Jr. of Indian Medical Association, Vol. 93, No. 3, March 1995, p 122.
37. Rao, Sreedhar, Soloman, Nathan, Miller, Scott, Dunn, Eddy. Scintigraphic differentiation of bone infarction from osteomyelitis in childern with Sickle cell disease. J. Pediat. 1985, 107 : 686-88.
38. Reynolds J. The Roentgenological features of Sickle cell disease and related hemoglobinopathies. Springfield, ILL: Chas C. Thomas 1965 : 99-105.
39. Robert A.R., Hilburg L.E. Sickle cell disease with salmonella osteomyelitis. J. Pediat.1958, 52: 170-75.
40. Sadat Ali, Mir, Sankaran-Kutty, Kannan-Kutty. Recent observations on osteomyelitis in Sickle cell disease. Internat. Orthop.1985, 9: 97-99.
41. Searle J.F. Anaesthesia in Sickle cell states. Anaesthesia 1973, 28 : 48.
42. Specht, E.E. Hemoglobinopathic salmonella osteomyelitis. Orthopedic aspect. Clin. Orthop. 1971, 79: 110-18.
43. Wigh R., and Thompson H.J., Jr. Cortical fissuring in osteomyelitis complicating Sickle cell anemia. Radiology 1950; 55 : 553-56.

9

Pathological Fractures of Long Bones in Patients with Sickle Cell Haemoglobinopathy

Pathological fractures are infrequent presentation of Sickle cell haemoglobinopathy resulting secondary to bone marrow hyperplasia, cortical thinning, atrophy of trabeculae, bone infarcts and osteomyelitis. A study of 46 patients among sicklers is presented with pathological fractures in various long bones affecting 61 bones .It was commonly observed in second decade in males. In one group (Non-infective) comprising of 34 patients the main reason of fracture was osteoporosis secondary to hyperplasia of red marrow resulting into wide medullary cavity, thin cortices and atrophy of trabeculae. In another group (Infective) of 12 patients the pathological fracture was following necrosis, infarction and osteomyelitis. Aspiration of pus, pus and blood culture clinched the diagnosis of infective group. By and large patient requires conservative treatment. Multiple pathological fractures and malunion resulting in deformities was observed in high percentage of patients.

SYMPTOMATOLOGY

All these patients mainly reported for the pain in bones and joints, swelling over the bones, frequent recurrent infections and loss of function of the involved extremity. A few had difficulty in walking and painful limp. Few patients reported for deformity following malunion. All these patients were thoroughly examined and investigated in detail. Total 46 patients of pathological fractures, affecting 61 bones were detected and studied with an average follow up of 8 years. There were 31 males and 15 females, ranging from 4 years to 25 years. The following table shows the age and sex distribution of pathological fractures in 46 patients.

Table 9.1. Age and Sex distribution

Age group	*Males*	*Females*	*Total*
04-10	07	04	11
11-15	11	05	16
16-20	07	03	10
21-25	06	03	09
Total	31	15	46

Amongst the patients of pathological fractures, in 34 cases there was no evidence of osteomyelitis where as in 12 patients there was evidence of bone infarction and osteomyelitis. In all these patients there was bending, angulation and deformity secondary to displacement or overriding of the fractured fragments. 40 patients were diagnosed during the acute phase of fracture where as 6 patients were diagnosed after the malunion.

CLINICAL MANIFESTATIONS

Most of the patients reported with history of fever, malaise, cough with expectoration, severe joint and bone pains with either localised or generalised tenderness of 3-10 days history. Deformity with restricted range of the movements of the involved joint and painful extremity was always seen.

All the patients were subjected to skeletal survey, routine blood chemistry which revealed leukocytosis, raised erythrocyte sedimentation rate. Haemoglobin levels found to be below 7-8 gm% and sickling test (Daland & Castle 1948) and haemoglobin electrophoresis were done in all the patients. Sickling was always positive and the various electrophoretic patterns observed in these 46 patients with osteomyelitis were as follows :

Table 9.2. Haemoglobin Electrophoresis Patterns

Pattern	*No. of patients*
SS	24
AS	16
SF	06

Sickle cell disease (SS) formed the major group i.e. 50%. Radiographs of affected part showed definite evidence of pathological fracture with generalised osseous changes. Pathological fractures in Sickle cell disease are thought to be due to cortical bone infarction as the primary process with or without super added osteomyelitis. Radionuclide scan studies may not be useful to differentiate the bone infarction from osteomyelitis. Because of non availability of the scan in our Institute and since most studies showed no firm establishment to confirm the diagnosis or differentiate these two groups of pathological fracture with scans either of technetium 99 or gallium (Rao et al 1985) I have not subjected any patient to this costly investigation. Spontaneous fractures are commonly observed in patients of Sickle cell haemoglobinopathy following minor trauma because of the thin bone cortices, marrow hyperplasia and atrophy of bony trabeculae (Fig 9.1 & 9.2). These cases of pathological fractures were divided into two groups (infective and non-infective). In 34 patients there was no evidence of osteomyelitis where as 12 patients had a definite evidence of bone infarction and osteomyelitis (Figs. 9.3 and 9.4). Aspiration of pus, positive pus and blood cultures helped to clinch the diagnosis of osteomyelitis and to differentiate from bone infarction on seven occasions. Based on physical and clinical findings the preliminary diagnosis of osteomyelitis was done and confirmed with pus and blood culture reports in these seven patients.

ETIOPATHOLOGY OF SKELETAL CHANGES

Skeletal changes occur mainly due to severe bone marrow hyperplasia and vascular insufficiency resulting in thrombosis and infarction (Caffey et al 1957, Barton C.J. et al 1962, Edward O'Hara A. 1967, Givner L.B. et al 1981, Keeley et al 1982, Koren A. et al 1984). Vascular insufficiency is triggered off by crowding of sickle cells, anoxia, reflex vasospasm, increased viscosity, capillary stasis and resultant ischaemic necrosis.

Associated bone infection is quite common, leading to osteomyelitis and sequestration (Johnston R.B. 1974, Launder W.J. 1979, Onwubalili J.K. 1983, Mallouh et al 1985). Osteoporosis, infarction and sequestration resulted in pathological fractures in 12 patients of osteomyelitis (Figs. 9.5 and 9.6).

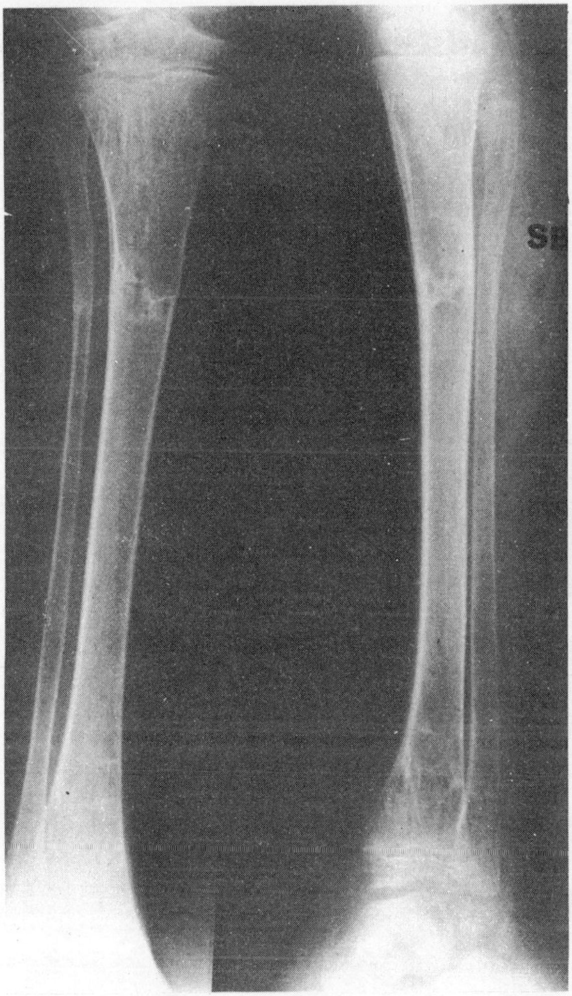

Fig. 9.1

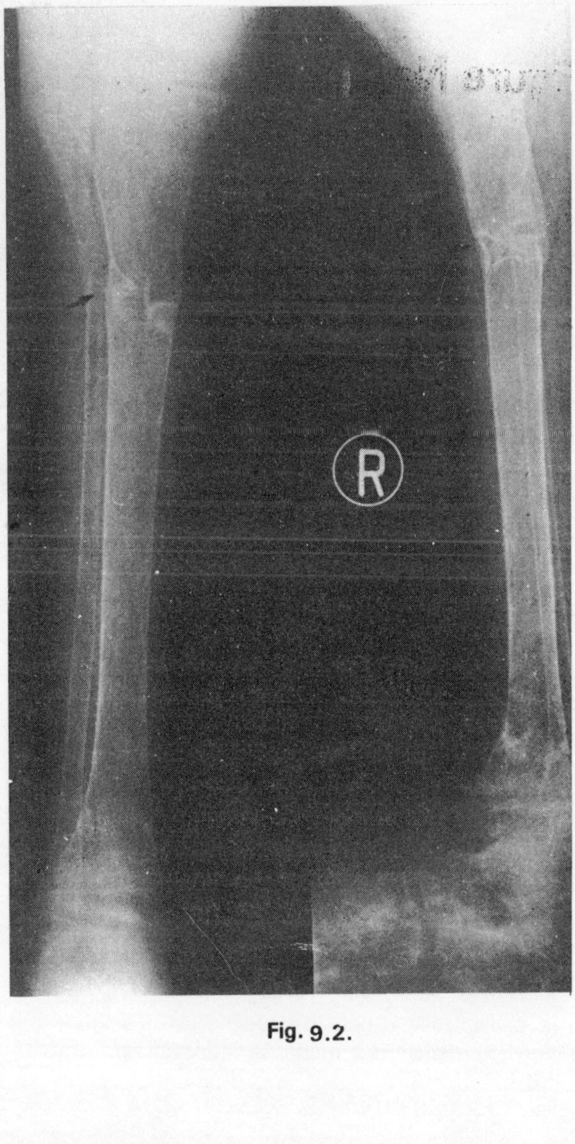

Fig. 9.2.

Fig. 9.1 & 9.2. X-rays of both Tibia showing marked osteoporosis, thin bone cortices, marrow hyperplasia and subperiosteal fracture at the upper one third and lower one third on right side and upper third on left side. Fracture in this case occurred with trivial trauma.

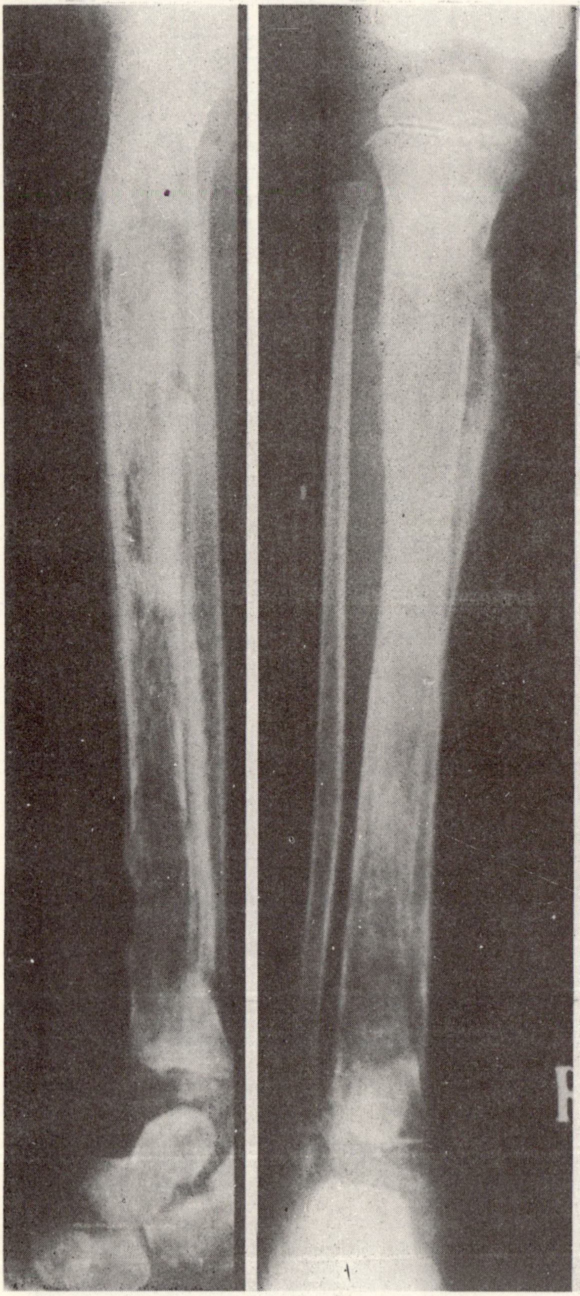

Fig. 9.3. X-ray of the Tibia showing a pathological fracture at both ends with changes of infarction, Osteomyelitis with new bone formation. Note the diaphyseal infarct which is sequestrated. Fracture is undisplaced mainly because of profuse new bone formation as a response to infarction.

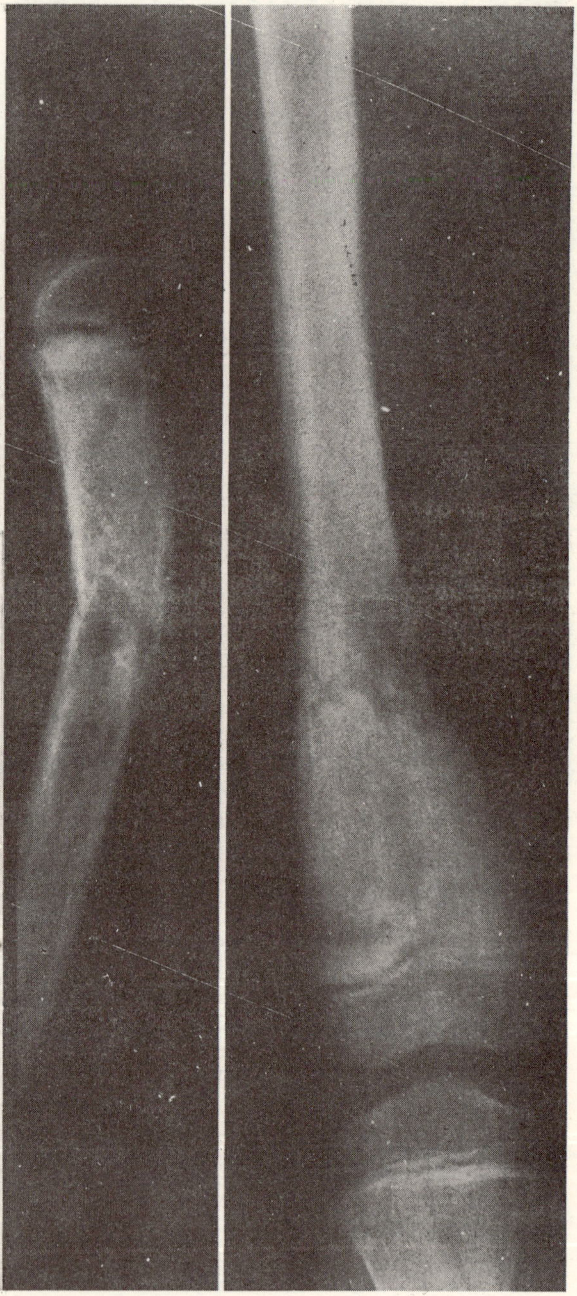

Fig. 9.4. X-ray of the Femur showing rarefaction and minimal changes of Osteomyelitis with pathological fracture.

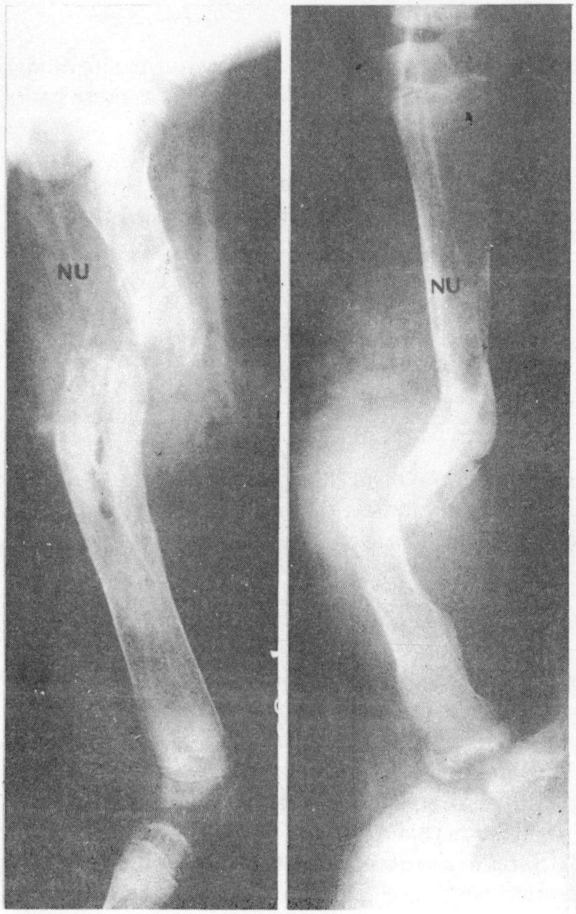

Fig. 9.5. X-ray of Femur and hip joint showing classical changes of Osteomyelitis with diaphyseal sequestration, profuse involucrum formation and pathological fracture neck Femur with coxa vara deformity.

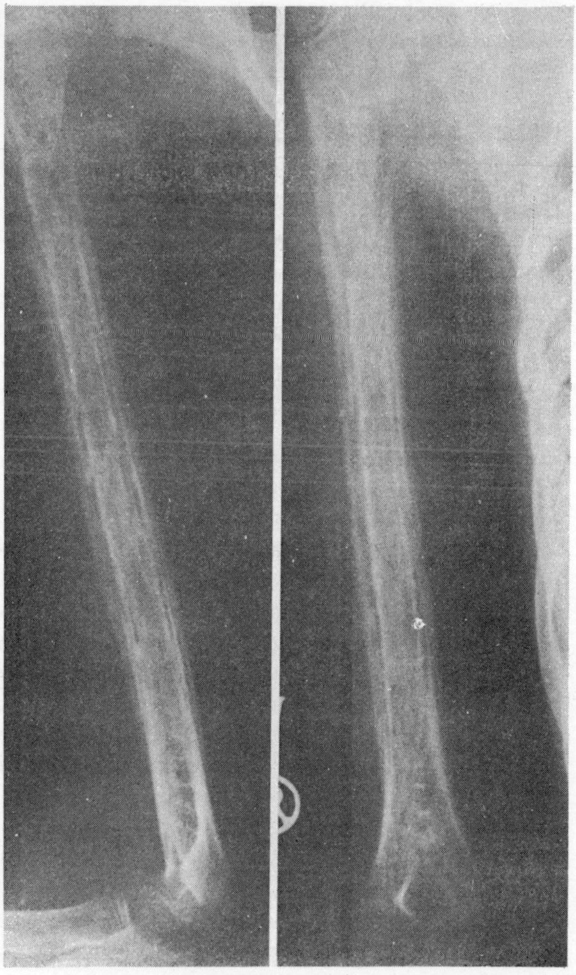

Fig. 9.6. X-ray of Humerus showing pathological fracture at the upper end. Note the diaphyseal sequestrum following infarction and typical radiological appearance of bone within bone formation and osteomyetitis.

OBSERVATIONS

Generalised osseous changes take place as microvascular circulation of bones is a favourite site of sickle cell to harbour. The pathological fractures were observed in 46 patients affecting 61 bones in these patients of Sickle cell haemoglobinopathy.

Table 9.3. Affection of various bones of pathological fractures in sickle cell Haemoglobinopathy

Affected Bone	*No. of Bones*
1. Tibia-fibula	22
3. Femur	17
4. Humerus	13
5. Radius-Ulna	09
Total no. of bones affected	61

Changes were seen in multiple sites involving more than one bone in 6 patients making the total of 61 bones in 46 patients with the 13% incidence of multiple pathological fractures. The highest incidence being observed in tibia (22). Bending, deformity and angulation was seen as a final outcome in 9 patients (Figs. 9.7, 9.8 and 9.9).

RADIOGRAPHIC CHANGES

Long bones in the patients of Sickle cell haemoglobinopathies usually reveal widening of medullary cavity, fine trabeculations, cortical thinning and osteoporosis. Infarcts of the marrow in the shafts and ends of long bones causing necrosis, lysis, fibrosis and sclerosis were observed in our study similar to findings reported by Almklov J.R. et al 1950, Barton C.J 1962, Reynolds J. 1965 and Aksoy M. et al 1966. In fact osteonecrosis of femoral head (224 patients) and humeral head (178 patients)observed in this large series of Sickle cell haemoglobinopathy, though not included in this report are the examples of epiphyseal fractures observed in this sickling disorder (Fig 9.10). Similarly rarefaction with compression fractures of vertebrae which were observed in more than 48 patients were also excluded from this study.

Fractures affecting the metaphyseo-diaphseal region were frequently seen in this group of pathological fractures. Radiographs in one group (Non-infective) demonstrated varying degrees of osteoporosis mainly because of the hyperplasia of bone marrow resulting into wide medullary cavity, cortical thinning and atrophy of trabeculae. This resulted into pathological fracture especially with angulation and deformity which was observed in majority of patients. On many occasions fractures were subclinical, subperiosteal with minimal angulation or displacement (Figs. 9.11 and 9.12).

In another group (Infective) of patients there was dense amorphous serpiginous medullary calcification especially at the ends of long bones because of infarcts. Many infarcts were seen in diaphyseal region which were cortical or medullary (Fig. 9.13). Cortical thickening, localised or generalised was observed in some long bones as a manifestation of subcortical infarction. Roentgen appearance of diaphyseal bone infarcts may show variety of appearances like subperiosteal new bone formation, localised osteolysis, mottled appearance, lysis with sclerosis (Fig.9.14) and at times sequestration. Fractures were seen at the sites of infarction which resulted in angulation, displacement and overriding. In few cases changes of superimposed osteomyelitis were seen. Chalky densities in medullary cavity, concentric layers of new bone formation along the cortices and exorbitant subperiosteal new bone formation in addition to pathological fractures were seen.

Radiographic changes varied from mild to severe form in addition to the fracture, but massive destruction was usually seen in this group of patients. The periosteum was elevated, irregularly thickened, cortex within cortex, bone within bone and bone around bone appearance, cortical fissuring, lysis, fragmentation of necrotic cortex, sclerosis, bone abscesses and large sequestras have been observed (Caroll D.S. et al 1949, Barton

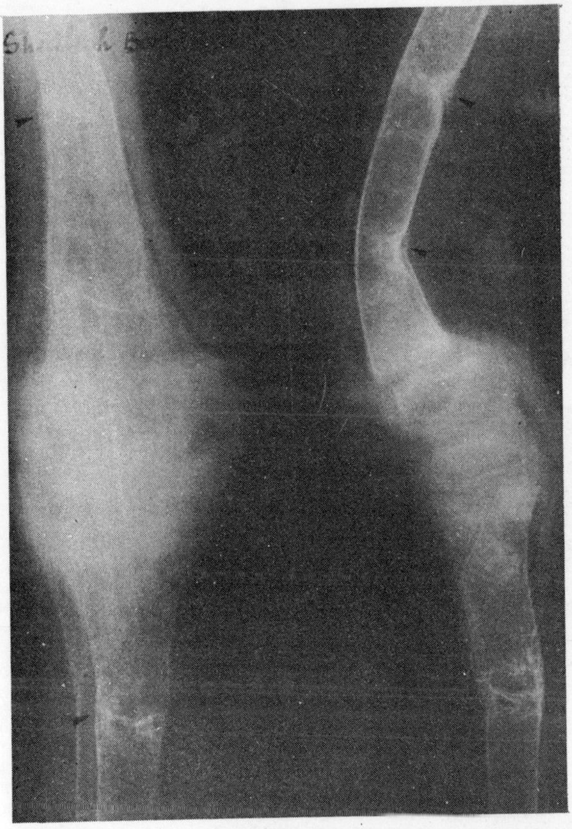

Fig. 9.7. X-ray of lower extremity showing distal Femur and proximal Tibia with knee joint having classical changes hyperplasia of bone marrow, thin bony cortices with multiple pathological fractures affecting distal Femur and proximal Tibia. Same patient had pathological fracture of both Tibia (Figs. 9.1 and 9.2), Radius-Ulna and Humerus.

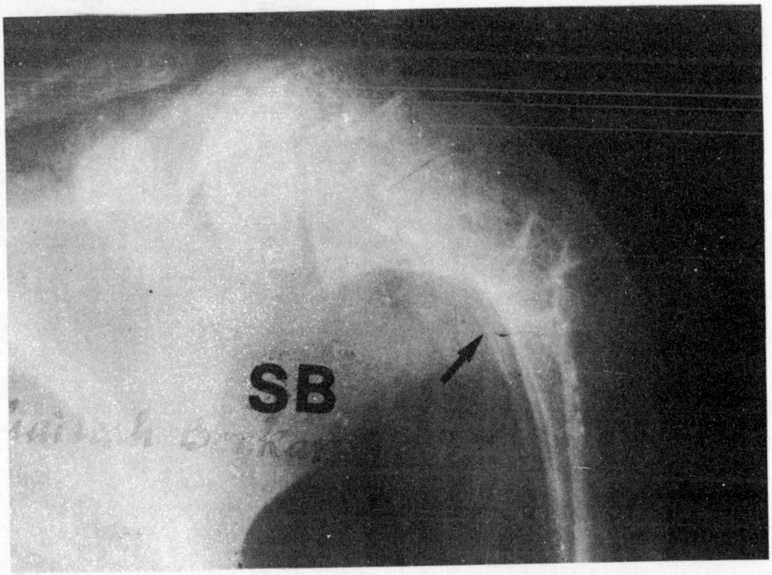

Fig. 9.8. X-ray of shoulder showing classical changes of sickle cell haemoglobinopathy. X-ray shows residual bending deformity following malunion at the level of metaphyseal-diaphyseal region.

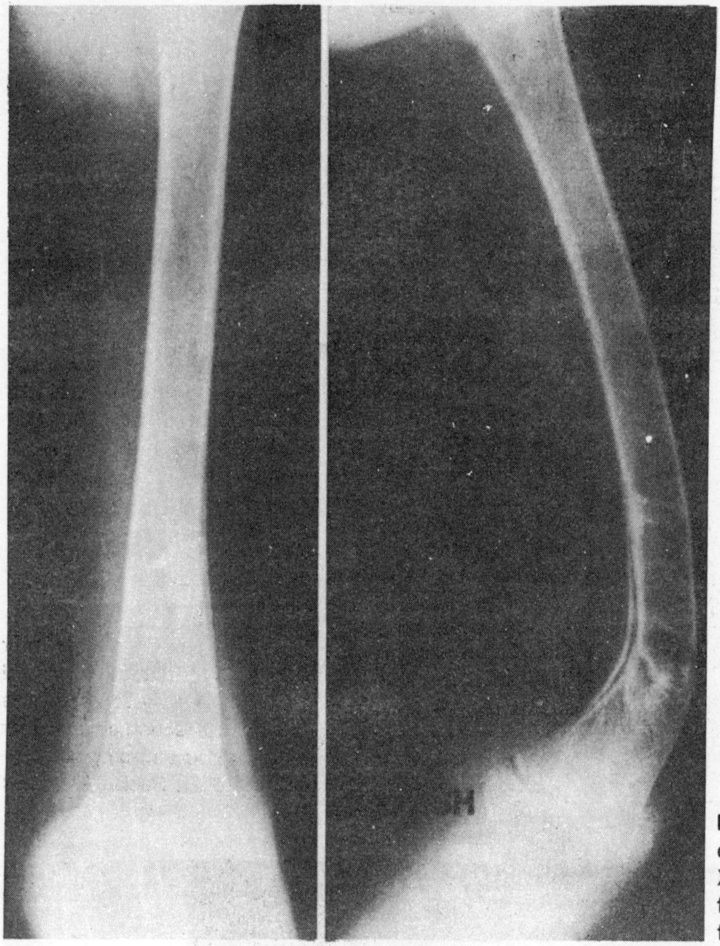

Fig. 9.9. X-ray of Femur showing classical changes of sickle cell haemoglobinopathy. X-ray shows bending deformity of lower fourth with periosteal new bone formation following a pathological fracture.

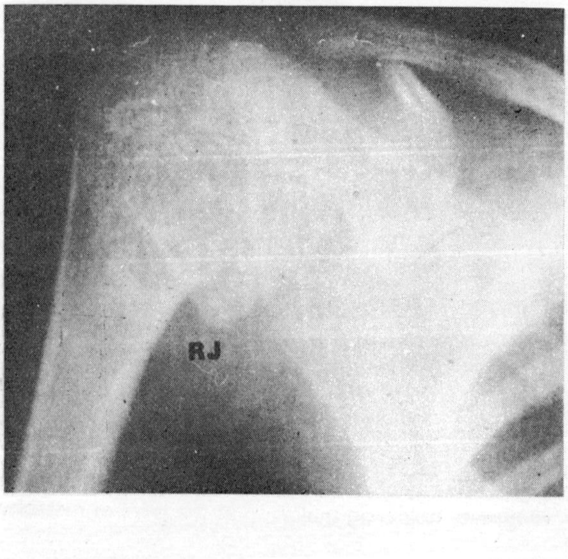

Fig. 9.10. X-ray of shoulder showing marked Osteoporosis in a patient of sickle cell disease with pathological fracture in metaphyseal region.

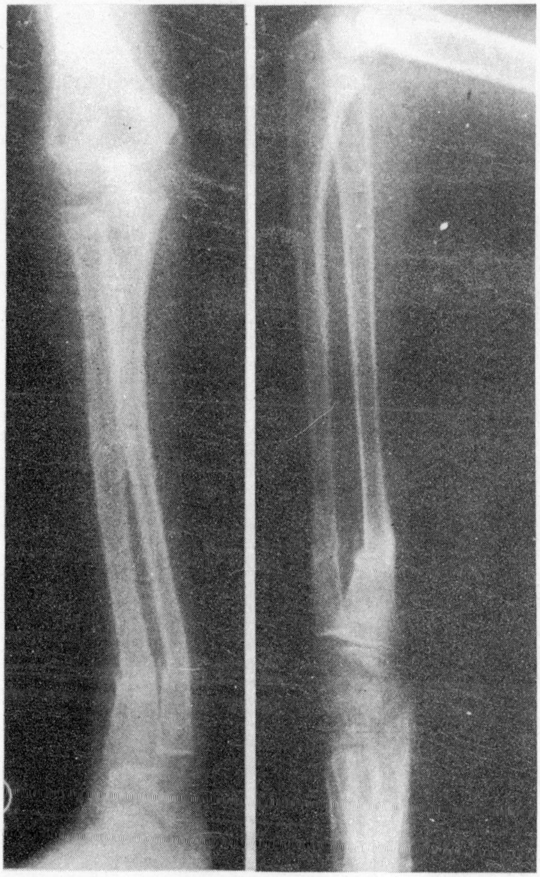

Fig. 9.11. X-ray forearm showing marked rarefaction with subperiosteal fracture of Radius and Ulna at lower one third with angulation.

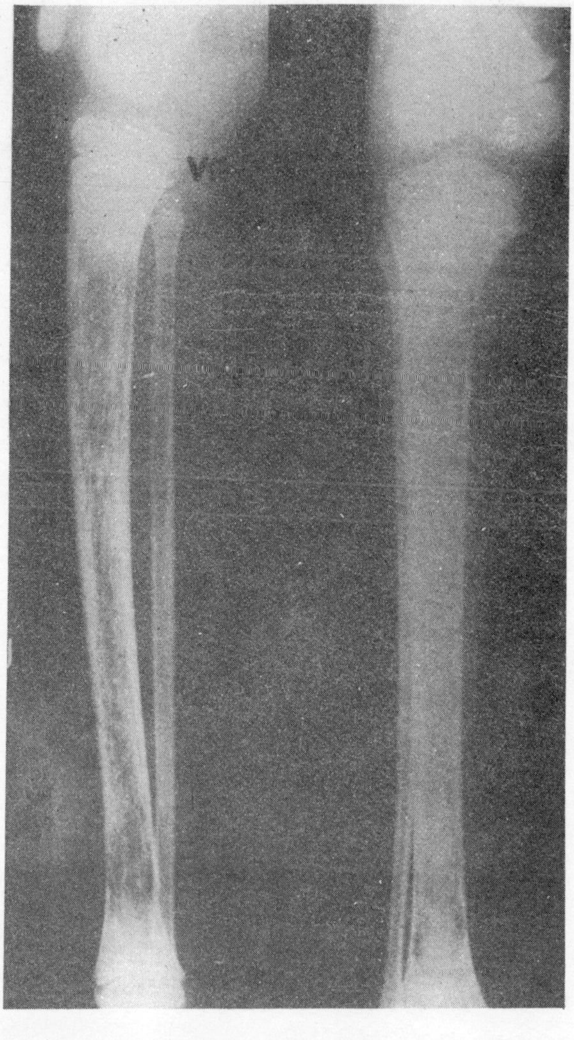

Fig. 9.12. X-ray Tibia AP and lateral showing classical diaphyseal infarct. There is cortical break at upper one fourth medially.

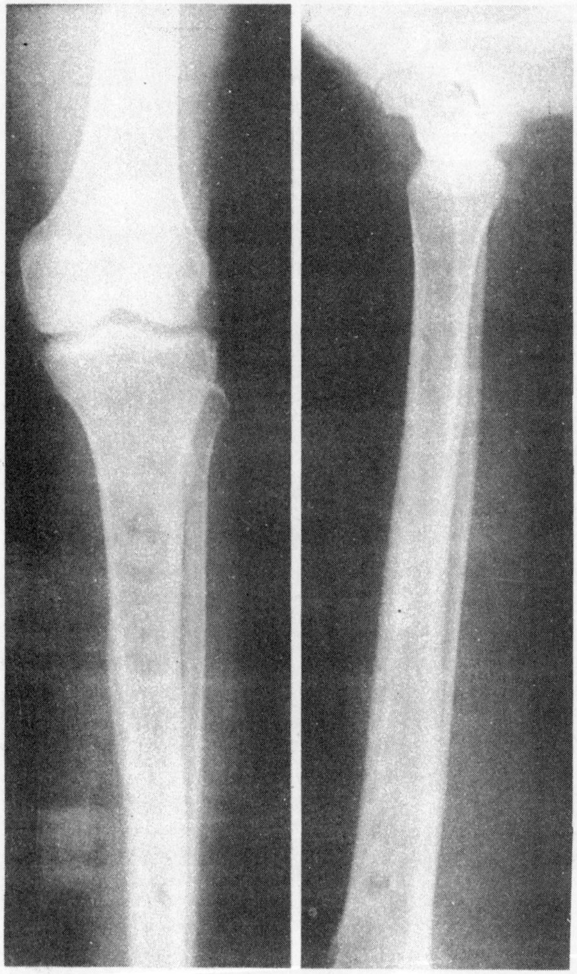

Fig. 9.13. X-ray of Tibia showing intramedullary Osteolysis with periosteal reaction suggestive of infarction. This patient is prone for pathological fracture if not immobilised.

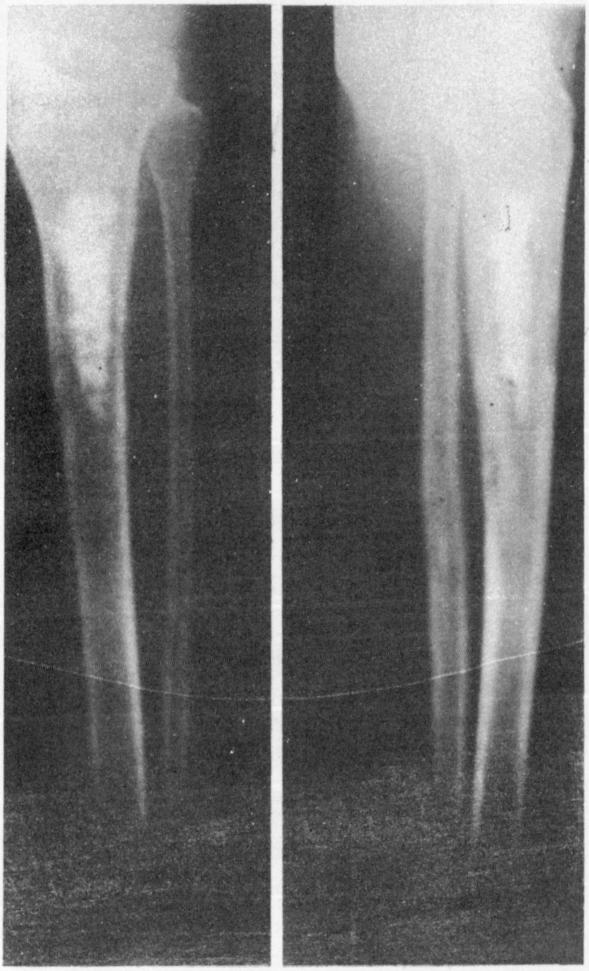

Fig. 9.14. X-ray of Tibia showing a classical big medullary infarct with marked rarefaction. This patient is very prone for pathological fracture if not protected.

C.J. et al 1962, Hewett B.V. et al 1964, Edward O'Hara A. 1967,Gardner R.V. 1985, Ebong W.W.1987, Ben Dridi et al 1987).

In some cases partial premature fusion of epiphysis was seen affecting the lower end of tibia—fibula, lower femoral epiphysis and upper humeral epiphysis in addition to generalised osteoporosis.

MANAGEMENT

Once the diagnosis of pathological fracture with Sickle cell haemoglobinopathy was suspected, the treatment was directed towards giving immediate relief to the patient. Splintage, traction or plaster slab was given depending upon the respective bone and its fracture and subsequently investigated to find out infective or non-infective pathology. In large percentage (34 patients, non-infective group) of patients the fracture was undisplaced and it only required correction of axial deformity which was achieved by traction or manipulation. Almost all the fractures were treated conservatively in this group which had fractures mainly because of osteoporosis. Sometimes reduction and correction was necessary before plaster immobilisation. Where as in another group of patients (12 patients, Infective group) the fracture occured through infarcts and osteomyelitic bone. Out of these 12 patients, 2 patients had discharging sinuses and the fracture occurred during the management of osteomyelitis.These two patients required only wide drainage of pus and fracture was treated by traction. Whereas on 5 occasions the pus was aspirated from the site of the fracture since the suspicion of infection was very high and one could confirm the micro-organism in these cases.On 3 occasions repeated attempts failed to aspirate any pus. Whereas in 2 patients it was felt that one should avoid aspiration since it might introduce outside infection in a patient with diaphyseal cortical infarcts.In these 5 patients bone marrow studies from iliac crest showed definite evidence of necrosis and infarction like the studies reported by Charache S. and Page D.L. 1967. However these 5 patients responded nicely to long-term therapy of antibiotics in addition to conservative treatment and did not require any surgical exploration. In all these 12 patients of infective pathology the treatment succeeded in achieving the union of the fracture.

DISCUSSION

Pathological fractures in patients with Sickle cell haemoglobinopathy though not common are seen in many patients in this region of Central India. Fractures earlier were thought to be uncommon in infarcted areas (Diggs 1967, Middlemiss and Raper 1966) and now are recognised to be very common (Bohrer 1970). Bones are markedly porotic in Sickle cell haemoglobinopathy and incidence of pathological fracture is expected to be very high since there is associated malnutrition in these patients belonging to specific community under consideration.

The most commonly affected bones were Tibia—Fibula, Femur, Humerus and Radius-Ulna in that order of frequency in this series. It is very obvious that the incidence should be more in the weight bearing bones, since the porotic bones do not sustain the weight (Dines et al 1976). Osteoporosis is frequently seen in these patients because of hyperplasia of red bone marrow resulting into widening of medullary cavity, thinning of cortices and atrophy of bony trabeculae (Diggs 1967, Golding et al 1959, Cassebaum and Patterson 1965). There was high incidence of angulation and deformity in the extremities because of malunion, since in high percentage of patients there was a subclinical fracture and patient reported late. The same state of high percentage was observed in the study of Currarino and Erlandson 1964 in B-Thalassemia but not in Sickle cell haemoglobinopathy. Pathological fractures are not necessarily the complications of cortical thinning and hyperplasia of bone marrow alone, but also occur secondary to necrosis following bone infarcts and osteomyelitis (Bohrer 1970,71). Fractures in Sickle cell disease are thought to be due to cortical bone infarction as the primary process with or without super added osteomyelitis. There could be a combination of osteoporosis, infarction and osteomyelitis (O'Hara 1967).

Basic radiological features of infarction are rarefaction and subperiosteal new bone formation (Edeiken et al 1967) which are also the classical features of osteomyelitis. It is presumed that frequent occurrence of osteomyelitis in Sickle cell disease is due to prior infarction of bone providing a fertile site for secondary infection. Hence there is always a difficulty in diagnosing the presence of infarct without any evidence of infection. Presently there is no completely reliable radiological criteria to rule out the presence of osteomyelitis in patients with bone infarcts or to diagnose primary infarcts in patients with osteomyelitis (Cockshott 1963, Edeikin et al 1967, Bohrer 1971, Moseley 1974). Actual aspiration of pus from the site of pathological fracture as observed in 5 patients is the most reliable clinical method to confirm the diagnosis of osteomyelitis. This type of aspiration may not be feasible in all patients with radiological evidence of diaphyseal infarcts, because one is likely to introduce secondary infection. However every attempt of pus aspiration and blood culture should be made wherever there is a suspicion of infection on clinical grounds. Without negative aspiration there is no way to be certain about the presence of only infarction since the radiological criteria to differentiate are still lacking. In some cases premature closure of epiphysis resulting into various deformities was observed. Most frequently it was observed in epiphysis of lower tibia - fibula, lower femoral and upper humeral epiphyses. These type of changes are rarely seen in Sickle cell disease but are frequently seen in B-Thalassemia (Currarino and Erlandson 1964, Diggs 1967, Dines et al, 1976 Exarchau et al 1984). The incidence of complications of pathological fractures in Sickle cell haemoglobinopathy is about 5% in patients with osseous manifestations in this series. It was commonly seen in second decade and in males. In 6 patients the patient had multiple pathological fractures. There was high percentage of 20% (9 patients) residual deformity especially angulation and bending deformity.

SUMMARY AND CONCLUSION

Pathological fractures though infrequently seen in Sickle cell haemoglobinopathy, were seen in 46 patients. These patients were divided into 2 groups. Aspiration of pus and identification of microorganisms was a definite method of confirming the diagnosis in the infective group. However negative aspiration was in favour of Sickle cell infarction causing pathological fracture. Most of the fractures were because of porotic bones requiring conservative treatment, though in few patients residual deformity was observed.

REFERENCES

1. Almklov, J.R., Hansen, A.E., and Schneider, M. : Long bone involvement in Sickle cell anemia. Pediatrics 1950; 5 : 204-209.
2. Aksoy, M., Camli, N., and Erdem, S. : Roentgenographic bone changes in chronic iron deficiency anemia. Blood 1966; 27 : 677-686.
3. Barton C.J. and Cockshott W.P. Bone changes in hemoglobin S-C disease. Amer. J. Roentgenol, Rad. Therapy and Nuclear Med. 1962; 88 : 523-32.
4. Ben Dridi, M.F., Oumaya A., Gastli H., Doggaz,C., Bousnina S., Fattoum S., Ben Osman R., Gharbi H.A. : Abnormalities of the skeleton in patients with Sickle cell anemia. A study of 222 cases in Tunisia. Pediat. Radiol., 1987, 17 : 293-302.
5. Bohrer S.P. Acute long diaphyseal infarcts in Sickle cell disease British Journal of Radiology 1970, 43: 685-97.
6. Bohrer S.P.: Fracture complicating bone infarcts and/or osteomyelitis in Sickle cell disease Clin. Radiol., 1971, 22 : 83-88.
7. Caffey I. Cooley's Anaemia. A Review of roentgenographic findings. American Journal of Roentgenography 1957, 78: 381.
8. Carroll D.S., Evans J.W. Roentgen findings in Sickle cell anemia. Radiology 1949; 53 : 834-844.
9. Cassebaumm W.H. and Patterson A.H. Fractures of distal femoral epiphysis Clin. Orth. 1965 41: 79-91.
10. Charache S., Page D.L. Infarction of bone marrow in Sickle cell disorders. Annals of internal medicine 1967, 67: 1195-1200.
11. Cockshott W.P. Haemoglobinopathies Br. Jr. of Radiology 1963, 36 : 19
12. Currarino C. and Erlandson M.E. Premature fusion of epiphysis in Cooley's Anaemia Radiology : 1964, 83 : 656
13. Daland G.A. and Castle W.B. A simple and rapid method for demonstrating the sickling of red blood cells; the use of reducing agents. J. Lab. Clin. Med. 1948, 33 : 1082-1088.

14. Diggs L.W. Bone and Joint lesions in Sickle cell disease. Ciin. Orth. 1967, 52:119-43
15. Dines M.D., Canale C.V., Arnold D.W. Fractures in Thalassaemia. J. Bone Joint Surg. 1976, 58-A: 662
16. Ebong, W.W. Septic arthritis in patients with Sickle cell disease. British J. Rheumatol. 1987, 26: 99-102.
17. Edeikin J., Hodes P.W., Libschit H.I., Wills M.H. Bone Ischaemia. Radiological Clinics of North America 1967: 5, 515-529
18. Edward O'Hara A. Roentgenographic osseous manifestations of the anemias and the leukemias. Clin Orth and Related Research 1967, 52 : 63 - 82.
19. E. Exarchou., C. Politou, E. Vretou, D. Pasparkis, G. Madessis and A.Caramerou. Fractures and epiphyseal deformities in B-Thalassaemia Clin. Orth. 1984, 189 : 229 - 33
20. Gardner, R.V. Salmonella vertebral osteomyelitis and epidural abscess in a child with Sickle cell anemia. Pediat. Emerg. Care, 1985, 1 : 87-9.
21. Givner L.B., Luddy R.E., Schwartz A.D. Etiology of osteomyelitis in patient with major Sickle cell hemoglobinopathies. J. Pediat., 1981, 99: 411-13.
22. Golding J.S.R., Maclever J.E. and Went L.N. Bone changes in Sickle cell anaemia and its genetic variants. J. Bone Joint Surg. 1959, 49-B 711
23. Hewett, B.V., and Nice, C.M. Radiographic manifestation of Sickle cell anemia. Rad. Clinics N.A. 1954; 2 : 249-59.
24. Johnston, R.B. Jr. Increased susceptibility to infection in Sickle cell disease. Review of its occurrence and possible causes. Southern Med. J. 1974, 67:1342-48.
25. Keeley Kathcrine and Buchanan, G.R. Acute infarction of long bones in childern with Sickle cell anemia. J. Pediat.1982, 101: 170-75.
26. Koren A., Garty I., Katzuni E. Bone infarction in childern with Sickle cell disease. Early diagnosis and differentiation from osteomyelitis. European J. Pediat. 1984, 142: 93-97.
27. Launder W.J. Musculoskeletal manifestations of the hemoglobinopathies. Orthop. Rev., 1979, 8(9): 111-18.
28. Mallouh, Ahmad, Talab, Younis. Bone and Joint infection in patients with sickle cell disease. J. Pediat. Orthop.1985, 5: 158-62.
29. Middlemiss J.H., Raper A.B. Skeletal changes in haemoglobinopathies. J. Bone Joint Surg. 1966 48 - B: 693-702.
30. Mosclcy J.E. Skeletal Changes in Anaemias. Seminars on Roentgenology 1974 vol IX, 3: 169-84
31. Onwubalili J.K. Sickle cell disease and infection. J. Infect. 1983, 7: 2-20.
32. Rao, Sreedhar, Soloman, Nathan, Millcr, Scott, Dunn, Eddy. Scintigraphic differentiation of bone infarction from osteomyelitis in childern with Sickle cell disease. J. Pediat. 1985, 107 : 686-88.
33. Reynolds J. The Roentgenological features of sickle cell disease and related hemoglobinopathies. Springfield, ILL: Chas C. Thomas 1965 : 99-105.

10

Hand-Foot Syndrome in Patients with Sickle Cell Haemoglobinopathy

Sickle cell dactylitis — Hand-foot syndrome is a frequently misdiagnosed condition occurring in infants and young children with Sickle cell disease. On many occasions this is the earliest and only clinical manifestation. This syndrome is clinically presented as swelling of hand and feet of acute onset. It usually occurs before the age of 5 years and is commonly seen in infants. The clinical picture of acute swelling of both hands and feet is accompanied by severe anaemia, fever and leucocytosis and may be associated with crisis or respiratory infection.

Skeletal manifestations were seen in 944 patients, 46 out of which had Hand foot syndrome. All the 46 patients were admitted in the stage of Sickle cell crisis. The workup of these patients involved haematological investigations and radiology of the involved part.

OBSERVATIONS

All these children were very sick and most of the time in Sickle cell crisis. The radiological picture of this syndrome is quite characteristic and is commonly observed between 7-14 days after the onset of symptoms. After the onset of swelling of hands and feet (Figs. 10.1 and 10.2) the earliest radiological change is appearance of sub-periosteal new bone formation in one or multiple metacarpals or phalanges. There is cortical thinning and there are multiple irregular intramedullary deposits, areas of spotty destruction and periosteal destruction is commonly seen (Figs. 10.3, 10.4 and 10.5). Usually the symptoms are bilateral and at times symmetrical. The smaller bones of the hands and feet becomes rectangular in outline and shape. Since the lesion usually causes periosteal elevation because of subperiosteal new bone formation, radiolucent areas intermingled with areas of increased density it gives "moth-eaten" appearance (Fig. 10.6).

Hand-foot Syndrome presents as mottled, lucent and sclerotic patches seen in shafts of metacarpals, Metatarsals, phalanges with periosteal changes (Figs. 10.7 and 10.8).

Watson and Burko 1963 designated "Hand-Foot Syndrome" as painful swelling of hands & feet seen in thrombotic crisis in young children. The clinical manifestation described were seen only in children under 6 years age. At the onset the child usually had concomitant respiratory infection & fever. There was puffiness of dorsum of hand and feet and tender fusiform swelling of phalanges.

The first case of dactylitis in a child with Sickle cell anaemia was reported by Danford and associates in 1941. In 1960, Smith used the term "Hand-Foot Syndrome" in describing this acute swelling in hand and feet of children with Sickle cell disease. The lesion is frequently mistaken for acute osteomyelitis.

The true incidence of sickle cell dactylitis is not clear. It is occurring in 10 to 20 per cent of children

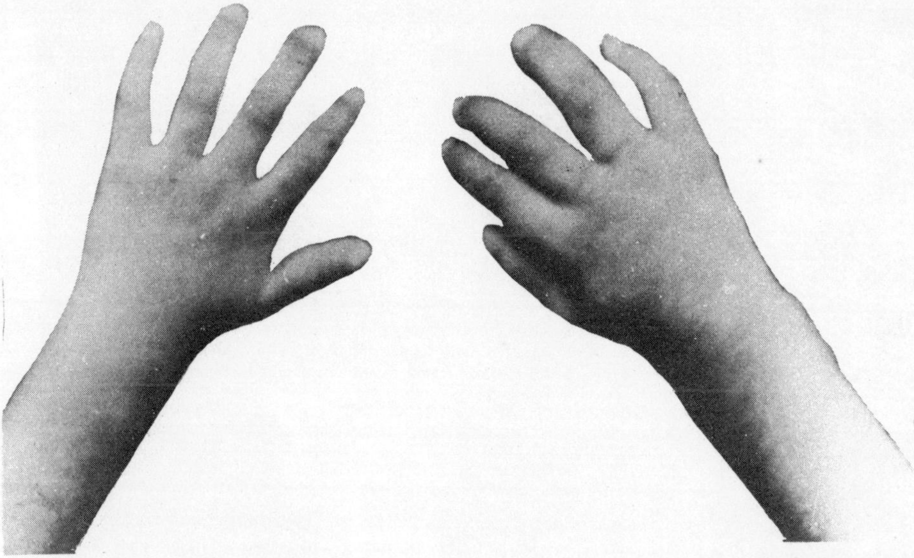

Fig. 10.1. Clinical photograph of a three years old child of Sickle cell disease with S-S pattern showing marked swelling of both the hands with fusiform swelling of fingers. Patient was admitted with the acute illness in the stage of sickle cell crisis.

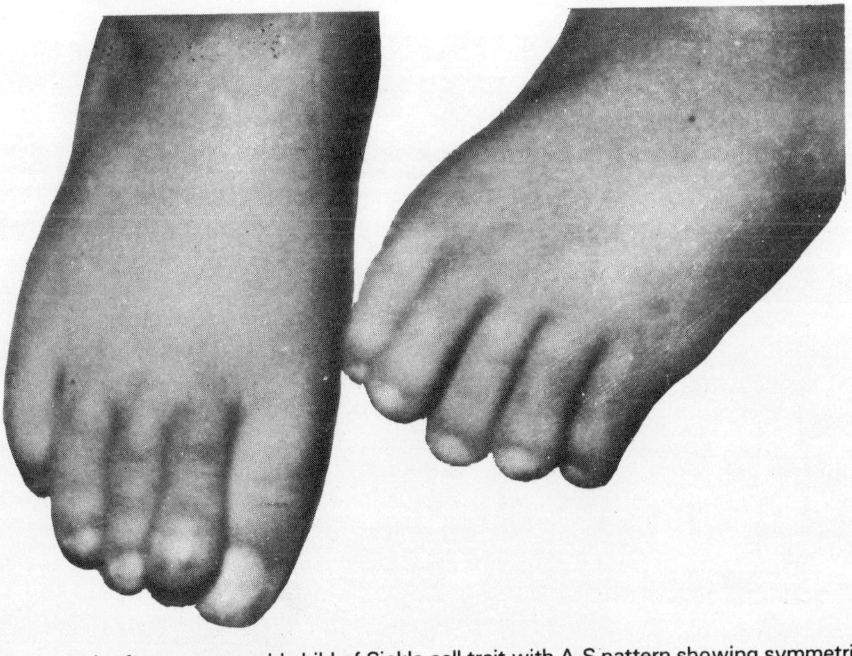

Fig. 10.2. Clinical photograph of a two years old child of Sickle cell trait with A-S pattern showing symmetrical swelling of both feet. Patient had a severe anaemia, was in poor general condition, debilitated, dehydrated and was admitted in crisis.

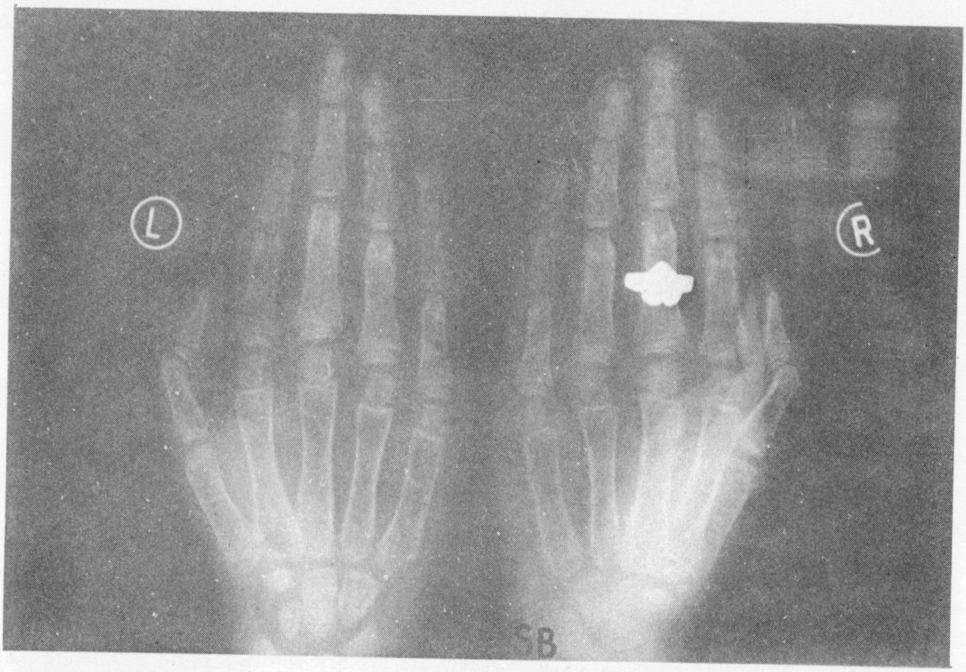

Fig. 10.3. X-ray of both hands showing typical radiological features of hand-foot syndrome. There is cortical thinning of metacarpals, phalanges with areas of intramedullary deposits and rectangular shape of metacarpals.

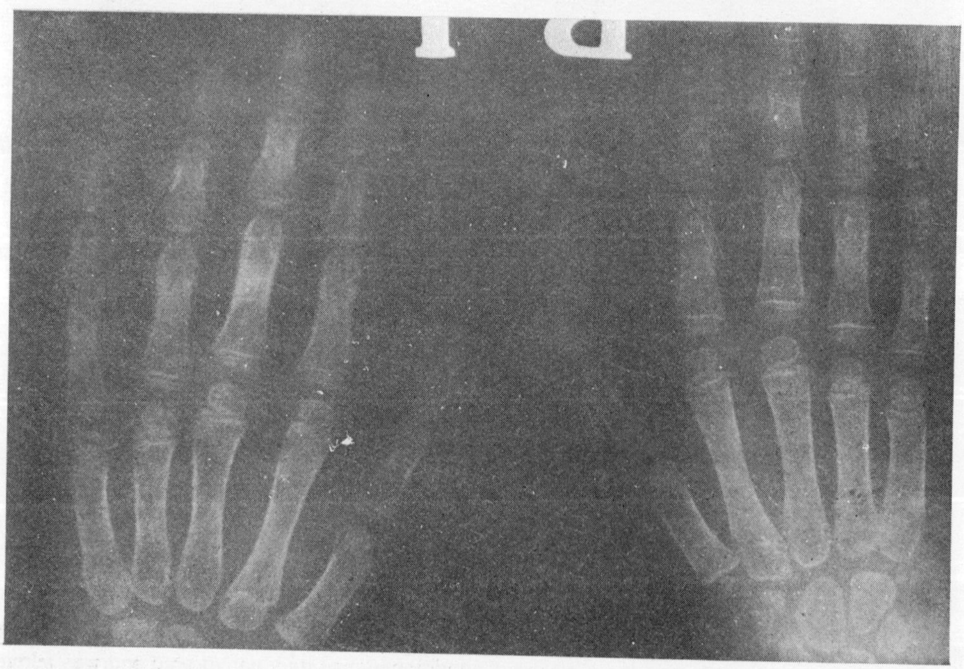

Fig. 10.4. X-ray of both hands showing intramedullary deposits with spotty destruction and cortical thinning.

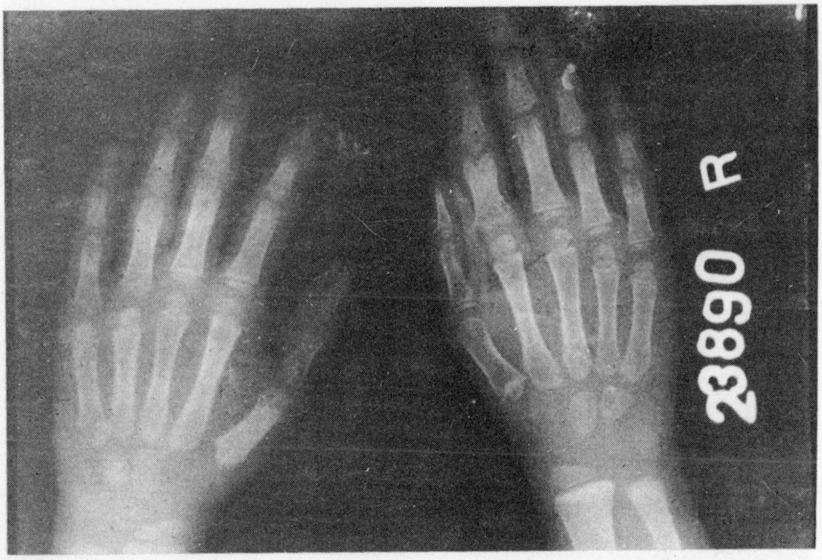

Fig. 10.5. X-ray of both hands showing spotty areas of intramedullary deposits and destruction with subperiosteal new bone formation.

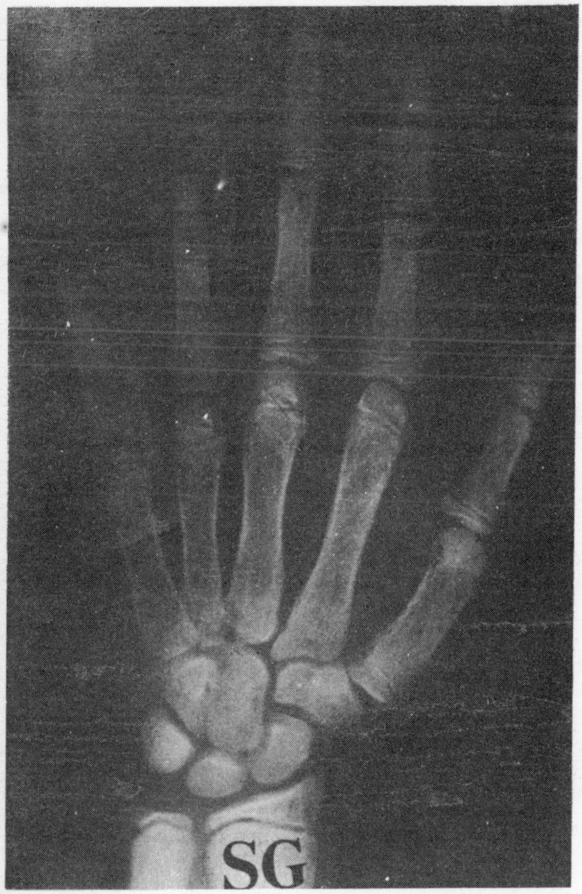

Fig. 10.6. X-ray of the hand showing fine and prominent trabeculations with intramedullary deposits and the moth- eaten appearance.

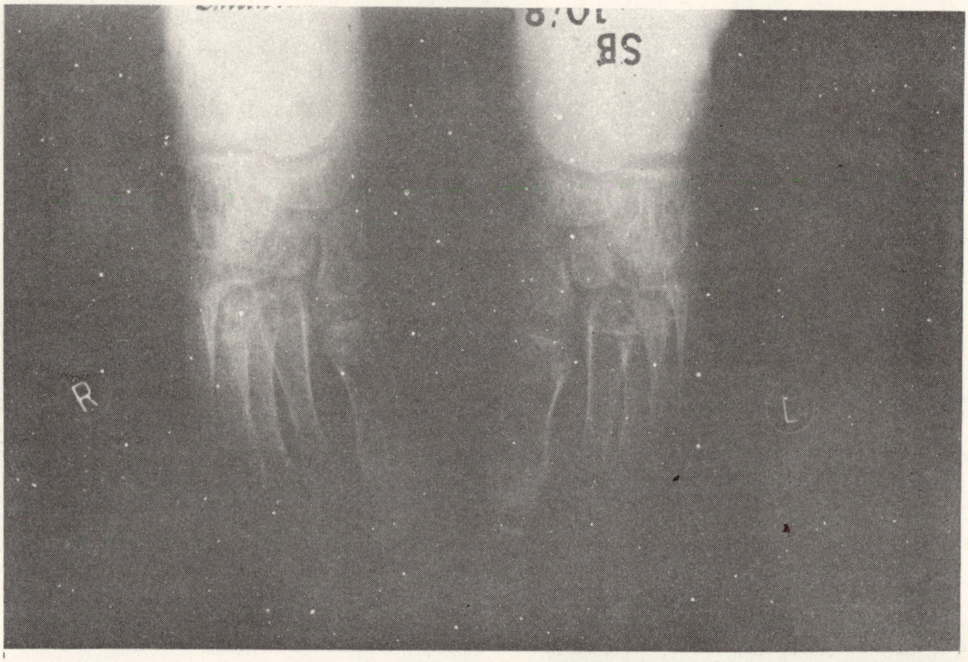

Fig. 10.7. X-ray of both feet in a young boy of 2 years with classical features of hand-foot syndrome showing marked cortical thinning, porosis and prominent trabeculations.

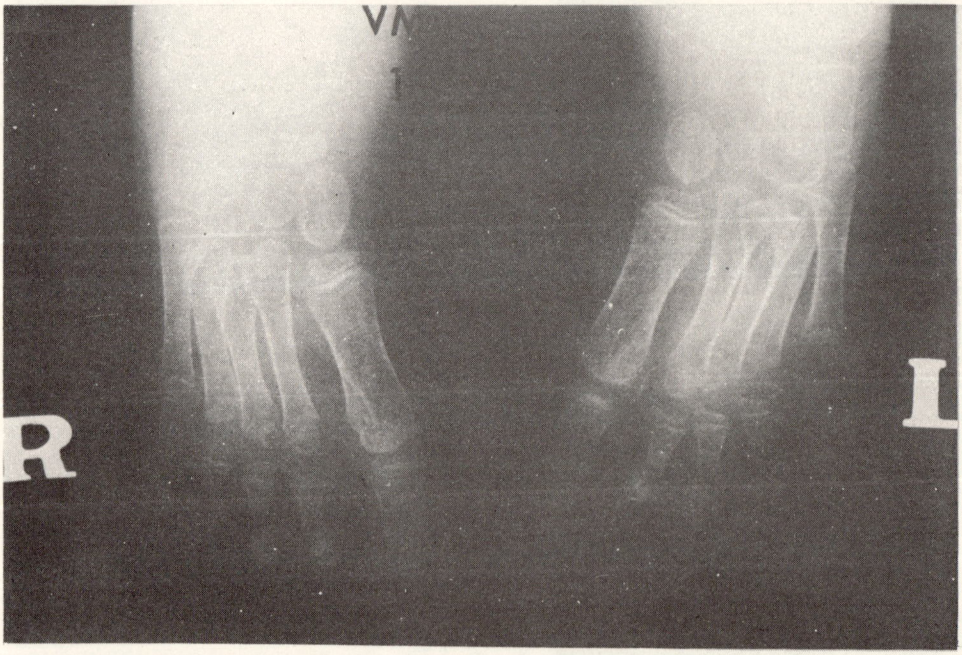

Fig. 10.8. X-ray of both feet in a young child with S-S pattern showing thinning of cortices with areas of intramedullary deposits and spotty destruction.

with Sickle cell disease. Dactylitis occurs most frequently in first four years of life. No instants have been reported in children older than 7 years. The onset is usually acute and is characterised by painful swelling of hand, feet, accompanied by fever, leucocytosis and anaemia. The clinical symptoms in this syndrome are self limiting and spontaneous improvement should be expected without any medical or surgical treatment. The roentgenographic features are usually noted between 7 to 15 days after the onset of clinical symptoms. Initially there is only soft tissue swelling in the affected extremity. X-ray pictures seem to follow two distinct patterns, the earliest change is appearance of subperiosteal new bone in one or more metacarpals or phalanges. This results in the rectangular outline of the involved bone (Fig.10.3). The second change is cortical thinning and irregular intra-medullary density in the involved bone. The radiological changes are completely reversible within 6-20 weeks.

The exact pathological process responsible for this acute syndrome remains somewhat unclear. Cockshott 1958, Diggs 1965, supported the theory of sickle cell thrombosis from abnormal RBCs with subsequent obstruction of flow and hypoxia resulting in cell death in the metaphyseal area of involved bone, whereas Ivy & Howard, 1953, thought that irregular densities within the medullary area of bone is best explained by marrow hyperplasia.

CLINICAL FEATURES

All the patients were admitted in crisis and it was the first manifestation of the disease in 14 cases (Babhulkar et al. 1995). The presentation was of acute onset with symmetrical swelling of hand and feet. Fever of varying degrees was a constant feature. The children were debilitated , with poor general condition and at times dehydrated. The disease took an average of 21 days to resolve. Hand-Foot Syndrome was seen in 46 patients (0.62%) in the study of 7380 cases of Sickle cell haemoglobinopathy. The maximum number of patients (29) were 2-3 years of age. All patients were below 5 years of age. There were 27 males and 19 females. Haemoglobin electrophoresis was ''SS'' in 12 patients, ''As'' in 24 and ''ASF'' in 10 children.

RADIOLOGY

The radiological changes are characteristic and were seen after an average of 10 days of onset of symptoms. After the onset of swelling, the earliest change is the appearance of subperiosteal new bone formation in one or multiple bones of hand or feet. There is cortical thinning and multiple irregular intramedullary deposits, areas of spotty destruction and periosteal new bone formation. Since the lesion usually causes periosteal elevation and new bone formation, radiolucent areas intermingled with areas of increased density it gives a "moth-eaten appearance".

The small bones of hands and feet become rectangular in outline and shape. These changes are seen in association with the classical changes described earlier.

MANAGEMENT

All the patients in this study were treated by conservative means.The drug treatment included analgesics, antibiotics, folic acid, zinc and soda-bicarbonate and supportive treatment with splints. Patients required correction of fluid imbalance and on rare occasions blood transfusions.

DISCUSSION

Danford and associates in 1941 reported the first case of dactylitis in a child of Sickle cell anaemia. Tori (1954) reported destruction and periosteal reaction in metacarpals of both hands in a patient of Sickle cell anaemia. Smith (1960) used the term 'Hand-Foot Syndrome' to describe the acute swelling in hands and feet of children with Sickle cell disease.

Watson J et al (1963) reported Hand foot syndrome as a common initial manifestation of Sickle cell disease usually in children. Since the early reports only few studies have appeared in the literature (Macht

& Roman 1948, Ivy & Howard 1953, Rowe & Haggard 1957, Victor & Imperiale 1957, Lambotte 1962, Porter & Thurman 1963, Diggs 1965, Worrall & Butera 1976).

The true incidence of Hand-foot syndrome is not clear. It has been reported to occur in 10-20% of patients of Sickle cell disease with orthopaedic manifestations (Macht & Roman 1948, Porter & Thurman 1963, Worrall & Butera 1976). Most of the patients are below 4 years of age and it has not been reported after the age of 7 years (Watson J. et al 1963).The low incidence in this study may be due to the fact that the patients included were the ones who were treated by the orthopaedician. The age distribution observed is comparable to the studies reported earlier.

The clinical symptoms in this syndrome are self limiting, the duration may vary from several days to a month (Danford et al 1941, Ivy & Howard 1953, Rowe & Haggard 1957, Watson J. et al 1963, Worrall & Butera 1976).

Skeletal changes in Sickle cell haemoglobinopathies occur mainly because of hyperplasia of bone marrow and vascular insufficiency resulting in thrombosis and infarction. Hyperplasia of erythrocytes increases the viscosity of blood leading to stasis and thrombosis in the micro circulation and eventually infarction and secondary infection.

The exact pathological process responsible for Hand-foot syndrome remains unclear. Cockshott (1958) and Diggs (1965) were of the opinion that thrombosis due to Sickle cell disease leads to obstruction of microcirculation and hypoxic cell death in the metaphyseal area of the bone. Ivy & Howard (1953) thought that increased density within the medullary area seen in Sickle cell disease is explained by marrow hyperplasia.

Weinberg and Currarino (1972) reported histopathologic features observed at autopsy of a child with Sickle cell dactylitis. The changes observed included extensive infarction of the marrow, medullary trabeculae and inner layers of the cortical bone. This was associated with circumferential periosteal elevation and subperiosteal new bone formation.

The radiologic changes of this disease are completely reversible and may take between 6 weeks to 8 months (Danford et al 1941, Victor & Imperiale 1957, Cockshott 1958, Moseley 1959, Watson J. 1963). The clinical and radiological features are characteristic but at times may pose a diagnostic problem. Hand-foot syndrome may be the earliest and the only clinical manifestation of Sickle cell haemoglobinopathy. Hand-foot syndrome is self-limiting condition requiring only supportive treatment and preventive therapy to avoid secondary infection.

CONCLUSION

This study highlights the diagnostic clinical and radiological features of Hand-foot syndrome. Hand-foot syndrome is often misdiagnosed. The importance of this condition lies in the fact that it may be the earliest and the only manifestation of Sickle cell disease and may be mistaken for osteomyelitis. It requires only conservative treatment, the changes being completely reversible. Hand-foot syndrome is a benign self limiting condition, usually seen during the period of Sickle cell crisis in young children. It is commonly seen during the attack of Sickle cell crisis in the age group of 2-3 years. It was observed between 1-5 years of age, commonly in males, and is rarely seen after 6 years of age. Radiological picture is very classical showing subperiosteal new bone formation in one or multiple bones of hand or feet with cortical thinning and areas of spotty destruction and periosteal new bone formation.

REFERENCES

1. Babhulkar S.S., Ketan Pande,Sushrut Babhulkar. Hand foot syndrome in Sickle cell haemoglobinopathy JBJS -1995 77B, 310-12 March '95.
2. Cockshott W.P. - Dactylitis and growth disturbances. J. Fac. Radiologists 1958, 9: 211
3. Daland G.A. and Castle W.B.: A simple and rapid method of demonstrating sickling of red blood cells, use of reducing agents. J. Lab. Clin. Med. 1948; 33 : 1082-8

4. Danford L.W., Marr R., Elsey E.C-Sickle cell anaemia with unusual bone changes. American J. Roentgen. 1941, 45 : 223.
5. Diggs L.W., Sickle cell crisis. American J. Clin. Path. 1965, 44:1.
6. Ivy R.E. and Horward F.H. Sickle cell anaemia with unusual bone changes. J. Paediat. 1953, 43:312
7. Lambotte C.: Hand Foot Syndrome in Sickle cell disease. Am. J. Dis. Child. 1962, 104: 200-201
8. Macht S.H.and Roman P.W.:The Radiologic Changes in Sickle cell anaemia. Radiology 1948, 51: 697-707
9. Moseley J.E. : Patterns of Bone Changes in Sickle cell crisis. J. Mt. Sinai Hosp. 1959, 26:424-439
10. Porter F.S. and Thurman W.G.: Studies of Sickle cell disease. Diagnosis in infancy. Am. J. Dis. Child. 1963, 106: 35-42.
11. Rowe C.W. and Haggard M.I. Bone infarcts in Sickle cell anaemia. Radiology 1957, 68 : 661-668
12. Smith W.S. Sickle cell anaemia and Salmonella osteomyelitis. Ohio Med. J. 1960, 49 : 692
13. Tori G. Clinical and Radiological observations on 102 cases of Sickle cell anaemia. Radiol. Clin. 1954, 23:87
14. Victor A.B. and Imperiale L.E. The Pulmonary and small bone changes in infants with Sickle cell anaemia. New York State J. Med. 1957, 57: 1403-1408.
15. Watson J., Burco H., Megas H and Robinson M.- The Hand Foot Syndrome in Sickle cell disease in young children. Paediatrics 1963, 31: 975.
16. Weinberg A.G. Currarino G.: Sickle cell dactilytis. Histopathologic observations. Am. J. of Clincal Pathology 1972, 58 : 518-523
17. Worrall V.T. and Butera V. : Sickle cell dactilytis J. Bone Joint Surg. 1976, 58 A :1161-1163.

11

Vertebral Changes in Sickle Cell Haemoglobinopathy

In this large study of patients of Sickle cell haemoglobinopathy, skeletal changes were seen only in 12.7% cases, much less in comparison with other workers. Less percentage is mainly because of illiteracy and lack of awareness about the condition. However, the main reason was, the cases were detected at the door-steps and in an asymptomatic condition.

Generalised changes like osteoporosis, coarse trabeculations and concave vertebrae dominate the picture. I attribute this, probably to associated nutritional anaemia and multiple deficiencies.

The changes of coarse trabeculation and compression fractures were seen in 48 patients. The fish vertebra deformity was seen in eight patients and kyphoscoliotic deformity in seven children.

In case of vertebral involvement analgesics, rest and spinal support was main treatment given to these patients. High doses of Vit. D, calcium and anabolic hormones were given as symptomatic treatment. Most of the patients required spinal support. In case of T.B. spine - Anti-tubercular drugs were given and regular treatment of Pott's spine was carried out.

Vertebral changes are infrequently seen in this disorder. Minor variations in normal anatomical structures are not uncommon, such lesions are usually caused by compression of weakened bone which has been subjected to the stresses of weight bearing. Under such circumstances the damaged vertebrae as viewed on X-ray assume one of the three basic shapes—flat, wedge, bi-concave, depending upon the site and force of the impact on these delicate vertebrae.

The vertebral changes were divided in two groups :

A. Generalised vertebral changes

B. Osteonecrosis of vertebral end plates

A. GENERALISED CHANGES IN VERTEBRAE

Following radiological changes were observed in 48 patients of Sickle cell haemoglobinopathy (Fig. 11.1, 11.2) (Table 11.1).

— Increased translucency and coarse trabeculations.

— Flattening of vertebral bodies.

— Increase in width in relation to height.

— "Fish vertebra deformity".

— Kypho-scoliotic deformity.

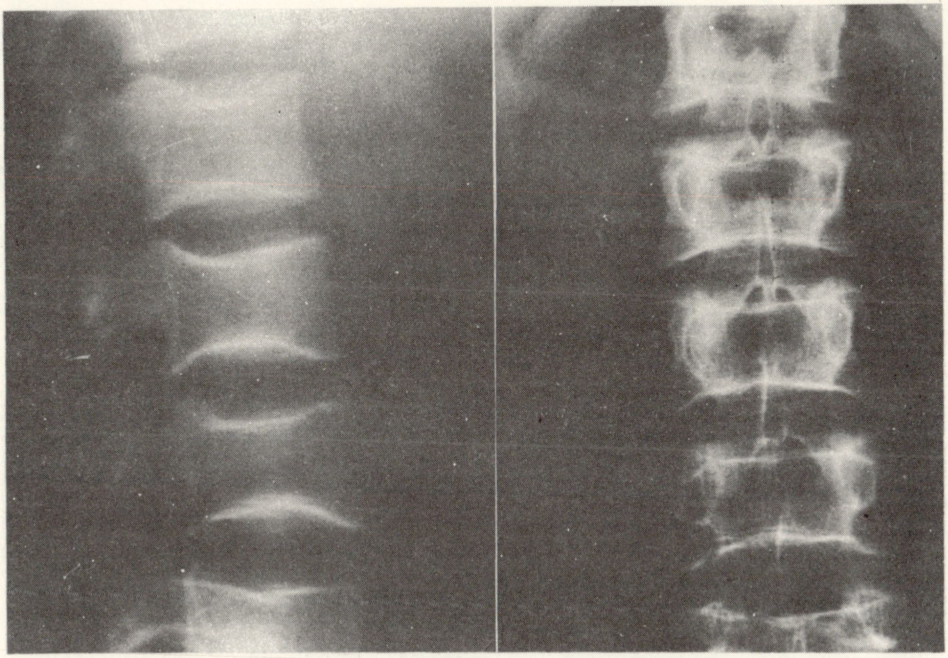

Fig. 11.1

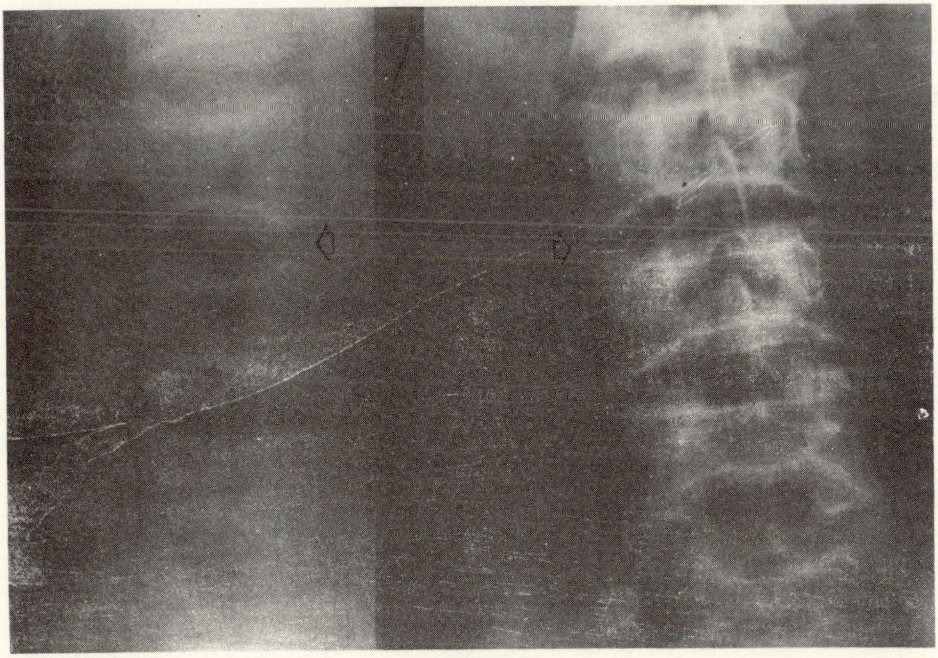

Fig. 11.2

Fig. 11.1 & 11.2. X-ray of lumbar spine. A.P. and lateral view showing osteoporosis with ballooning of disc spaces and changes like cod fish vertebra with deformation of vertebral body.

— Compression fractures.
— Secondary associated T.B. spine.
— Generalised osteoporosis.

Table 11.1. Percentage of radiological changes in spine

Radiological findings	*No. of patients*	*Percentage of involvement*
1. Increases translucency and coarse trabeculation	in all	100%
2. Flattening of vertebral bodies	in all	100%
3. Increase in width in relation to height	14	30.75%
4. "Fish vertebra deformity"	12	23%
5. Kypho-scoliotic deformity	7	15.38%
6. Compression fractures.	16	38.46%
7. Secondary association T.B. spine	12	25%

There was increased translucency, coarse trabeculation and osteoporosis. Spine showed the appearance of biconcave vertebrae (fish mouth appearance) because of porosis where the entire disc surface of vertebral body showed the changes from anterior to posterior corner. The height of vertebrae was reduced and width - height ratio was changed (Fig. 11.2). Rarely there was flattening and compression of vertebral body, at times giving rise to kyphoscoliotic deformity.

There was kyphoscoliotic deformity secondary to multiple compression fractures and osteoporosis. T.B. spine was infrequently seen in association with this disorder. It was observed in twelve patients and on one occasion there was skipped lesion. Probably these patients are very prone to catch the infection & incidence of tuberculosis is very high in these diseased patients (Figs. 11.11, 15.7-15.10).

B. OSTEONECROSIS OF VERTEBRAL END PLATES

Osteonecrosis of vertebral end plates is a rare presentation following vaso-occlusive phenomenon seen in patients of Sickle cell haemoglobinopathy. Thirty six such cases were studied in a duration of 25 years. A stagewise radiological interpretation is assessed and evaluated in detail. Hypothesis for the etiopathology of this peculiar pathognomonic feature following vascular insult and ischaemia in patients of Sickle cell haemoglobinopathy is explained.

SYMPTOMATOLOGY

Amongst these, 36 patients had changes of osteonecrosis of vertebral end plates. These changes of osteonecrosis were frequently seen in Sickle cell disease patients (SS). In addition to these 36 patients other vertebral changes were seen in 48 more patients which included increased translucency, coarse trabeculation, flattening of vertebral bodies, biconcave vertebrae (fish vertebrae), kyphoscoliotic deformity and compression fractures.

In this study the youngest patient was 12 years and 32 years was the oldest with equal incidence in both the sexes.

CLINICAL FEATURES

Usually patient reports for backache and deformity of spine. The onset of pain might be sudden without any relation to any stress, weight lifting or trauma. At times the clinical changes are detected during regular periodical check up in sickle cell centre. The changes of osteonecrosis were frequently observed in adolescents and young adults, in group of Sickle cell disease (SS) patients and are infrequently seen in

Sickle cell trait (AS) patients. The epiphyseal vertebral end plate changes were not noticed in any children and were not seen in patients less than 12 years of age.

All patients were investigated by sickling test (Daland & Castle 1948) and haemoglobin electrophoresis in addition to routine blood investigations. Out of 36 patients of osteonecrosis of vertebral end plates SS pattern on electrophoresis was found in 28 patients and AS pattern in 8 patients (Sickle cell disease formed the major group i.e., 80%).

RADIOGRAPHIC FEATURES

In all these 36 patients radiographic changes were peculiar and identical. The changes were frequently noticed in thoracic and lumbar region especially in the adjoining disc surface of vertebral body. Normal rectangular shape of the vertebrae was changed and peculiar shape of vertebral body was noticed (Fig. 11.3). The changes were very obvious in the centre of vertebral end plates close to intervertebral disc spaces. The changes were mirror image changes on the disc surface of vertebral body changing the vertebral configuration which showed central depression with an abrupt transition to the more normal shape of vertebral body in the periphery (Figs. 11.4 and 11.5). There was no collapse of the vertebral body but simply a failure of growth in the central portion of growth plate. The probable sequence of changes is bone infarct in the centre of metaphyseal region of vertebral body which becomes sclerosed and fragmented (Figs. 11.6-11.9). Subsequently there is growth arrest and localised central collapse of vertebral end plate giving rise to "step off" deformity. There was reactive sclerosis parallel to the end plates in some vertebral bodies as a straight zone of condensation 1-2 mm below the vertebral end plate in the centre of involved centrum (Fig. 11.9). This zone of condensation resembles short growth arrest line observed commonly in distal femur. This zone of condensation of the vertebral end plates causes squaring of vertebral body and at times gives the appearance of "Bone within bone" (Fig. 11.10). This central cup depression called as "step off'' or H vertebrae, might look like dome, might be asymmetrically irregular or flattened at the top giving the profile of truncated triangle. These changes are different from fish mouth vertebrae in which smooth biconcave depression of end plates extends from corner to corner of vertebral body usually secondary to osteoporosis. Associated tuberculous infection is infrequently seen. There is typical destruction of adjoining disc surfaces of vertebral body with loss of intervertebral space giving typical appearance of Pott's spine (Fig. 11.11).

ETIOPATHOLOGY OF OSTEONECROSIS

Though these changes were attributed as ischaemic changes secondary to vaso-occlusion following increased viscosity, thrombosis and infarction but it could also be because of vascular compression from overactive marrow (hyperplasia). Nowhere in literature these vertebral changes were labelled as changes of osteonecrosis in patients of Sickle cell haemoglobinopathy.

As per observation of these patients, it is felt that these are classical changes of osteonecrosis of vertebral end plates akin to the changes seen in long bones and osteonecrosis of femoral head and humeral head (Fig. 11.12). The major portion of the blood supply of vertebral body to the extent of 75% which is mainly involving the central core comes from the nutrient vessels which is a branch from ventral tributary of spinal branch, which itself is a dorsal branch of a segmental artery. Rest of the 25% of blood supply belonging to the peripheral zone comes from periosteal vessels which are the branches from segmental artery and are small and multiple (Hollinshead et al 1985). The ischaemia is produced because of vaso occlusion of major nutrient artery of vertebral body which affects the central part of growth plate of vertebra since periphery continues to grow at normal rate because of supplementary periosteal blood supply (Fig. 11.13). In Sickle cell disease blood containing long, multipointed, curved and rigid sickled cells are more viscid and flow less readily through terminal vessels. Utilisation of oxygen by living blood cells and by endothelial tissue cells favors an exaggeration of sickling which increases viscosity and sludging of RBCs.

Chronic stasis of blood in capillaries and defective oxygenation leads to thrombosis, infarction in various tissues. Sickle cells which are mechanically more fragile are phagocytosed more readily and are subjected to haemolysis in the circulating blood. This ischaemia is produced because of sludging of RBCs and

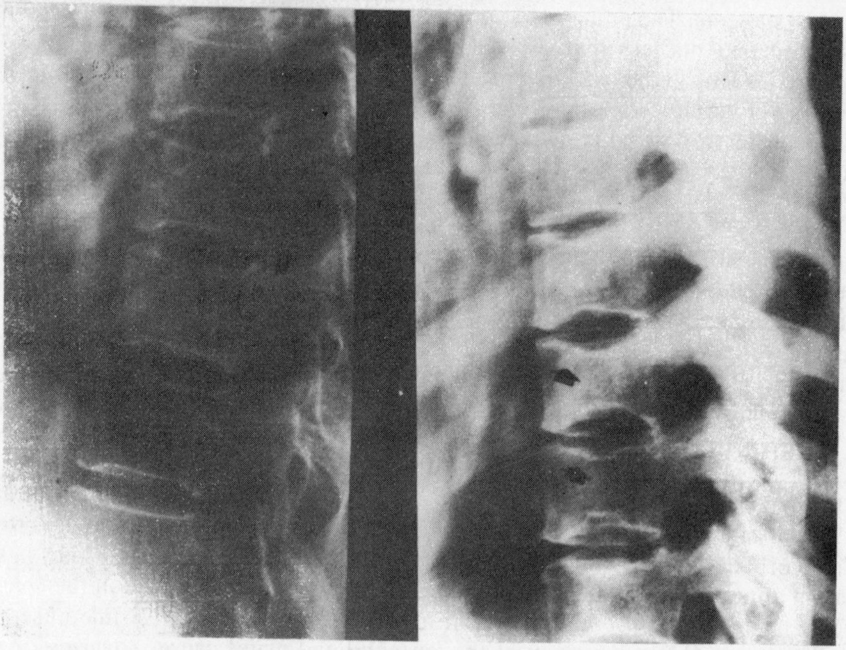

Fig. 11.3. X-ray of thoracic spine showing typical "step off" deformity in the centre of vertebral body with normal appearance at the periphery (Early changes).

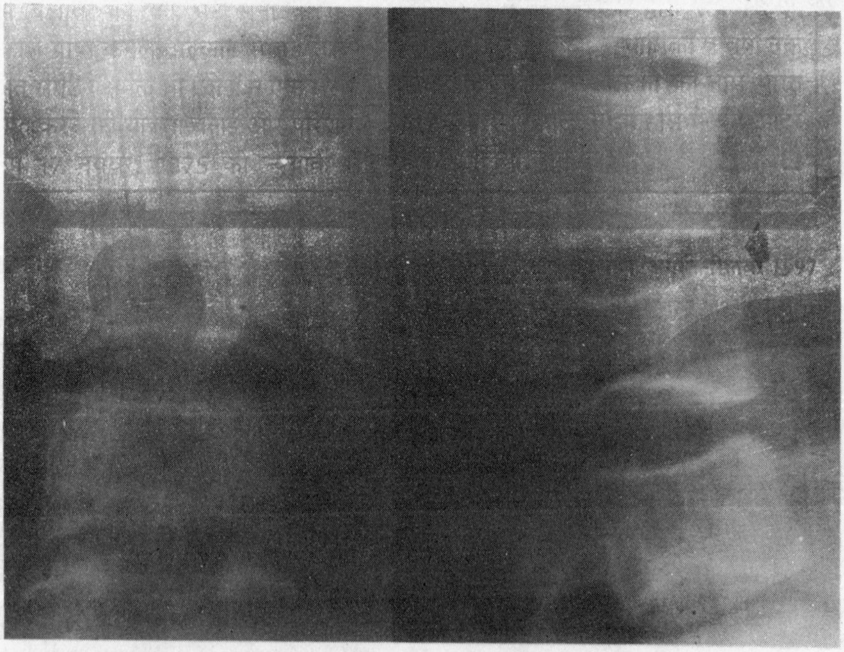

Fig. 11.4. X-ray of another patient showing advanced central cupping (step off deformity) showing mirror image central depression, fragmentation, collapse of vertebral end plates with normal periphery.

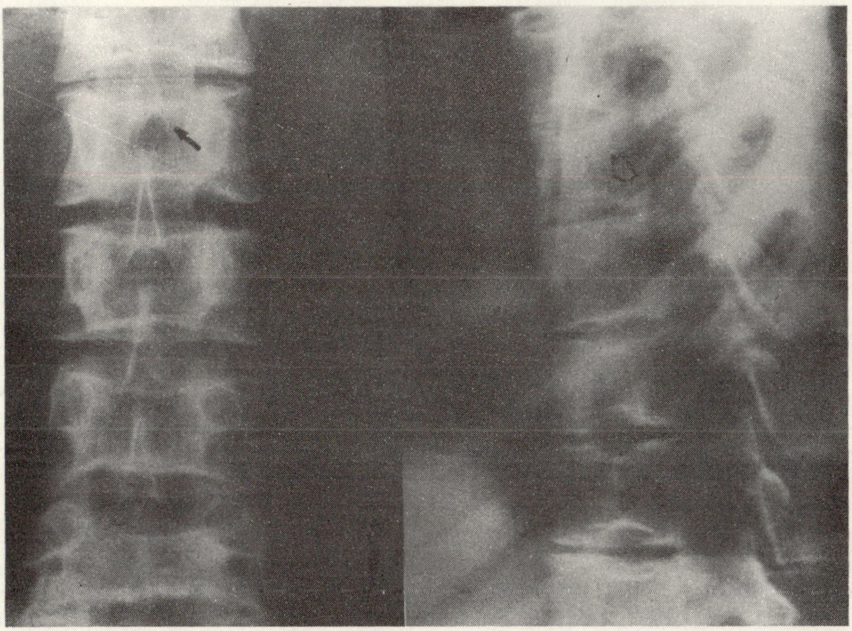

Fig. 11.5. X-ray lumbar spine A.P. & lateral views showing development of step off deformity - Early changes close to the arrow and advanced central cupping in the next disc space.

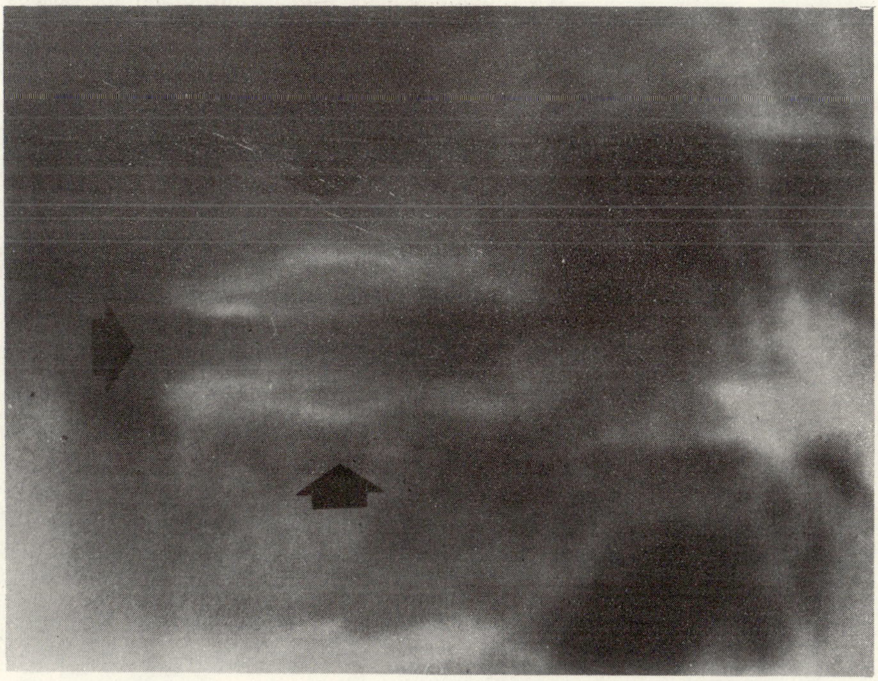

Fig. 11.6. X-ray Lumbar spine lateral view showing infarcts in the centre close to arrow.

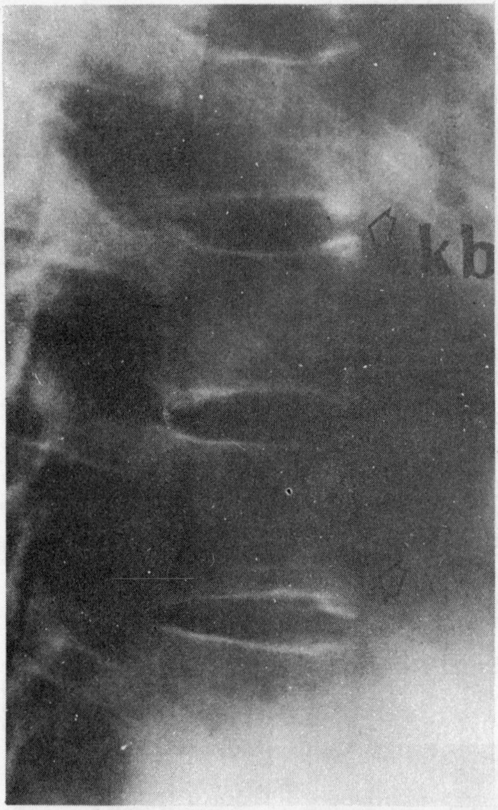

Fig. 11.7. X-ray Thoracic spine lateral view. Lower arrow showing bone infarct in the centre of vertebral end plate with fragmentation and collapse. These are early changes before developing step off deformity.

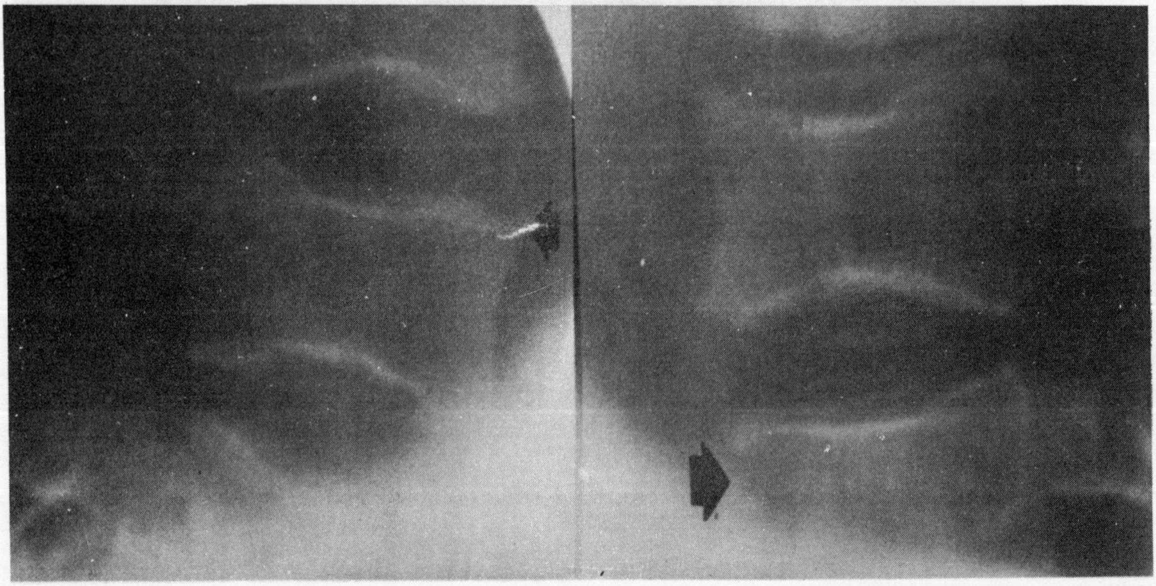

Fig. 11.8. Localised view of intervertebral disc space showing early changes of fragmentation of vertebral end plates.

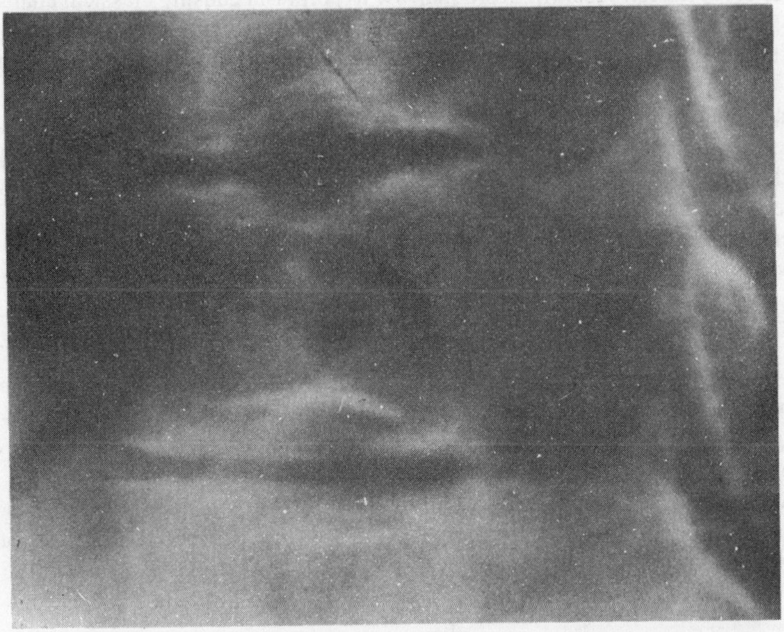

Fig. 11.9. Localised lateral view of spine showing straight zone of condensation 1-2 mm away from the vertebral end plate of involved vertebrae—an early presentation before developing step off deformity.

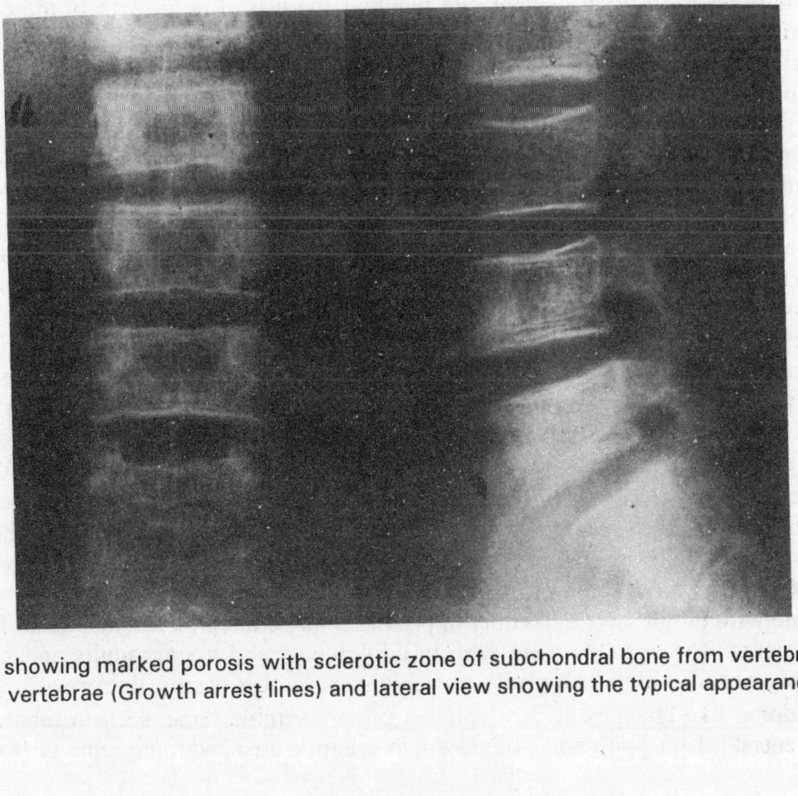

Fig. 11.10. X-ray showing marked porosis with sclerotic zone of subchondral bone from vertebral end plate nicely seen in L4 and L5 vertebrae (Growth arrest lines) and lateral view showing the typical appearance of "Bone within the Bone".

increased vascular compression resulting from marrow hyperplasia causing classical changes of osteonecrosis like in femoral head and humeral head. There might be bone infarct, followed by classical changes of osteonecrosis in the form of spotty irregularities, increased densities, subsequent fragmentation and collapse of end plates (Figs. 11.6-11.10). Since the symptoms are few the fragmentation of vertebral epiphysis is not properly seen as the X-rays are usually done late during the stage of revascularisation and repair process. However in case the patients of Sickle cell disease are followed roentgenographically, proper sequence of radiological changes can be observed and many times at different vertebral levels on the same skiagram (Fig. 11.14). Weight transmission through these vertebral bodies might also play the significant role in flattening the vertebral end plates and in its repair process. Basically all the changes of epiphyseal growth arrest are following ischaemia which resulted in osteonecrosis.

MANAGEMENT

These patients require follow up and general line of treatment for Sickle cell disease. No specific treatment is required for changes of osteonecrosis. Supportive treatment for porosis in the form of vitamin D, calcium, anabolics and in grossly porotic bones with compression spinal support may be necessary. Systemic treatment by soda bicarbonate, zinc, folic acid and correction of fluid imbalance is required.

In the cases where there was associated secondary TB infection, treatment on the lines of Pott's disease—anti-tubercular treatment, rest and spinal support, is necessary. Rarely surgical decompression may be necessary, if there is associated neurodeficit which is not responding to conservative treatment.

DISCUSSION

Reynolds in 1966 hypothesised that essentially stasis and ischaemia retard the growth in central portion of vertebral cartilaginous growth plate in sickle cell disease. The periphery of growth plate with different blood supply continues to grow at normal rate whereas there is slow growth in the centre of vertebral body because of compromised vascular supply to the major nutrient feeding artery of vertebral body. Periphery of vertebral body receives supplementary blood supply from periosteal feeding vessels whereas centre depends on major nutrient artery. In a stage of vaso-occlusion as by sludging in patients of Sickle cell disease peripheral growth continues whereas the centre would have ischaemic retardation of vertebral growth plate. This results into classical step off sign and these central end plate depressions or cupping are due to growth arrest. Reynolds (1973, 1977) compared these cartilaginous growth plate of vertebral body to the epiphyseal plate of long bones which when injured in toto resulted in odd shaped epiphysis and cupped metaphysis with greater growth peripherally. It is clear from these radiological pictures that the changes are result of vascular insult which results in osteonecrosis of vertebral end plates. Though Reynolds (1978) thought this to be ischaemic he never postulated these as changes of osteonecrosis. I feel that changes of osteonecrosis (avascular necrosis) which are commonly seen in femoral head and humeral head are identical to these changes of osteonecrosis of vertebral end plates as observed by me with probably by the same etiopathological process. This step off sign was also observed in Gaucher's disease (Hansen & Gold 1977, Moseley 1974, Schwartz A.M. et al 1979). It was also seen in patients of Thalassemia major and Hereditary spherocytosis (Cassady J.R. et al 1967, Reynolds J. 1977).

In the presentation of step off sign the vascular supply of end plate plays important role since it is simply a failure of growth. The squared appearance of vertebral body is due to straight zone of condensation which resembles short growth arrest lines seen in long bones. This type of epiphyseal growth disturbance was reported by Currarino & Erlandson (1964) in Thalassemia major showing premature closure of portion of epiphyseal plate with progressive deformity in proximal humeral epiphysis and distal femoral epiphysis of adolescent patients. The changes were seen in adolescents and young adults and not in children in our series possibly because blood supply to the epiphysis is best during the growth.

Cupping or dome-like changes in cartilaginous plate resemble those seen in tubular bones of hand which is due to central infarcts with arrest of growth in sclerotic area and more rapid growth in the marginal

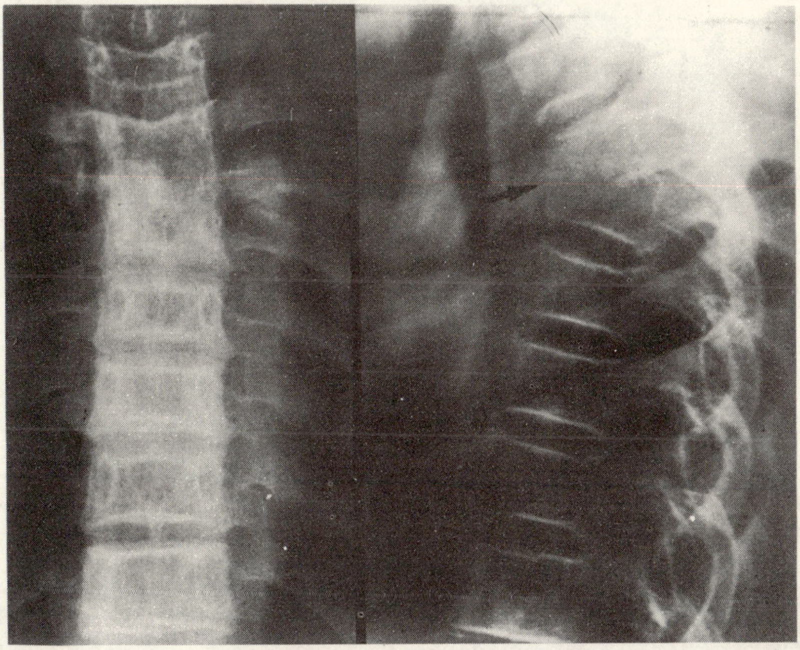

Fig. 11.11. Typical Pott's spine appearance of destruction with loss of disc space in the upper portion with typical changes of step off deformity in the vertebrae.

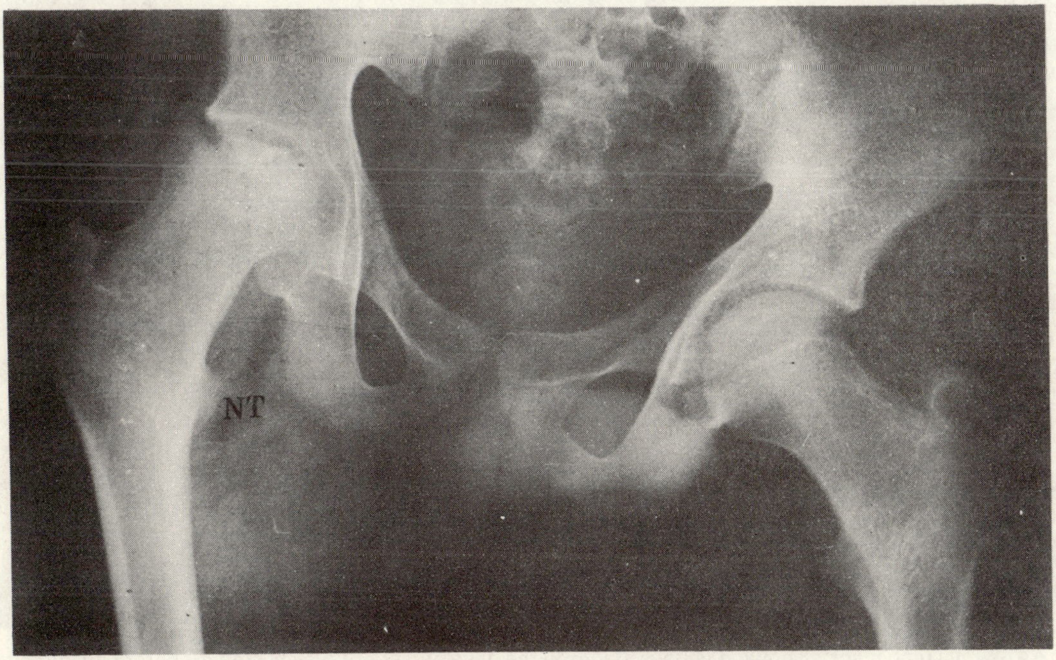

Fig. 11.12. X-ray showing typical changes of osteonecrosis of Femoral head with central collapse.

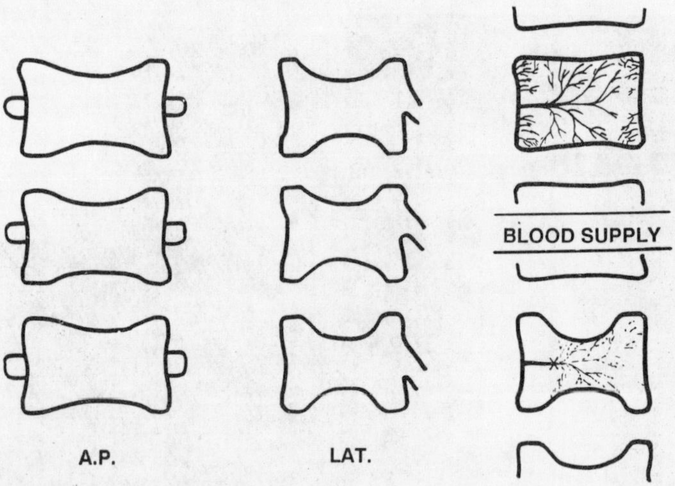

Fig. 11.13. Diagrammatic representation of the hypothesis for step off deformity and diagrammatic picture showing the vascular supply of vertebral body.

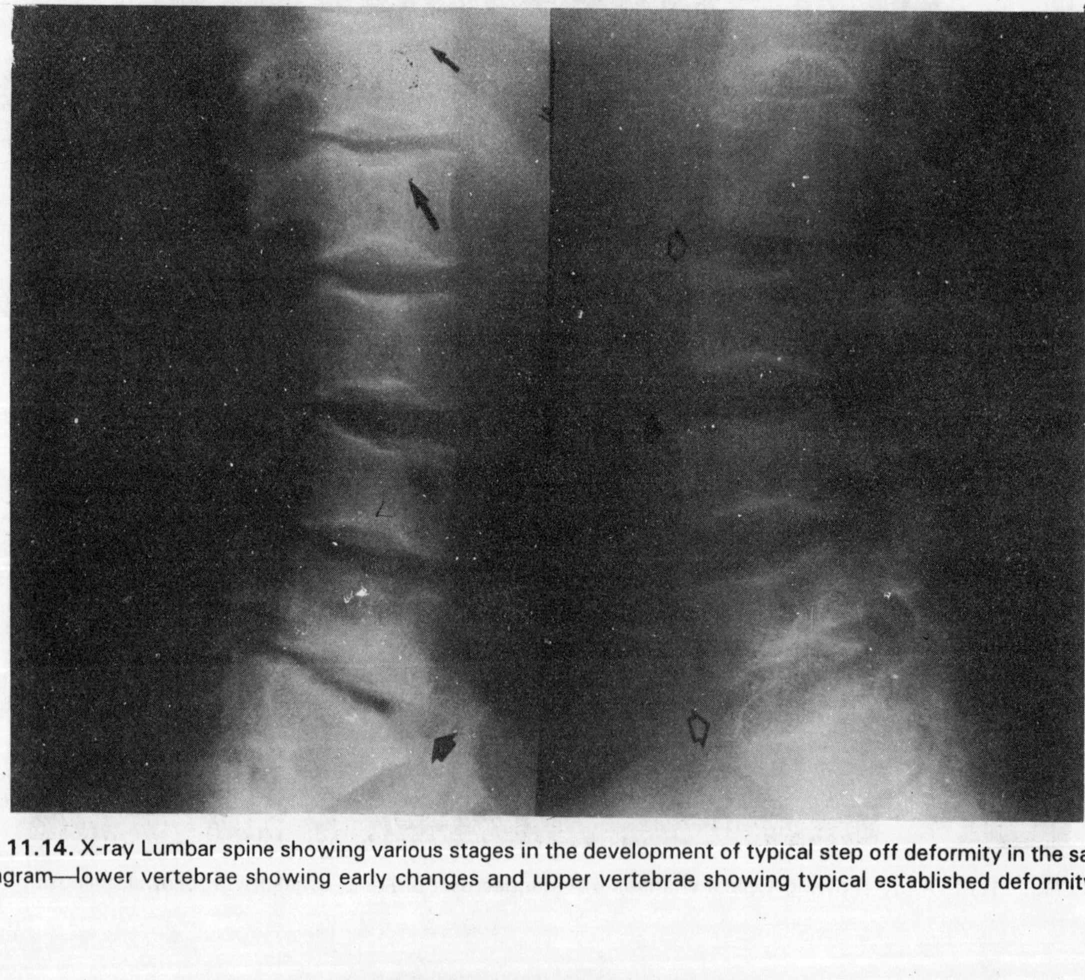

Fig. 11.14. X-ray Lumbar spine showing various stages in the development of typical step off deformity in the same skiagram—lower vertebrae showing early changes and upper vertebrae showing typical established deformity.

bone which has better blood supply (Diggs L.W., 1967). These epiphyseal infarcts give a classical appearance of combination of sclerotic and lucent changes in long bones (Bohrer S.P. 1974), femoral head, humeral head and tubular bones of hand and foot (Babhulkar S.S. et al. 1995).

Etiology of these osteonecrotic changes is ischaemic and the vascular insult in these patients of Sickle cell disease is not clearly understood. Accepted explanation is hypoxia induces sickling which leads to sludging of RBCs and vascular stasis which may cause thrombosis and infarction. Ischaemia partly could be because of hyperplasia of bone marrow causing vascular compression. Bone infarcts by itself have no roentgenographic changes unless the infarct is revascularised. Reossification is accompanied by deposition of new bone on the framework of dead bone. These reossified bones may not be strong and usually collapses and it looses its growth potential.

CONCLUSION

Sickle cell disease being a multi-system genetic hereditary chronic disease, early detection and awareness of its sequelae is necessary. Vertebral changes though not frequent can be easily diagnosed especially osteonecrosis by its classical radiological appearance.

The hypothesis of osteonecrosis of vertebral end plate is put forward according to the anatomical arrangement of vertebrae and etiopathology of Sickle cell disease based on the study of patients of vertebral changes in Sickle cell haemoglobinopathy. This probably explains the appearance of typical radiological changes observed at our centre.

Patients require protection and supportive treatment. Basic effort and treatment is directed towards avoidance of unphysiological condition and hypoxia, so that patients do not go into crisis and thus hyperplasia of marrow is minimal and its ischaemic complications like osteonecrosis are rare. A genetic and marriage counselling alone would help in dilution of the disease.

REFERENCES

1. Babhulkar S. S., Pande K.C., Babhulkar S. : Hand foot syndrome in Sickle cell haemoglobinopathy JBJS (Br.) 1995, 77B : 310-12.
2. Bohrer S.P. : Growth disturbances of the distal femur following Sickle cell bone infarcts and/or osteomyelitis. Clinical radiology 1974, 25 : 221-35.
3. Cassady J.R., Berdon W.E., Baker D.H. : The "typical" spine changes in Sickle cell anemia in a patient with thalassemia major (Cooley's anemia) Radiology 1967, 89 : 1065-8.
4. Currarino & Erlandson. Premature fusion of epiphysis in Cooley's anemia Radiology 1964, 83 : 655-64.
5. Diggs L.W. : Bone and joint lesions in Sickle cell disease Clin Orth 1967, 119-43.
6. Daland & Castle W.B.: A simple and rapid method for demonstrating sickling of red blood cells : the use of reducing agents. J Lab. Clin. 1948, 33: 1082-8.
7. Hansen G.C., Gold R.H. : Central depression of multiple vertebral endplates : A pathognomonic sign of Sickle hemoglobinopathy in Gaucher's disease. AJR 1977, 129 : 343-4.
8. Hollinshead W.H., Rosse Cornelius. Textbook of Anatomy, 4th Edition. Harper & Row Publishers Inc., Philadelphia, 1985, 298-9.
9. Moseley JE : Skeletal changes in the anemias, Semin Roentgenol 1974, 9 : 169-84.
10. Reynolds J : A re-evaluation of the "fish vertebra" sign in Sickle cell hemoglobinopathy. AJR 1966, 97 : 693-707.
11. Reynolds J, Pritchard JA, Ludders D, Mason RA : Roentgenographic and clinical appraisal of Sickle cell beta-thalassemia disease. AJR 1973, 118 : 378-400.
12. Reynolds J : Radiologic manifestations of sickle cell haemoglobinopathy, JAMA 1977, 238 : 247-50.
13. Reynolds J, Jack A.P, Darrell Ludders, Ruble A. M. : Roentgenographic and clinical appraisal of sickle cell beta-thalassemia disease. Radiology, 1978, 118 : 378-97.
14. Schwartz Alan M., Marc J, Homer and Roy G.K., McCauley : "Step-off" vertebral body : Gaucher's disease versus Sickle cell haemoglobinopathy. AJR 1979, 132 : 81-85.

12

Growth Disturbances in Sickle Cell Haemoglobinopathy

Growth disturbances in Sickle cell haemoglobinopathy are produced due to damage to epiphyseal circulation and infarction in the form of epiphyseal shortening, variety of deformities of epiphysis & metaphysis. At times growth disturbance may be secondary to Sickle cell osteomyelitis damaging the epiphyseal plate. Golding et al (1959), out of a series of 51 cases reported 48 as showing growth disturbances. Middlemiss (1958) also reports such findings as coxa vara and vertebral changes with decrease in stature. Growth disturbance has also been a prominent feature of Cooley's anaemia, as pointed out by Caffey (1967).

Generalised bone growth retardation is seen in Sickle cell disease patients, since average haemoglobin content of blood is 7.5 gm% which affects various growth centres in the body.

Distal femur is the common site to observe for growth disturbances (Stanley Bohrer 1974) as a distinct consequence of acute long bone diaphyseal infarcts. The growth disturbance is seen in epiphysis (triangular, metaphysis cupped) along with growth arrest. This commonly results in coxa vara, vertebral changes with decrease in stature & kyphosis, shortening and delay in epiphyseal closure. Such changes are classically observed as growth disturbances in epiphyseometaphyseal region.

Seventy-six patients who had growth disturbances secondary to Sickle cell haemoglobinopathy were observed followed and treated in this 25 years duration.

MATERIAL AND METHODS

This is the study of 76 patients of growth disturbances in Sickle cell haemoglobinopathy amongst 7380 patients of Sickle cell haemoglobinopathy.

Table 12.1. Age and sex incidence

Age Group	*Sex (years)*	
	Male	*Female*
0-05	05	02
06-10	14	09
11-15	11	07
16-20	17	11
Total	47	29

There were 40 patients with affection of femur and tibia. Genu varum & valgum were the common presentation, as deformity around knee because of affection of growing ends (Figs. 12.1 and 12.2). Flexion angulation deformity of lower end femur and upper end tibia was observed in seven patients (Fig. 12.3). Coxa vara was seen in more than 50% patients with affection of femur. The valgus deformity of ankle was noticed in 4 patients.

Table 12.2. Bone involvement

	Bone Involved	*No of Patients*
1.	Femur	26
2.	Tibia	14
3.	Spine	12
4.	Humerus	06
5.	Radius/Ulna	08
6.	Multiple bone involvement	10
	Total	76

The affection of thoracolumbar spine was seen in 12 patients, with mainly kyphoscoliotic deformity and stunted growth. There was affection of concomitant surfaces of central portion of epiphyseal endplates showing typical step off deformity on X-ray, which was noticed in 36 patients. This step off deformity was noticed only on X-ray, but per se it never caused any kyphoscoliotic deformity clinically.

OBSERVATIONS

The region of knee is the commonest site in the long bones for the development of epiphyseometaphyseal growth disturbances and the metaphyseal channel defects. This is because of the fact that, it is one of the most active regions for enchondral bone growth and is subjected to stresses of weight bearing. The distal femoral growth plate accounts for about 70% of final length of femur.

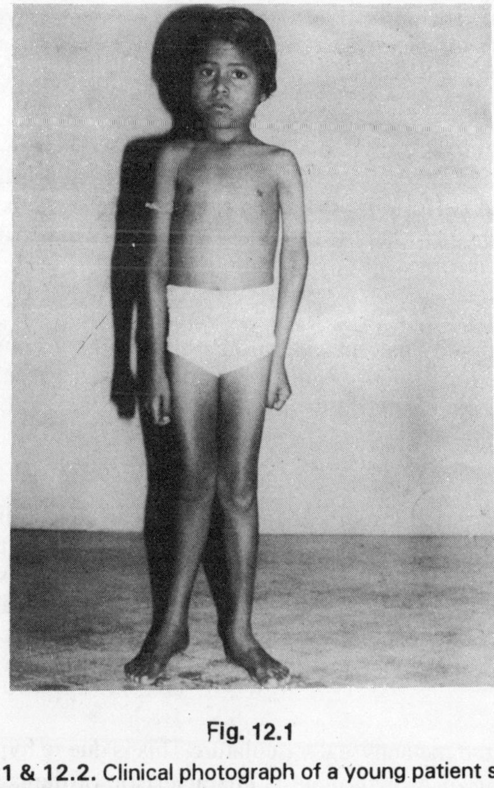

Fig. 12.1

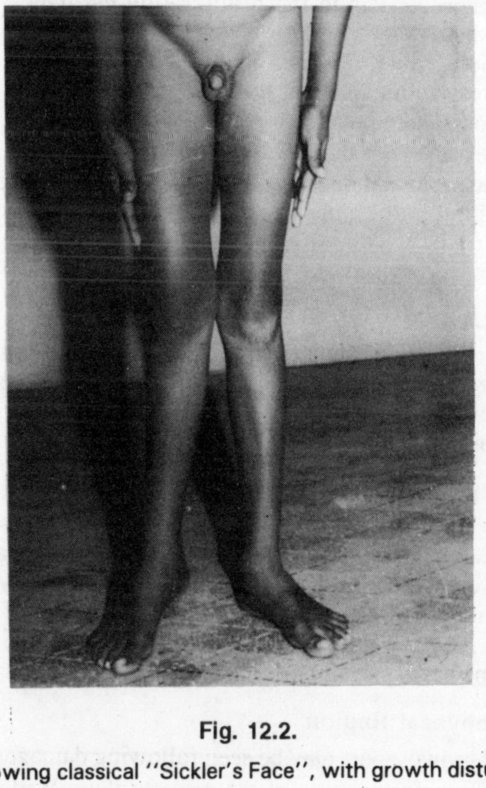

Fig. 12.2.

Fig. 12.1 & 12.2. Clinical photograph of a young patient showing classical ''Sickler's Face'', with growth disturbance showing genu valgum deformity.

The blood supply of the epiphyseal ossification centre of the distal femur is entirely from the medial and lateral genicular branches of the popliteal artery. These medial and lateral genicular arteries feed, on an average, 35 evenly distributed smaller vessels which enter from the sides, and the central intercondylar or the middle genicular arteries which enter between the condyles. These latter vessels may enter the bone through the central fovea between the cruciate ligaments or be evenly distributed and enter through 15 to 20 smaller foramina. In the foetus and the newborn, these vessels nourish the growing epiphysis and communicate across the cartilaginous growth plate with the metaphyseal vessels. Between the ages of one to three years, the developing cartilage becomes an effective barrier to all epiphyseometaphyseal vascular communications.

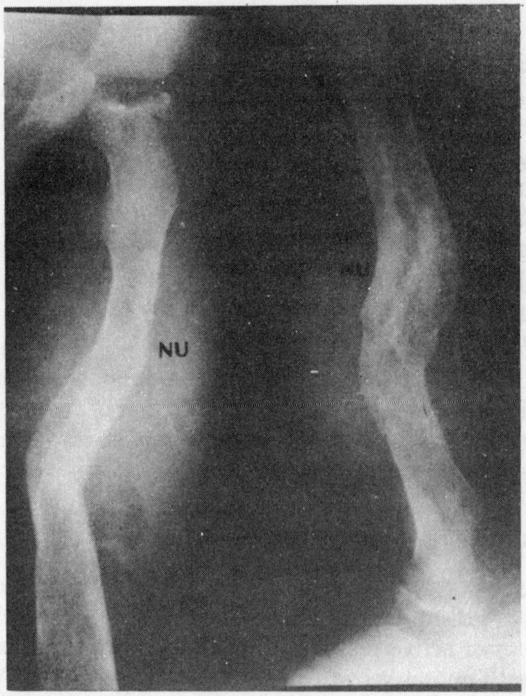

Fig. 12.3. X-ray of a young boy with S-S pattern who had osteonecrosis of left femoral head with osteomyelitis and growth disturbance secondary to epiphyseal arrest, deformity and shortening.

In the cartilaginous growth plate, vessels from epiphyseal side penetrate the bony plate of the epiphyseal ossification centre and terminate at the level of germinating cartilage cells in the growth plate. Nutrition is thus carried distally in the zone of chondrogenesis to the proliferating cartilage cells, the columns and the hypertrophic cells by diffusion, which depends upon the intermittent compressive mechanical forces upon the epiphyseal ossification center.

Vessels from the metaphyseal side of the cartilaginous growth plate support the osteogenesis (matrix calcification, cell degeneration and vascular invasion). The terminal branches of the nutrient artery supply the central portion of this side of the growth plate and perforating metaphyseal periosteal vessels support the periphery. Circumferential arteries of small caliber surround the periphery of the growth cartilage and connect the epiphyseal and metaphyseal circulation during and beyond infancy.

DISCUSSION

The growth disturbances in Sickle cell haemoglobinopathy patients are commonly observed between the age group of 8-10 & 15-16 years. The main reason for growth changes is compromised vascularity to the developing portion of bone and the changes can be easily described according to the various parts of growing bones (Figs. 12.4 and 12.5).

Epiphyseal Region

Severe vascular deprivation produces arrested or decreased growth of the dividing cartilage cells which causes eventual shortening of the bone if vascular supply is not established. There may be ingrowth of new vessels from the metaphyseal side and bony fusion. The periphery suffers the least because of the separate circulation to this region. Hyperaemia of the perichondral ring of vessels may be a factor related to the increase in growth peripherally. Damage to the cartilage cells is irreparable. Apparent regeneration in some cases probably is due to temporary vascular insufficiency rather than complete cartilage cell death.

Metaphyseal Region

Initial growth spurt may be seen following damage to the metaphyseal vasculature.This is due to hyperaemia on the epiphyseal side of the growth plate. Widening of growth plate is characteristic of damage to the

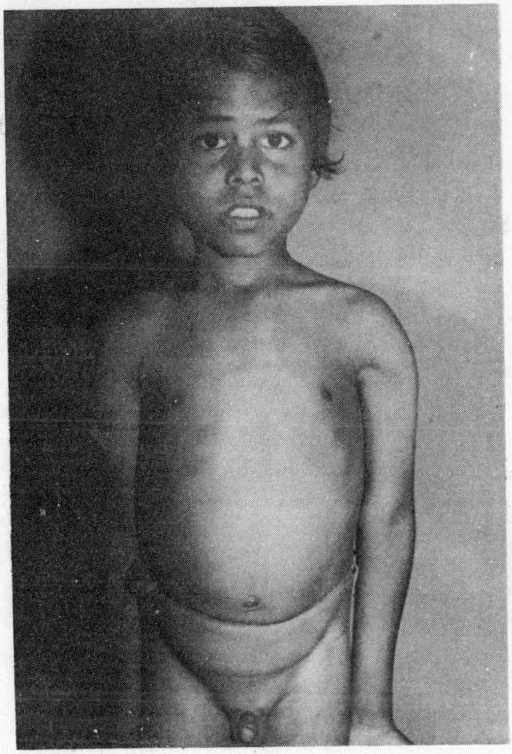

Fig. 12.4. Clinical photograph of (Fig. 12.1) showing deformity of left arm because of epiphyseo-metaphyseal growth arrest of left humerus with deformity.

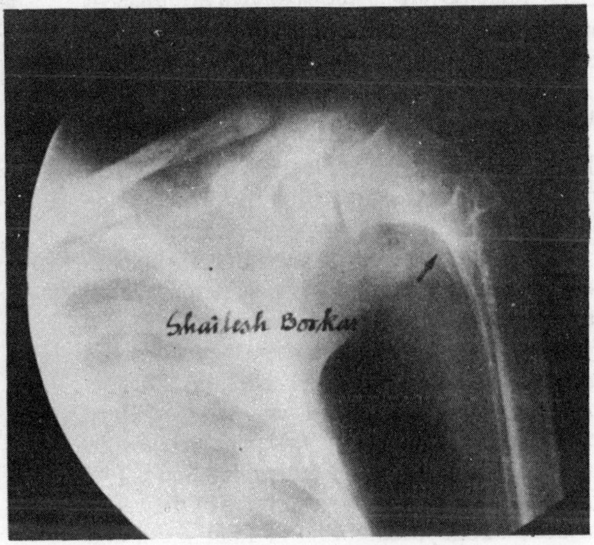

Fig. 12.5. X-ray left shoulder showing bending deformity secondary to epiphyseo-metaphyseal growth irregularity and arrest.

metaphyseal vessels. If metaphyseal circulation is not re-established, vessels from the epiphyseal side extend to the metaphysis and lead to fusion. If the metaphyseal circulation is re-established, rapid calcification occurs, beginning at the periphery. A central uncalcified zone of hypertrophic cells may persist.

Growth disturbance of the epiphyseometaphyseal region

Growth disturbances in this region occur because of infarction of the central portion of cartilaginous growth plate. Osteonecrosis of vertebral end plates lead to deformities in the vertebra like the step off deformity and fish mouth vertebra, radiologically. At times it can lead to clinically overt kyphoscoliotic deformity. The osteonecrosis of femoral head leads to deformities like coxa vara, collapse of the head, subluxation of the hip joint.

Hands and feet are the common sites for epiphyseometaphyseal growth disturbance in Sickle cell haemoglobinopathy patients. Cockshott (1961, 1963) believed that ischaemia on the metaphyseal side of the growth plate was responsible for the development of variety of deformities of the epiphysis, collectively termed as "cone shaped epiphysis". Although epiphysis are most commonly conical in shape (Projected as a triangle on the radiograph), they can assume other shapes such as a cylinder with parallel sides extending into the shaft with a transverse end—"Peg-in-hole" deformity.

The overgrowth deformities of the epiphyseal ossification center are associated with adjacent metaphyseal growth defects such as an inverted "V", a "cup" or a "hole" into which the triangular or elongated epiphysis fits.

Similar cone-shaped epiphysis may be seen around the knee in variety of diseases such as tuberculosis of the hip, polio, vitamin A poisoning, slipped capital femoral epiphysis, osteomyelitis and congenital dislocation of hip etc., where immobilisation with resultant vascular stasis, thrombosis and local oligaemia is the proposed cause. Epiphyseometaphyseal growth disturbances in the knee are relatively rare in patients of Sickle cell disease.

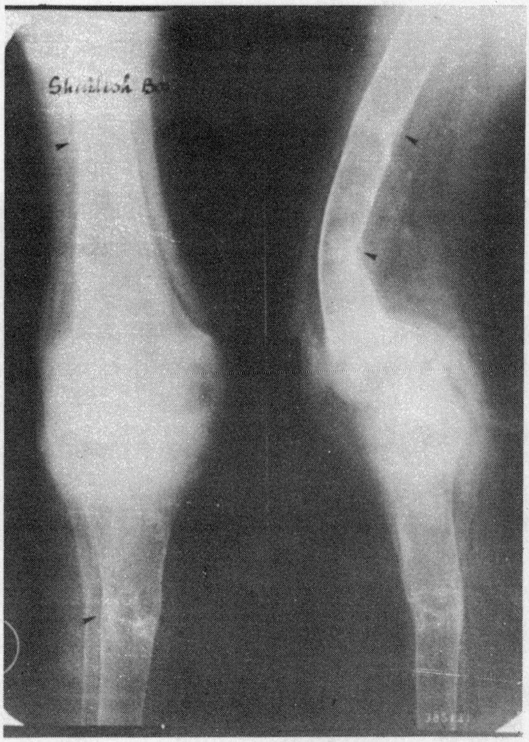

Fig. 12.6. X-ray of lower femur and tibia fibula showing marked porosis, with bending deformity with doubtful subperiosteal fracture and resultant shortening and growth disturbance.

Metaphyseal channel defects

These may present as a variety of elongated radiolucencies extending from the growth plate into the shaft. Some channel defects may simply be the result of architectural alteration of metaphyseal trabecular pattern. This may also develop after sickle cell infarcts or osteomyelitis. Enlow (1963) states that in the area where the metaphysis grades into the diaphysis, cancellous bone is often less widely distracted and the medullary cavity becomes essentially void of *trabeculae*. In *osteoporois*, it is the trabecular bone that is lost first (Nordin 1971) and irrespective of the cause of bone atrophy, resorption of finer mesh and cross bracing trabeculae occurs first than the broader weight bearing trajectory ones.

Many of the fine trabeculae may disappear completely. In the distal femur, longitudinal weight supporting trabeculae become more prominent especially in the metaphyseal region, where the straight cortical margins of the diaphysis begin to flare to meet the broader diameter at the growth plate.

Similarly appearing channel defects in the distal femur may be seen following healed rickets, paraplegia, following steroid therapy etc.

Channel defects may co-exist with epiphyseometaphyseal growth disturbances or occur without them. They are not neccesarily the direct result of ischaemia alone. They are probably the result of combination of factors, metaphyseal central nutrient artery ischaemia, an altered trabecular pattern from the bone atrophy and/or the structural response of the bone to the longitudinal stresses.

CONCLUSIONS

Patients with Sickle cell anaemia classically develop short tubular and long bone diaphyseal infarcts at an early age. The distal metadiaphyseal segment of the femur is the most common site of the localised long bone infarcts. In spite of common occurrence of such infarcts, epiphyseometaphyseal growth disturbances are not common.

Even though 80% of the metaphyseal blood supply comes from the central nutrient artery, experimental occlusion of this artery alone does not produce cortical bone infarction because a very effective collateral circulation develops from the perforating peripheral vessels in older animals. If the nutrient artery is interrupted and the periosteum is stripped from the cortex, cortical infarction will occur but the metaphysis immediately adjacent to the growth plate is spared because of extra rich collateral circulation supplied by the perforating metaphyseal vessels in this region.

These observations account for the relative rarity of epiphyseometaphyseal growth disturbances at the knee following infarcts in Sickle cell anaemia and the fact that when seen, the acute episode occurred at a very early age when the periosteal and the perforating metaphyseal circulations are not well developed.

Osteomyelitis, especially *Staphylococci* and *Salmonella* are common complications of sickle cell bone infarcts. In such cases subperiosteal edema and medullary pus draining subperiosteally may play an important role in stripping the periosteum with its potential collateral circulation and allowing bone infarction to take place by severely compromising the circulation to the metaphyseal side of the growth plate.

Bone infarcts probably predispose patients of Sickle cell anaemia to a variety of epiphyseometaphyseal growth disturbances and metaphyseal channel defects through a variety of mechanisms.

The resorption of the necrotic trabeculae following the revascularisation of the infarcted area, osteoporosis, periods of growth arrest, predisposition to osteomyelitis and altered chondrogenesis and chondrogenesis due to ischaemia are main reasons for growth disturbances.

REFERENCES

1. Bohrer S.P. (1974): Growth disturbances of the distal femur following Sickle cell bone infarcts and/or osteomyelitis. Clin.Radiology 25:221-225.
2. Caffey J. (1967) : Paediatric X-ray diagnosis. 5th edition Year Book Medical Publication, p. 770.
3. Cockshott W.P. (1961) : Haemoglobinopathies. Tropical Radiology Ed.
4. Cockshott W.P.(1963) : Dactylitis and growth disturbances, British Journal of Radiology. 36, 19-26.
5. Golding J.S.R., Maclver J.E., Went L.N. (1959). The Bone changes in Sickle Cell Anaemia and its genetic variants J. Bone Joint Surg. 41-B: 711-718
6. Johnson A., Jackson M.A., Ferguson A.D., Scott R.B. (1966) Studies in Sickle cell anaemia - Pathological aspects of osseous changes. Journal of National Med. Asso. , 58, 4:239-244.
7. Middlemiss J.H. (1958) : Sickle cell anaemia J. Fac. Radiologist 9: 16-24, 1958.
8. Reynolds J. The Roentgenological features of Sickle cell disease and related haemoglobinopathies Springfield, Charles C Thomas, 1965.
9. Nordin B.E.C. (1971): Clinical significance and pathogenesis of osteoporosis. British Med. Journal, 1: 571-576.

13

Sickle Cell Arthropathy (Joint Manifestations in Patients with Sickle Cell Haemoglobinopathy)

Sickle cell arthropathy is an infrequent presentation of Sickle cell haemoglobinopathy resulting from, vascular insufficiency, thrombosis and infarction secondary to sickling phenomenon. A study of 46 such patients among sicklers is presented with changes in various region affecting 67 joints. Recurrent episodes of arthritis and effusion were commonly seen. Soft tissue swelling in the vicinity of involved joint was the commonest radiological feature. Joint fluid aspiration which was routinely done was always non-inflammatory and was supposed to be secondary to vascular occlusion following sickling in the articular end, synovium and periarticular tissue. Synovial biopsy showed focal lining cell proliferation, congestion of vessels and thrombosis with minimal mononuclear cell proliferation. The management of this disorder is simple and requires conservative treatment. Management to prevent Sickle cell crisis is necessary, since joint manifestations are associated with crisis in 60 percent of occasions of Sickle cell arthropathy.

SYMPTOMATOLOGY

All these patients mainly reported for the pain in bones and joints, swelling over the bones and frequent recurrent infections. A few had difficulty in walking and painful limp. Total 46 patients of Sickle cell arthropathy affecting 67 joints were detected and studied with an average follow up of 8 years. There were 27 males and 19 females, ranging from 4 years to 45 years. The following table shows the age and sex distribution of Sickle cell arthropathy in 46 patients.

Table 13.1. Age and sex distribution

Age group	*Males*	*Females*	*Total*
04-10	07	05	12
11-20	11	08	19
21-30	05	03	08
31-40	03	02	05
41-45	01	01	02
Total	27	19	46

Table 13.2. Affection of different joints

Joints involved	*No.*
Knee	21
Hip	09
Elbow	13
Ankle (Foot)	07
Wrist	04
Shoulder	11
Sacroiliac joints	02
Total	67

Most of the patients reported for arthralgia and painful joint effusion resulting into inability to walk. In majority of the patients joint manifestations were accompanied by some symptomatology and clinical evidence of Sickle cell crisis. Many patients gave the history of repeated hospitalisation in the past and recurrent episodes of arthritis and joint effusions. Presentation was commonly seen affecting 1-2 joints in the same patient, usually the larger joints of lower extremity and knee was the commonest joint to be involved. In about 20% of patients (9 patients), multiple joint involvement was seen.

CLINICAL MANIFESTATIONS

Most of the patients reported with history of fever, malaise, cough with expectoration, severe joint and bone pains with either localised or generalised tenderness of 3-10 days history. Range of the movements of the affected joint was restricted and painful. More than 60% patients were admitted into the hospital during the stage of crisis. Most of the patients were admitted with recurrent episodes of arthralgia, joint effusions and arthritis. About 25% of patients reported with acute symptoms of pain, swelling, warmth, tenderness affecting one joint only, with fever. Few patients reported with history of chronic symptoms of larger joint with flexion deformity especially of the knee and the elbow. Effusion of joint and synovial thickening around knee and elbow was frequent presentation in about 20 patients, though commonest presentation of arthropathy consisted of transient non-inflammatory effusion which is often associated with crisis. Commonest joint to be affected was knee followed by elbow (Figs. 13.1-13.4).

Persistent chronic synovitis with deformity and restricted movements of knee, elbow and shoulder was observed in 12 patients. Amongst these 46 patients only 3 patients had hyperuricaemia in whom serum uric acid level ranged from 9 mg% to 11 mg% but had never a presentation like acute gouty arthritis or tophi formation. Rarely the joint swelling was associated with leg ulcerations seen in Sickle cell disease (Fig. 13.5).

Secondary arthritis of hip and shoulder secondary to osteonecrosis of femoral head and humeral head are excluded from this study. (For that matter pain in the hips and shoulder secondary to osteonecrosis are not included). Similarly the patients of hand foot syndrome (Babhulkar et al 1995) seen in 46 patients and associated tuberculous arthritis seen in 24 patients, were also not included.

INVESTIGATIONS

All the patients were subjected to routine blood chemistry which revealed leukocytosis, raised erythrocyte sedimentation rate. Haemoglobin levels found to be below 7-8 gm% and reticulocyte count raised over 8-10%. Sickling test (Daland & Castle 1948) and haemoglobin electrophoresis were done in all the patients. Sickling was always positive and the various electrophoretic patterns observed in these 46 patients with joint arthropathy are as follows :

Table 13.3. Haemoglobin patterns seen on electrophoresis

HB pattern	*No. of patients*
SS	14
AS	20
SF	08
ASF	04

Joint aspiration was always done and sent for microscopic, histopathological examination and culture-sensitivity test. The transudate has been always non-inflammatory. The aspirated fluid was clear and amber

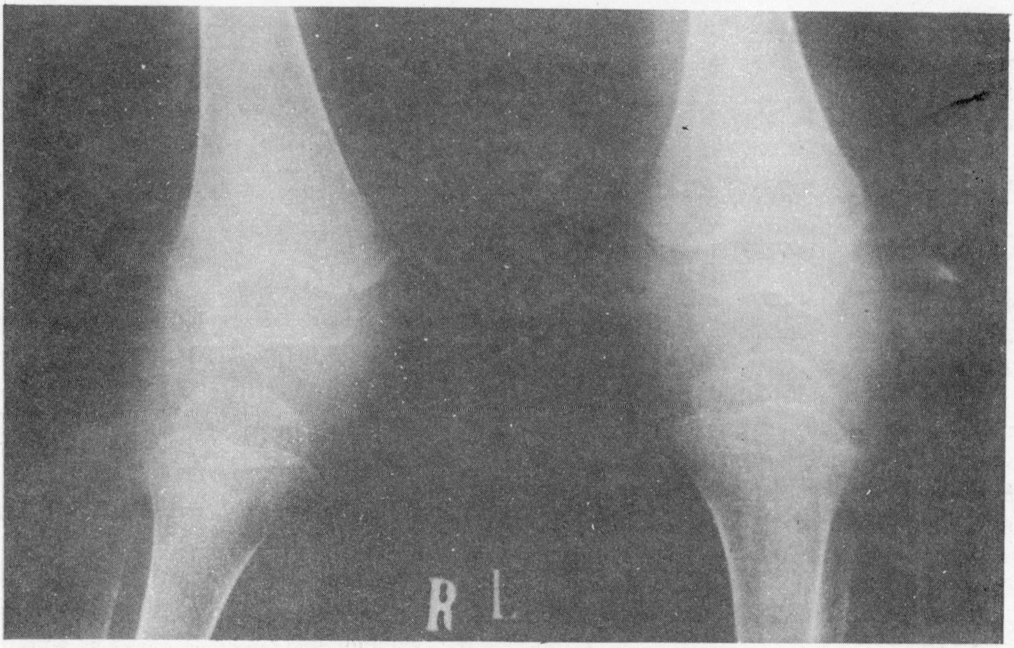

Fig. 13.1

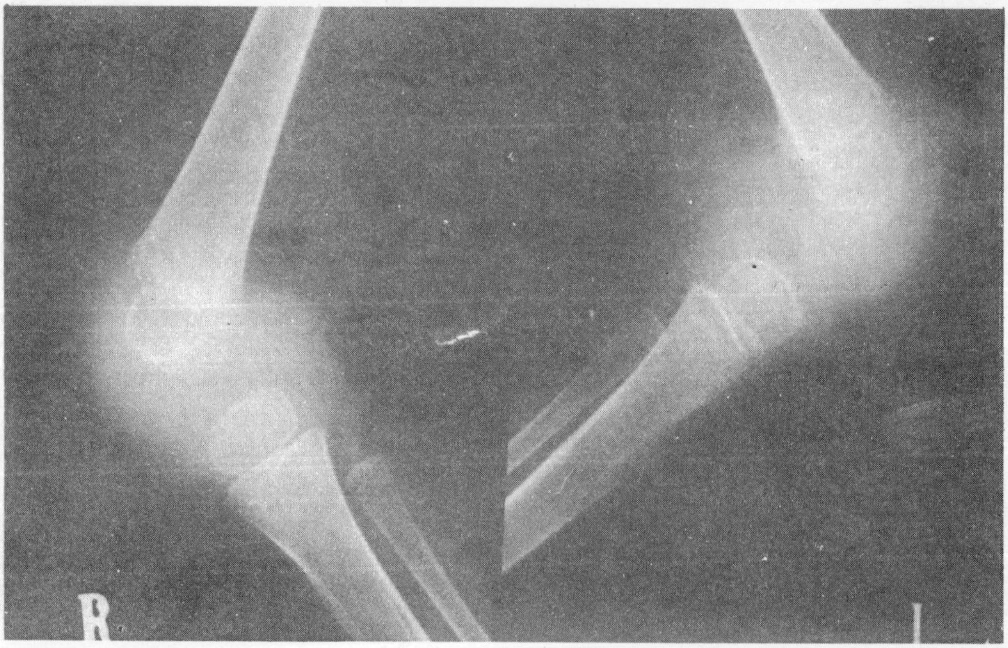

Fig. 13.2.

Fig. 13.1 & 13.2. X-ray of both knees A.P. and the lateral views showing soft tissue swelling. Patient had flexion deformity with bilateral effusion.

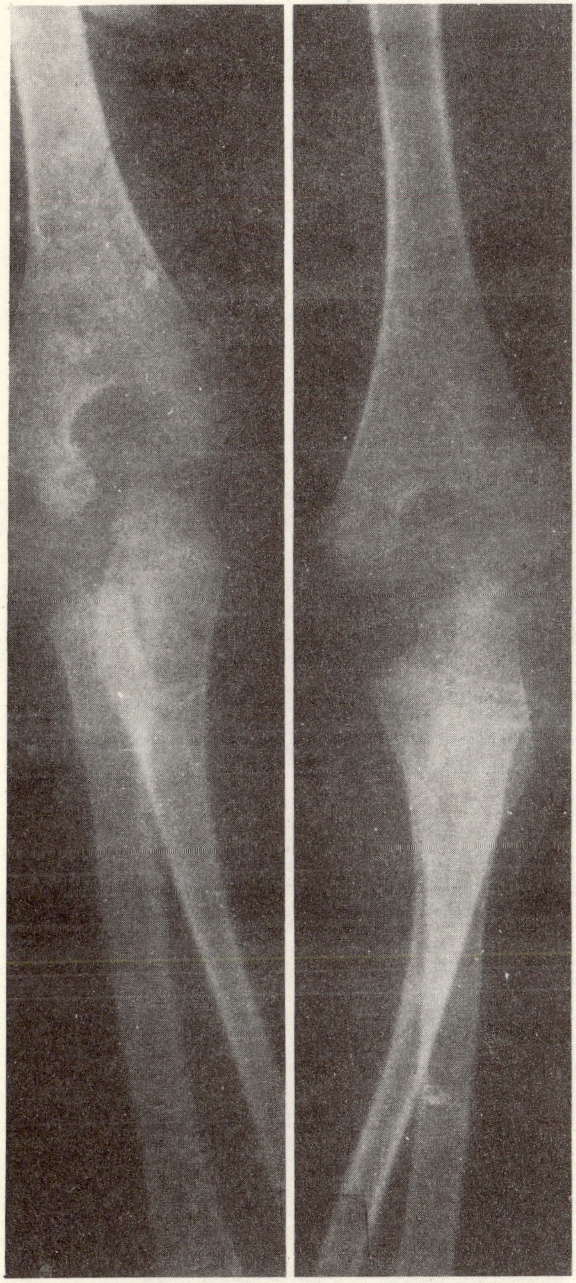

Fig. 13.3

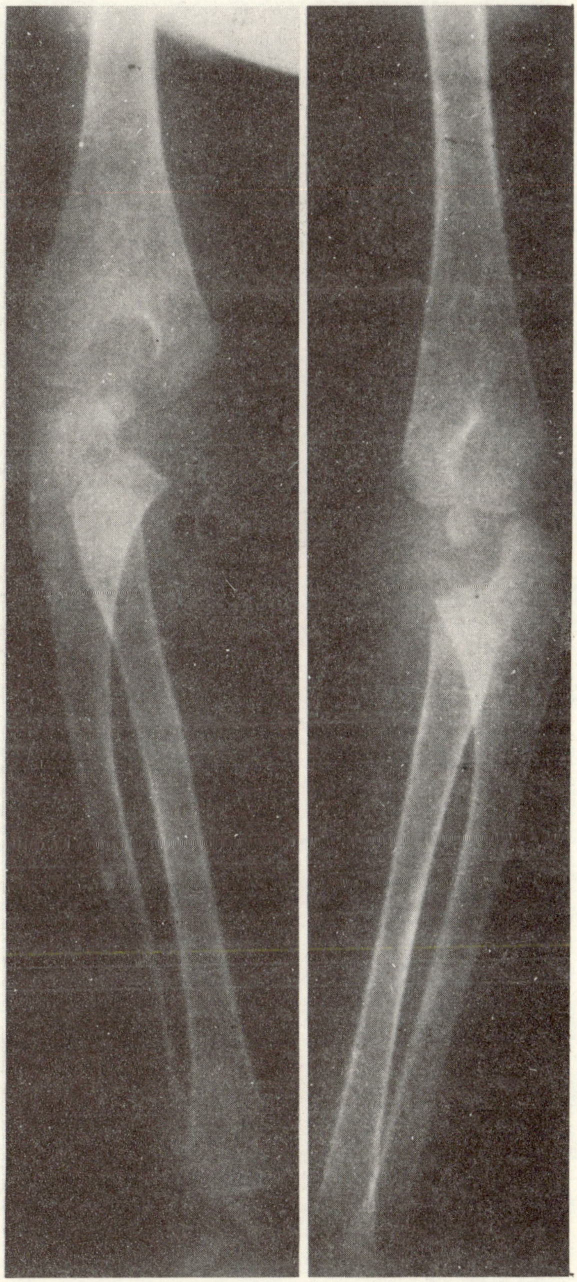

Fig. 13.4

Fig. 13.3 & 13.4. X-ray both elbows A.P. and lateral views showing soft tissue swelling secondary to synovial effusion.

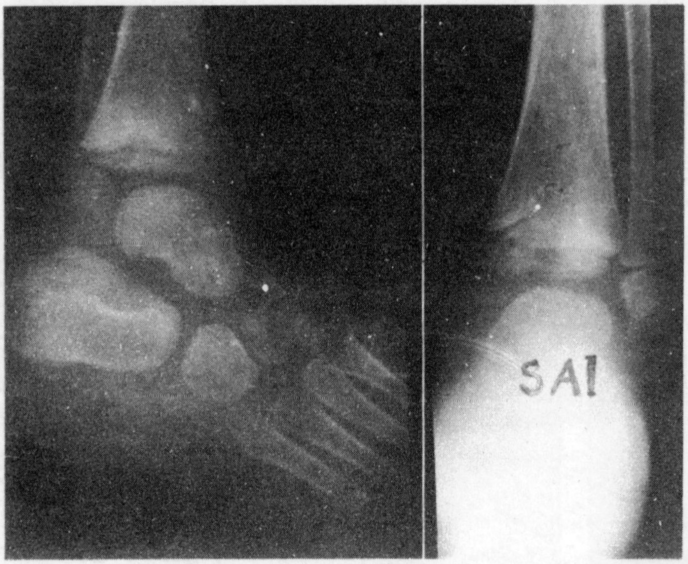

Fig. 13.5. X-ray of the patient of leg ulcerations showing soft tissue swelling with changes of Osteomyelitis in distal Tibia. Clinical photograph of patient shown in Figs. 15.5 and 15.6.

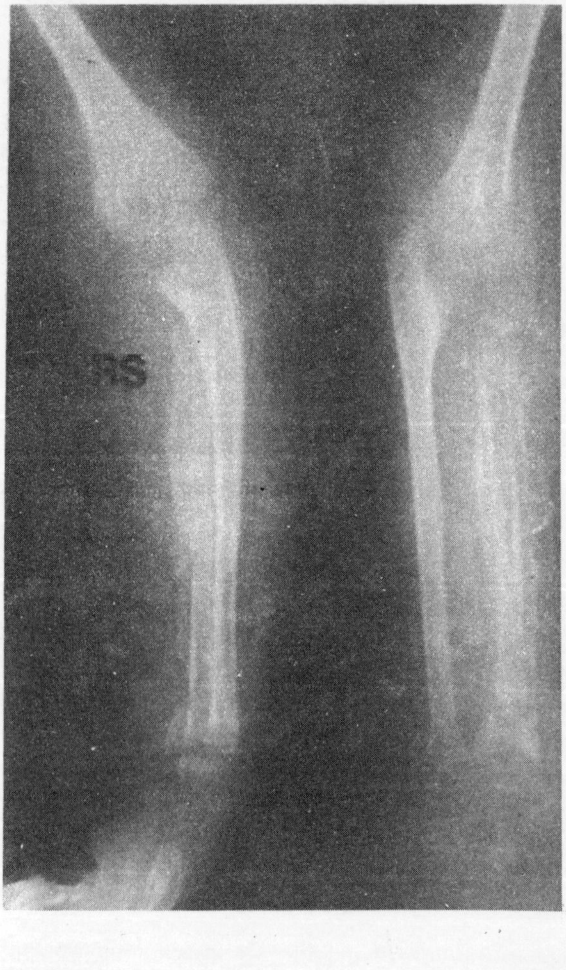

Fig. 13.6. X-ray left forearm with elbow showing changes of septic arthritis secondary to spread of inflammation from osteomyelipis of radius.

or yellow coloured of normal viscosity. In few patients there were plenty of RBC's in aspiration and sickling of erythrocytes was evident in these aspirations. Some of these patients had haemarthrosis, non-inflammatory synovitis and effusion. In all the patients aspirated fluid was sent for culture and sensitivity which never showed growth of any organisms. Synovial biopsy was done on 6 occasions which showed obliteration of small vessels in the synovium with abnormality showing focal lining cell proliferation, minimal mononuclear cell proliferation and congestion of vessels leading to thrombosis.

RADIOLOGY

Soft tissue swelling of the affected joint was a common radiological finding. Bone infarcts were frequently seen in the metaphyseal region. In few patients periosteal reaction was seen adjoining the joint especially in the ends of long bones. Periosteal elevation was commonly seen in the distal femur.

Changes of septic arthritis were observed in one elbow and two knees (Fig. 13.6). This was noticed secondary to osteomyelitis of radius and distal femur causing secondary spread into the joint. Sclerosis with erosion was observed in one sacroiliac joint in a patient without any affection of the lumbosacral spine.

Skeletal changes occur mainly due to severe bone marrow hyperplasia and vascular insufficiency resulting in thrombosis and infarction (Barton C.J. et al 1962, Edward O'Hara A. 1967, Givner L.B. et al 1981, Keeley et al 1982, Koren A. et al 1984).

Vascular insufficiency is triggered off by crowding of sickle cells, anoxia, reflex vasospasm, increased viscosity, capillary stasis and resultant ischaemic necrosis. This results into multiple bone infarcts mainly because of local damage to small vessels producing vascular occlusion. Transudate in the joints is secondary result of occlusive process probably in the articular end, synovium and periarticular tissue.

OBSERVATIONS

Generalised osseous and joint changes take place as microvascular circulation of bones is a favourite site of sickle cell to harbor. Sickle cell arthropathy was observed in 46 patients affecting 67 joints. Onset of arthritis was commonly observed in first and second decade as observed by Crout J.E. et al 1976. In many patients, the joint symptoms were associated with clinical features of Sickle cell crisis (Orozeo Aleala et al 1973, Schumacher et al 1973, Espinoza et al 1974, Hanissan et al 1974). Acute symptoms of pain, swelling, warmth, tenderness along with fever was observed in 12 patients. Knee joint was most commonly involved followed by elbow involvement. Few patients had persistent chronic synovitis and 3 patients had persistent bilateral knee effusion. Synovial aspiration and biopsy was done routinely but the transudate has been always non-inflammatory and in few patients there was haemarthrosis (Schumacher 1973 & 1977, Goldberg M.A.1973, Espinoza et al 1974, Crout J.E 1976). Synovial biopsy showed thrombosis in small obliterated vessels.

Persistent soft tissue periarticular swelling was a common finding though on number of occasions there was periosteal elevation and reaction in the vicinity of involved joint (Fig. 13.7), (Schumacher et al 1973, Espinoza et al 1974). There were bone infarcts at the ends of long bones causing irritation in the vicinity of joint and reactionary sympathetic effusion (Figs. 13.9 and 13.9). The cause of effusion is still not very clear but is supposed to be as a result of vascular occlusion in articular, periarticular and adjacent tissue causing secondary transudation in the joint (Casey et al 1970, Schumacher 1973 & 1977). The transudate has been always noninfective and the crystals were never found in the effusion even in those patients with hyperuricaemia (Aquiline et al 1958, Gold et al 1968, Ball et al 1970, Walker et al 1971, Schumacher et al 1973 and Espinoza et al 1974).

MANAGEMENT

Once the diagnosis of Sickle cell arthropathy was suspected in a patient, it is necessary to confirm the diagnosis by sickling test and pattern of haemoglobin electrophoresis. General treatment of Sickle cell disease to maintain a steady state of haemoglobin and avoidance of factors that are known to precipitate sickling and crisis like hypoxia, hypotension, acidosis, peripheral circulatory stasis, hypothermia, dehydration was instituted. Administration of soda-bi-carb, plenty of fluids, zinc and folic acid is necessary to prevent sickling.

Immobilisation, splintage or traction of the involved joint is necessary. Aspiration of the joint fluid for examination and culture is done routinely. Patient must be observed for development of pyogenic infection since the bony infarcts at times mimic an acute attack of pyogenic arthritis or acute osteomyelitis. It is necessary to exclude acute Gouty attack by estimating serum uric acid. Since the entity closely resembles the septic arthritis, aspiration of joint fluid and confirmation of non infective pathology is absolutely necessary. Repeated bacteriological examination is necessary especially in a patient with persistent synovitis and periosteal reaction in the vicinity of the joint. At times it is necessary to administer antibiotics as a precautionary measure. If the recurrent attacks of joint arthritis and effusion are frequent, use of NSAID's is advisable in addition to the treatment of Sickle cell crisis to keep the symptoms under control. Sometimes synovial biopsy is necessary to confirm the diagnosis or to exclude other forms of chronic synovitis.

DISCUSSION

Bone and joint pains are frequent presentations in Sickle cell haemoglobinopathy. In about 80% of patients symptoms of pain around bone and joints are predominant (Espinoza et al 1974). The incidence of Sickle cell arthropathy was about 10%. Joint manifestation was commonly seen in 1st and 2nd decade. Knee was the most frequently involved joint, followed by elbow. Simultaneous polyarticular involvement was seen in few patients (12% cases). Persistent bilateral knee effusion of chronicity was seen in 3 patients. The effusion was frequently seen in larger joints affecting the knee, elbow and ankle (Figs. 13.2-13.5, and 13.9). Synovial fluid which was routinely examined was non inflammatory and repeated bacteriological examination has been negative (Schumacher et al 1973 & 1977, Espinoza et al 1974). On few occasions synovial fluid showed sickled RBC's. Persistent soft tissue swelling was the most consistent finding on X rays. On many occasions bone infarcts were seen and sometimes periosteal reaction was observed at the ends of long bones in the vicinity of the involved joint. The biopsy showed histopathological abnormality of focal lining cell proliferation, minimal mononuclear cell proliferation, congestion and thrombosis of small blood vessels (Schumacher et al 1973 & 1977, Espinoza et al 1974). Even though the entity at times simulates septic arthritis especially with acute presentation, aspiration of non-infective synovial fluid rules out the diagnosis of septic arthritis. Septic arthritis of two knees and one elbow was observed by us following a spread of infection from osteomyelitis of radius and distal femur (Fig. 13.6). Acute arthritic presentation with hyperuricaemia was observed in this series in 3 patients who were given uricosuric drugs in addition to NSAID's, but urate crystals were not seen in the synovial fluid from these patients.

The commonest presentation was recurrent episodes of joint effusion and chronic synovitis. Joint effusion was frequently associated with other evidence of Sickle cell crisis (Espinoza et al 1974). The effusions are non-inflammatory despite the frequent occurrence of warmth and tenderness accompanied by fever. Bone infarcts in patients of Sickle cell haemoglobinopathy are caused by haemorrhage and local damage to small vessels producing vascular occlusion and secondary transudation in to the joint. Coincidental acute inflammation of the synovial membrane enhances the sickling phenomenon and produces the vascular occlusion secondary to increased viscosity and sludging of blood flow because of sickled erythrocytes. This produces thrombosis and ischaemia in the articular and adjacent tissues with secondary transudation in to the joint (Schumacher 1973 & 1977, Crout J 1976). Onset of inflammatory arthritis may induce sickling in the synovial membrane. An increase in the intra-articular temperature and decrease in the oxygen

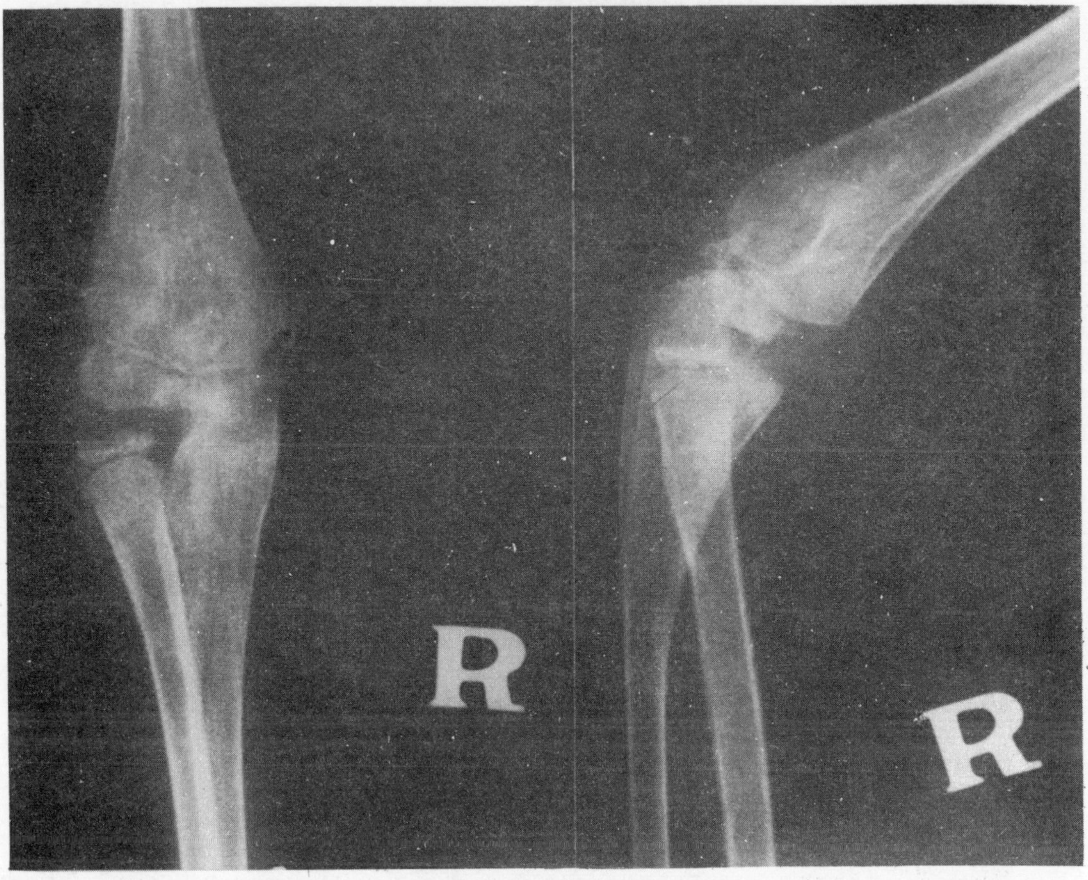

Fig. 13.7. X-ray of right elbow showing soft tissue swelling with periosteal reaction in distal humerus and proximal ulna.

tension is found in the synovial fluid which may enhance sickling phenomenon (Casey et al 1970).

Musculoskeletal pain of Sickle cell haemoglobinopathy has been primarily attributed to ischaemic damage secondary to occlusion of small vessels by sickled erythrocytes (Schumacher 1973, 1977). Chronic synovitis though seen less commonly in these patients of Sickle cell haemoglobinopathy , is associated with synovial thickening and formation of pannus on the articular surface which may lead to cartilage erosion. Sometimes these patients may present with attack of haemarthrosis, may be in several joints and are supposed to be secondary to sickling phenomenon in the synovium resulting in to bleeding disorders (Casey et al 1970).

SUMMARY AND CONCLUSION

Recurrent episodes of joint arthritis and effusion was frequently observed in this study. The joint effusion was commonly seen affecting the larger joints of lower extremities and was commonly observed in the second decade of life. Synovial transudation frequently seen in this disease is supposed to be secondary to the vascular occlusion following sickling phenomenon. These joint manifestations were frequently seen in association with Sickle cell crisis. Joint aspiration was always noninflammatory and synovial biopsy showed small obliterated thrombosed vessels but these were enough to cause effusion was not clear.

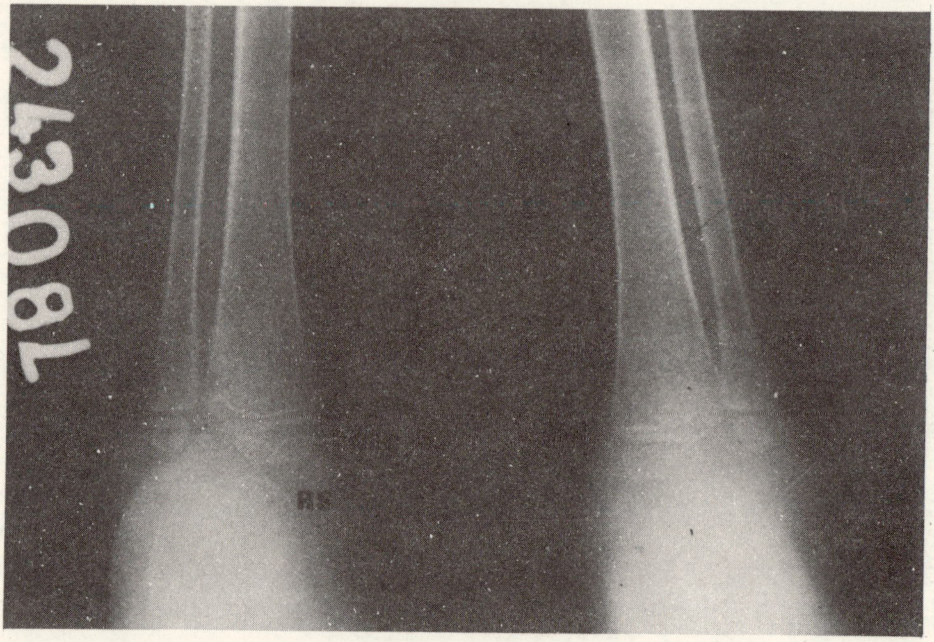

Fig. 13.8

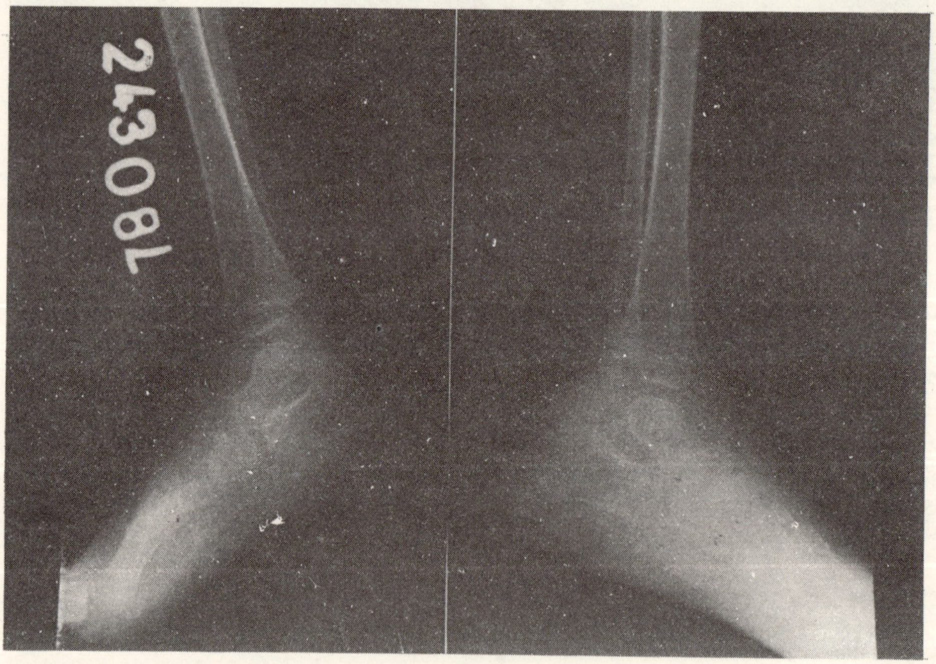

Fig. 13.9

Fig. 13.8 & 13.9. X-ray of both ankles A.P. and lateral views showing soft tissue swelling with evidence of synovial effusion only.

The management of this manifestation is simple. Repeated aspiration, immobilisation with splintage and traction and symptomatic treatment of NSAIDs is sufficient to control this condition. Treatment for the prevention of Sickle cell crisis is necessary.

REFERENCES

1. Aquiline J.I., Mornihan J.W., Bissel G.W., Talbott J.H. Gout in Sickle cell anaemia. Arch Interamerican Rheumatol. 1958, 1 : 708-713;
2. Babhulkar S.S., Pande K.C., Babhulkar Sushrut S. Hand Foot Syndrome in Sickle cell haemoglobinopathy. J. Bone and Joint Surg. March 1995 77-B:310-12.
3. Ball G.V., Sorrenson L.B. The Pathogenesis of hyperuricaemia and Gout in Sickle cell anaemia. Arthritis Rheum. 1970, 13 : 846-848.
4. Barton C.J., and Cockshott W.P. : Bone changes in hemoglobin S-C disease. Amer. J. Roentgenol 1962 ; 88 : 523-32.
5. Bohrer, S.P.: Fracture complicating bone infarcts and/or Osteomyelitis in Sickle-cell disease. Clin. Radiol., 1971, 22:83-8.
6. Casey D.F., Cathcart E.S. Haemarthrosis and Sickle cell trait. Arthritis Rheum. 1970, 13 : 882-886
7. Crout J.E., Mackenna C.H., Petit R.M. Symptomatic Joint effusions in Sickle cell-B-Thalassaemia disease - A Case report. JAMA 235.1976, No.17:1878-1879
8. Daland G.A. and Castle W.B.: A simple and rapid method for demonstrating sickling of red blood cells : The use of reducing agents J.Lab. Clin 1948 : 33, 1082-8.
9. Diggs L.W. : Bone and Joint lesions in Sickle cell disease Clin. Orth. 1967, 52 : 119-43.
10. Edward O'Hara A. : Roentgenographic osseous manifestations of the anemias and the leukemias. Clin Orth and Related Research 1967, 52 : 63 - 82.
11. Espinoza L, Spilberg I, Osterland C.K. Joint Manifestations of Sickle cell disease. Medicine 1974, Vol 53, No 4. 295-305.
12. Givner L.B., Luddy R.E., Schwartz A.D. : Etiology of osteomyelitis in patient with major Sickle cell hemoglobinopathies. J. Pediat., 1981, 99: 411-13.
13. Gold M.S., Williams J.C., Spivack M, Grann V. Sickle Cell Anaemia and Hyperuricaemia JAMA 1968, 206:1572-1573.
14. Goldberg M.A. Analysis of synovial fluid in Sickle cell anaemia with joint effusion. Southern Med. J. 1973, 66:956-958.
15. Hanissian A.S. and Silverman A. Arthritis of Sickle cell anaemia Southern Med. J. 1974, 67:28-32.
16. Johnston, R.B., Jr.: Increased susceptibility to infection in Sickle cell disease. Review of its occurrence and possible causes. Southern Med. J. 1974, 67:1342-48.
17. Keeley K., Buchanan, G.R. Acute infarction of long bones in childern with Sickle cell anemia. J. Pediat.1982, 101 No 2 : 170-5.
18. Koren A., Garty I., Katzuni E. Bone infarction in childern with Sickle cell disease. Early diagnosis and differentiation from osteomyelitis. European J. Pediat.1984, 142: 93-7.
19. Launder W.J. Musculoskeletal manifestations of the hemoglobinopathies. Orthop. Rev., 1979, 8(9): 111-8.
20. Mallouh, Ahmad and Talab, Younis. Bone and Joint infection in patients with Sickle cell disease. J. Pediat. Orthop. 1985, 5: 158-62.
21. Middlemiss J.H. and Raper A.B. Skeletal changes in the haemoglobinopathies. J. Bone Joint Surg. 1966, 48 - B: 693-702.
22. Onwubalili J.K.: Sickle cell disease and infection. J. Infect.1983, 7: 2-20.
23. Orozeo Aleala J. & Baum J. Arthritis during Sickle cell crisis. N. Eng. J. Med. 1973, 288 : 420
24. Schumacher H.R., Andrews R. and Mclaughlin G. Arthropathy in Sickle cell disease. Ann. Intern. Med. 1973, 78 : 203-211.
25. Schumacher H.R., Dorwart B., James Bond, Abbas Alavi, Miller W. Chronic Synovitis with early cartilage destruction in Sickle cell disease. Annals of Rheumatic Dis. 1977, 36 : 413-419.
26. Walker B.R. and Alexander F. Uric acid excretion in Sickle cell anaemia. JAMA, 1971, 215.

14

Sickle Cell Crisis

The word crisis was first used in association with Sickle cell anaemia in 1924 by Sydenstriker. Aches and pains make the life miserable in these patients of Sickle cell disorders. It affects and restricts not only the duration of life but also affects the quality of life. In spite of extensive research no definitive treatment is available for this genetic disorder.

The word crisis has its origin from Greek word "Crisis" which means "Turning Point" whereas dictionary definition of crisis is :

I. Obvious and striking change in symptoms observed by outward manifestations.

II. Painful paroxysmal disturbances of function.

Though Sydenstricker used first time word crisis, Graham (1924) described pains in the same year suggestive of Sickle cell crisis. Penbetty & Cooley 1955 discovered haemolytic crisis occurring in patients with Sickle cell anaemia with Streptococcal infection. However accepted definition and classification of Sickle cell crisis was given by L.W. Diggs in 1965.

The word crisis is defined as sharp turn or definite changes in the course of disease with development of new symptoms & signs.

L.W. Diggs (1965) divided crisis as follows :

1. Vaso-occlusive Crisis

(a) Capillary Stasis

(b) Venous Thrombosis

(c) Arterial Emboli

2. Heamatological Crisis

(a) Aplastic Crisis

(b) Haematolytic Crisis

There is often a combination of two or more of these types of crisis in a single clinical picture "Mixed Crisis".

Greenbourgh M.S. & Kass E.H. 1958 postulated that metabolic acidosis is initiative factor. Smith E.W. and Conley 1955 described common denominators as :

I. Sickled Erythrocytes

II. Increased Viscosity

III. Circulatory Stasis

IV. Hypoxia

V. Vasospasm

VI Dehydration
VII Concentration
VIII Acidosis

Diggs L.W. (1965) and later Felix I.D. et al. put schematic presentation of crisis with hypoxia and reduced pH being initiative factors and vicious circle starts from lowered oxygen tension which leads to Hb "S" crystallisation, increased blood viscosity, stasis and further hypoxia.

CLINICAL MATERIAL

Total 38 patients of Sickle cell crisis were detected who were repeatedly admitted in the hospital during the last 25 years, were studied and followed in detail.

Amongst 38 patients, twenty five were males and thirteen patients were females, mainly in the adolescent group (Table 14.1).

Table 14.1. Age, sex and electrophoresis

Age group in years	*Number of patients*	*Sex Male/Female*	*Hb electrophoresis SS/AS*
05-10	12	08/04	12/0
11-15	21	14/07	19/02
16-20	05	03/02	02/03
Total	38	25/13	33/05

Majority of the patients (33) were Sickle cell disease (SS pattern) and 5 patients were Sickle cell trait (AS pattern) in these group of Sickle cell crisis. While under physiological conditions true Sickle cell trait individuals should never have Sickle cell crisis, it is only precipitated whenever associated with some other pathology.

Most of these patients were admitted in the hospital during the attack of crisis and commonly the attack was observed in rainy season and wet spell of the year. Every patient was investigated for sickling, haemoglobin electrophoresis and detailed history regarding attacks of crisis, repeated hospitalisation, signs & symptoms to know the type of crisis. All these 38 patients were seen during the attack of crisis and followed subsequently. Emphasis was given mainly on pallor, icterus, lymphadenopathy and bone tenderness etc. In few females there was exacerbation of crisis with menarche and every month they started with new period of pains. The priapism was noticed on four occasions in adolescents and young adults. Leg ulceration was observed in three male adolescents in this group of Sickle cell crisis. This was mainly because of insufficiency of dermal circulation & increased frequency of exposure to injury. "Acute chest syndrome" characterised by fever, chest pain, leucocytosis was seen on six occasions. Chronic haemolysis also affected gall bladder. In this study three patients had Cholelithiasis in second decade which were symptomatic and all had visible stones on oral cholecystogram. In these 38 patients the attack of Sickle cell crises was noted on 142 occasions (Table 14.2).

Table 14.2. Types of Sickle cell crisis.

Type of Crisis	*No. of Crises*
Vaso-occlusive	88
Mixed	27
Haemolytic	19
Sequestration	07
Aplastic	01
Total No. of Sickle cell crises in 38 patients	142

As it is evident from Table 14.2, vaso-occlusive is commonest type of crisis and in mixed type also symptoms and sign of vaso-occlusive crisis predominates (Mixed episodes = Vasoocclusive + haemolytic). Vasoocclusive phenomenon is the commonest type that occurs in the course of disease and is responsible for most of the manifestations but also for morbidity and mortality which goes with Sickle cell anaemia. Vasooclussive phenomenon lead to ischaemia & infarction. This is responsible for "pains" in Sickle cell anaemia which was recognised earlier as cardinal manifestation of disease and till today it is so. "Pains" and "aches" mark the course of disease making life of the patient painful and crippling. This was described as "painful crisis" earlier.

Disability and morbidity was adjudged from total days spent by patient in hospital and loss of working days. Thirty eight patients spent total 502 days in hospital and on an average every patients spent 20 days in hospital.

Sicklers are plagued throughout their life with attacks of "Pains". Pain which is ischaemic in origin is very severe and agonizing, intolerable. What precipitates "crisis" is not known in most of the cases, however, infection is important known precipitating factor. Sickle cell anaemia is prone for infection with gram negative group of organisms specially salmonella group of organisms. They are also prone to develop pneumococcal infection and staphylococcal infection.

When a bone is affected in a crisis, the part becomes hot, swollen & tender. There is a fever and a moderate leucocytosis. This quite often occurs in the hands and feet of small children—Hand-Foot syndrome. Usually these bones show osteoporosis, widened trabeculae and the structure in general has a ground-glass appearance. However, if an infarct occurs, a layer of subperiosteal new bone is laid down which makes it look rectangular in shape (Babhulkar et al 1995, Carrol & Evans 1949). Within the bone the cortex loses its structure temporarily and small areas of transradiancy may be seen. The affected bone when the process is complete may be seen to have lost its normal waist and remains with parallel sides.

If a joint is affected, a large acutely tender effusion develops which is a deep yellow in colour and a glairy in consistency. There are a few red cells in the effusion and some of these will be seen to have sickled.

OBSERVATIONS

In this study males out numbered females (ratio 2:1), males having easy access to hospital, their exposure to known precipitating factors contributed to this, besides apathy and negligence on the part of fair sex to report to hospital. Patients reported mostly in second decade (mean age 12 years). Most of the patients were in school going age, adolescence (similar to the studies of Wethers D.L. 1982). Patients were symptomatic in preschool age and even earlier. "Vaso-occlusive crisis" or painful crisis was most common type of crisis followed by mixed type (Vaso-occlusive + haemolytic; haemolytic), sequestration and Aplastic crisis. Aplastic crisis is most rare type. "Vaso-occlusive" or painful crisis is commonest clinical presentation of Sickle cell anaemia with which patients are admitted to hospital or for which medical advise is sought.

Many precipitating factors have been identified of Sickle cell crisis e.g. infection, dehydration, stress (Diggs L.W., 1965; Smith E.W. and Conley, 1955; Felix I.D. et al., 1974). Infection per se is more important as sicklers are prone to infection by *Salmonella* group of organisms and gram-negative organisms, this was thought to be because of deficiency of Factor 'B' which in turn results in defective C3 essential opsonin against gram-negative organisms and pneumococci (W.A. Wilson, 1976).

DISCUSSION

The elongated, multi-pointed and rigid sickled erythrocytes cause an increase in viscosity and obstruct the flow of blood in capillaries, terminal arterioles and veins. Hypoxia due to stasis of blood , is associated with cellular injury, vasospasm, leakage of fluids and cells into perivascular spaces, haemoconcentration and fibrin formation. Localised sickling, temporary or partial, vascular occlusion and perifasicular occlusion cause oedema, pain and swelling of involved organs. Generalised sickling is associated with symptoms and unexpected death. Chronic anemia, stasis and hypoxia lead to endothelial proliferation, tissue injury and replacement of parenchymal cells by fibrous tissue. If ischaemia is severe and prolonged in a given anatomic site there is infarction and necrosis.

In general, the degree of anaemia, jaundice, frequency and severity of the vascular occlusive process are proportional to the percentage of Sickle cell haemoglobin that is present.

The fundamental abnormality resides in Sickle cell haemoglobin which is gene determined type of abnormal haemoglobin. In the deoxygenated state Hb "S" is relatively insoluble and forms needle like tactoids which distort shape of erythrocytes producing the characteristic Sickle cell deformity. Sickled erythrocytes are mechanically more fragile, phagocytosed readily and destroyed more rapidly in the circulation than are non sickled cells. The increased blood destruction is associated with jaundice of haemolytic type, hyperplasia of bone marrow, reticulocytosis and immature cells in peripheral blood. As a result of imbalance between the rates of blood formation and destruction there is varying degree of anaemia which for given individual tend to remain fairly constant. Clinical presentation depends on type of crisis the patients has, most common being vascular occlusive or painful crisis what is described as typical crisis in Sickle cell disease.

Diggs L.W. (1965) has reported vascular occlusive crisis as typical type of crisis that occurs in most of patients. He has described following variants of occlusive crisis and studied them in detail,

1. Hand-Foot Syndrome
2. Recurrent painful & febrile crisis
3. Hepatic crisis with regurgitant jaundice
4. Aseptic necrosis of head of femur/head of humerus
5. Acute chest syndrome
6. Priapism
7. Splenic infarcts
8. Cerebral cortical infarction with hemiplegia
9. Encephalopathies
10. Papillary renal necrosis with haematuria
11. Haematuria
12. Infarcts of other viscera
13. Venous thrombi
14. Pulmonary artery emboli
15. Fat emboli
16. Sudden & unexpected death.

Karayalcin et al (1975) in their series of 100 patients, reported highest number suffering from painful crisis.

The hand-foot syndrome, a common initial manifestation of Sickle cell disease during infancy refers to dactylitis resulting from symmetrical involvement of metacarpal and metatarsal bones (Babhulkar S.S., 1995). It is manifested as painful swelling of dorsum of hands and feet. Symptomatic painful crisis involving the joints and extremities usually begins in early childhood. Pain may be due to infarction of long bones and bone marrow or involvement of periarticular tissues.

Painful abdominal crises are due to infarction of areas of liver, spleen and lymph nodes. Pain is usually attributed to stretching of the capsule of these structures and sequestration.

The other type of crisis in Sickle cell is the hyperhaemolytic crisis, in which there is a sudden increased destruction of red blood cells associated with erythroid hyperplasia in bone marrow (Scott R.B., 1952). Hyperhaemolytic crisis may be accompanied by pain, fever, anaemia, normoblastemia, reticulocytosis and increased serum unconjugated bilirubin levels.

Aplastic crisis is a misnomer, since there is only an acute erythroblastopaenia (Miosch D.C., Baxter M.R. et al. 1957). Leukopaenia is quite uncommon and thrombocytopenia extremely rare. The most common symptoms in association with fever are pain, lethargy, anorexia, weakness, nausea, vomiting and headache. Most prominent physical findings include pallor, hepatosplenomegaly, lymphadenopathy and signs of upper respiratory tract infections (Kim K.Y., 1975; Karayalcin G., 1975).

Intravascular destruction of Sickle cells may occur at a fairly substantial pace in this disease. Given the stresses of the circulation, rigidity of deoxygenated cells and repetitive attacks of Sickle & unsickle cycles, fragmentation of cells is likely.

Both the configuration of cell membrane and the physical state of the cellular contents play a role in haemolysis. Documentation of increased plasma haemoglobin levels during the first few hours of painful crisis has recently been reported as evidence of accelerated haemolysis in "SS" patients in the associated defects of Glucose-6-Phosphate dehydrogenase deficiency. This has been shown to produce hyperhaemolytic crisis.

"Crisis" was seen mainly in patients with 'SS' haemoglobin. These patients seek medical attention off and on. Patient is able to describe this to its fullest clinical spectrum. It will be worthwhile to read "Sickler's Lament" which is composed by a sickler.

"Why do I have to be in pain
every day of my life . . . .
I wake up each day the pain appears
I go to sleep but it doesn't disappear
You have got " Sickle Cell" the G.P.'s say
There is nothing we can do for you today
I wish people can understand just how I feel
The sudden pain which makes me reel
You have got "Crisis" the houseman cry
But don't you worry
We won't allow you to die

(Courtesy : Sickle Cell Society, U.K.)

TREATMENT

The management aims at maintenance of a steady state of haemoglobin and avoidance of factors that are known to precipitate sickling like hypoxia, acidosis, hypotension, peripheral circulatory stasis, hypothermia, dehydration, respiratory depression.

During the period of crisis very active treatment by administration of I.V. fluids (low molecular weight Dextran), I.V. Soda bi-carb 33 mEq/kg/hour for 24 to 48 hours and maintenance of fluid balance.

Oral use of Zinc Sulphate 220 mg TDS along with Folic Acid, Vit. B_{12}, and Soda bi-carb.

Rarely packed red cells transfusion may be necessary which is not without any risk.

Whenever there is possibility of infection precipitating crisis, antibiotics were administered for a period of one week at least.

Tranquilisers, sedatives & analgesics were given where pains & aches were excruciating and intolerable during the acute episode.

After the acute crisis attack was over patients were monitored regularly and were kept on zinc sulphate, folic acid & soda bi-carb for long time. Patients were instructed to avoid situations which precipitates the sickling and crisis.

REFERENCES

1. Babhulkar S.S., Babhulkar Sushrut, Pande Ketan. Hand-foot syndrome as a Manifestation of Sickle cell haemoglobinopathy; J.B.J.S. (Br), 77-B, 310-12, Mar. 1995.
2. Diggs L.W. Sickle Cell Crisis. Amer, Jour. Clin. Path. 44: 1, 1965.

3. Felix I.D. and Konotey A. The Sickle cell disease. Arch. Int. Med. 133: 64, 1974.
4. Graham G.S. A case of Sickle cell anaemia with necropsy, Arch. Int. Med. 34: 778, 1924.
5. Greenburg M.S. and Kass G.H. Studies on the destruction of red blood cells XIII observations on the role of pH on the pathogenesis and treatment of painful crisis in Sickle cell disease. Arch. Int. Med. 101 : 355, 1958.
6. Karaylcin G. et al Sickle cell anaemia, Clinical manifestations in 100 patients with review of literature. Amer. Jour. Med. Sci. 269: 51, 1975.
7. Kim K.Y. et al. Pancytopenia in a patient with Sickle cell anaemia. Amer. Jour. Dis. Child 129: 1195, 1975.
8. Miosch D.C. Baxter M.R. and Lovin W.E. Arch. Int. Medicine 99 : 461, 1957.
9. Penbetty and Looley. Crisis in Sickle cell disease. Amer. Journ. Surg. 102: 645, 1955.
10. Scott R.B. Sickle Cell Crisis. Amer. Jour. Clin. Path. 44. No.8, 1952.
11. Smith E.W. and Conley C.L. Sicklemia and infarction of the spleen during aerial flight. Bull. John Hopkins Hops. 96 : 55, 1955.
12. Sydenstricher A.P., Mulherin W.A.R. and Houseal R.W. Sickle Cell Anaemia. Report of two cases in children and necropsy in one case. Amer. Jour. Dis. Child 26 : 132, 1924.
13. Wethers D.L. Porblems and Complications in the adolescent with Sickle cell diseaase ; The American Jouranl Paediatric Haematology/Oncology. Vol. 4, No. 1, 47-53, 1982.
14. Wilson W.A. Hugues. Salmonella infection in Sickle cell disease. B.M.J. 9 : 491, 1976.

15

Other Manifestations of Sickle Cell Haemoglobinopathy

1. SKULL CHANGES

The skull changes are usually in the form of thickening of outer table, widening of diploic space and marked osteoporosis (Figs. 15.1 and 15.2). Outer table is at times thinned out and when hyperplastic marrow perforates or destroys the outer table, it proliferates under the invisible periosteum and new bone is laid down perpendicular to the inner table giving "Hair on end" appearance (Figs. 15.3 and 15.4). Such changes were seen in 16 patients, most of the cases it was seen below the age of 12 years.

Skeletal changes in this disease are essentially related to vascular insufficiency, occlusion and resultant marrow hyperplasia and associated infections. Though major changes are observed in long bones and vertebrae, skull bones too share the burden and approximately represent 15 to 20 percent of the spectrum.

As a result of severe prolonged anaemia there is hypercellularity and marrow hyperplasia involving all the elements. This results in widening of medullary cavities and intertrabecular spaces and also rarefaction of remaining trabeculae.

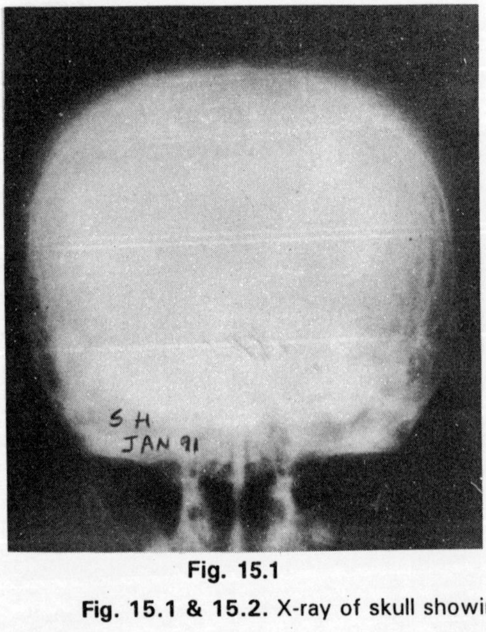

Fig. 15.1

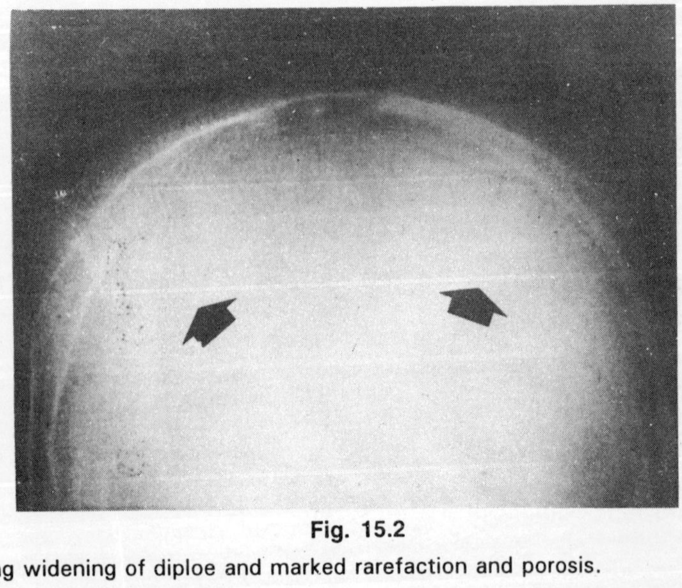

Fig. 15.2

Fig. 15.1 & 15.2. X-ray of skull showing widening of diploe and marked rarefaction and porosis.

In the skull bones, there is a diffuse widening of diploic spaces, associated with thinning of outer as well as inner table. It gives an appearance of coarse, granular osteoporosis of entire cranial vault, except the occiput which is spared. Changes are more prominent in frontal and parietal bones.

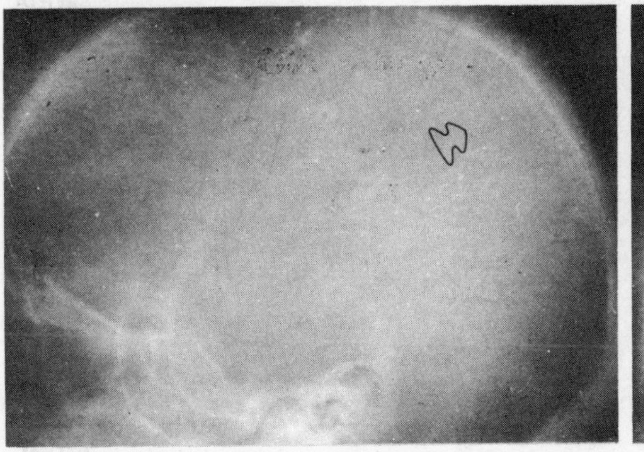

Fig. 15.3

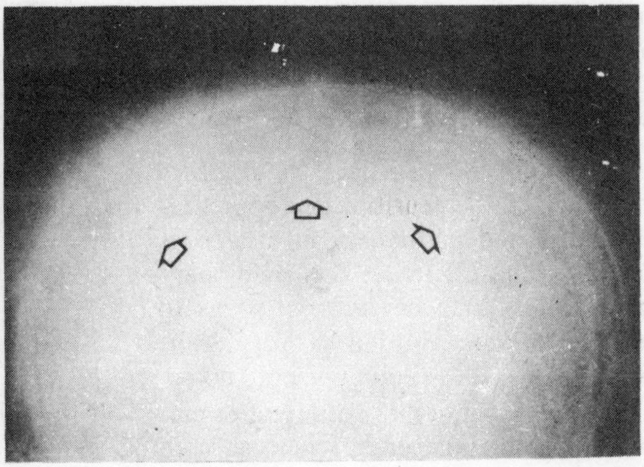

Fig. 15.4

Figs. 15.3 & 15.4. X-ray of skull showing classical "hair on end" appearance.

2. LEG ULCERATIONS

Leg ulceration is commonly seen in patients of Sickle cell haemoglobinopathy. To begin with there is hyperpigmentation, roughening and wrinkling of the skin at the site where ulcer is likely to appear (Fig. 15.5). It progresses further to nodular swelling associated with itching, pain and tenderness. Subsequently the skin is broken and the margins of the ulcer are somewhat elevated and hemorrhagic and gives the entire ulcerated area the appearance of crater (Fig. 15.6). A well circumscribed necrotic area appears in the region of medial malleolus and is suggestive of vascular obstruction. Later necrotic slough falls off leaving the ulcer crater. Ulcers in Sickle cell anaemia typically involve the lower thirds of legs around the malleoli and are usually covered by a thick yellow slough, and are seen in adolescent age groups. The physically active nature of adolescent males causes increased exposure to external injury. There is insufficiency of dermal circulation. Most of these patients had haemolytic jaundice in past. These ulcers are difficult to heal, possibly because of decreased oxygenation of the area and impediment in blood flow from sickled red cells.

These ulcers may form yellowish gray tissue owing to fibrin strands, cellular debris, bacteria, fungus and other micro-organisms. The floor of ulcer remains unhealthy for a long time and even after repetitive cleaning ulcer takes long time to assume a bright red colour.

Clinical Material

In this study we detected 12 patients who had ulcers over the legs in the region of medial malleolus. They gave the history of repetitive breakdown of ulcers which took a long time to heal.This was seen in the age group of 12-18 years in young males in Sickle cell disease patients only (SS).

TREATMENT

Various procedures have been advocated to achieve rapid healing of leg ulcers. Use of antibiotics, hyperbaric oxygen, sterile dressings and elastocrepe compression bandage. Hydrogen peroxide, boric acid and use of betadine solution are used for cleaning the ulcers.

The objectives of procedure are to reduce the pain and promote healing of ulcer. Healing of ulcer may be achieved but may not be permanent because of frequent recurrences. Rarely skin grafting might be required.

3. ACUTE CHEST SYNDROME

Its a complication of Sickle cell disease characterised by pleuritic chest pain, fever, rales and pulmonary infiltrates as seen on chest X-ray. The pulmonary involvement may be massive so as to readily kill the child in a very short period. The exact etiology is not known.

It was thought that variety of organisms might be the underlying cause of acute chest syndrome but till today careful undertaken studies of bacteriological and virological possibilities has been negative. Despite this every one still treats this disorder with antibiotics. Hypoventilation leading to atelectasis and pulmonary vascular occlusion remains an possible cause. In last 25 years I had seen 18 patients of Acute chest syndrome, out of which 11 patients were within the age 12 years and rest were adults. The incidence of ACS was higher in patients with homozygous Sickle cell disease than in traits.

The empirical treatment of ACS involves hydration, oxygen when needed and in many cases exchange transfusions. It is believed that drugs such as hydroxyurea or byurate which increases the concentration of foetal haemoglobin is likely to prevent the recurrent episodes of ACS.

4. ASSOOCIATED OSTEOARTICULAR TUBERCULOSIS

Bacterial infection is one of the major causes of morbidity and mortality in patients with Sickle cell disease. Patients with Sickle cell disease (SS Pattern) are more susceptible whereas Sickle cell trait seems to have lesser risk of infection.

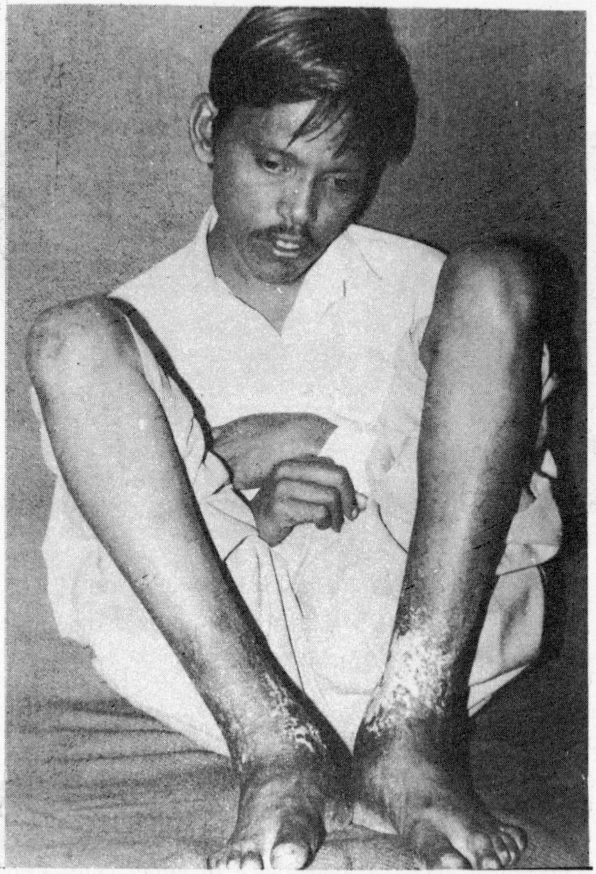

Fig. 15.5. Clinical photograph of a young sickler showing hyperpigmented patches over both ankles.

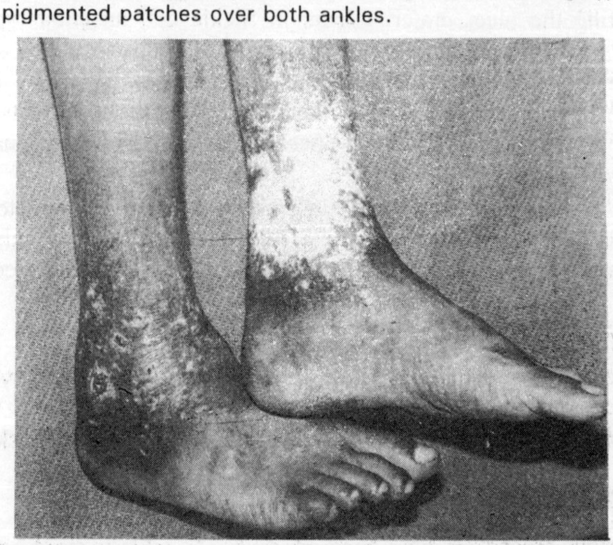

Fig. 15.6. Clinical photograph of same patient's feet showing leg ulceration.

Bacterial infection occurs when the defence mechanism of body fails. This type of falure is seen in patients of Sickle cell haemoglobinopathy for several reasons, and one of the most important of which is functional asplenia. There is decreased function of the spleen and very little amount of antibodies are found in these patients of Sickle cell haemoglobinopathy. Because of repeated episodes of sickling within the sinusoids of spleen, autosplenectomy usually occurs.

Another important reason is decreased opsonization in affected individuals, particularly to Pneumococci and other microorganisms. An opsonphagocytic defect due to an abnormality of the alternative complement pathway and deficiency of specific circulatory antibodies is observed which increases the possibility of infection.

The extraordinary susceptibility of patients with Sickle cell disease to osteomyelitis is well documented. The incidence of osteoarticular tuberculosis is also very high in these individuals of Sickle cell haemoglobinopathy patients.

Clinical Material

Twenty four patients of osteoarticular tuberculosis affecting various bones & joints were detected during last twenty-five years. Fifteen patients had Pott's spine affecting thoracolumbar spine out of which three patients had Pott's paraplegia (Figs. 11.11 and 15.7-15.10). The other joints involved by tubercular infections were hip, (Fig. 15.11) sacroiliac joint, knee, elbow and wrist joints (Table 15.1). These three patients required surgery for decompression.

Table 15.1. Details of Osteoarticular Tuberculosis with Sickle Cell Disease

Sr.No. Site	*No. of patients*
1. Tuberculosis of Spine	15
Lumbar (10)	
Thoracic (05)	
2. Tuberculosis of Hip	04
3. Tuberculosis of Sacroiliac Joint	02
4. Tuberculosis of Knee	01
5. Tuberculosis of Elbow	01
6. Tuberculosis of Wrist	01
Total	24

By and large, these patients had poor resistance and they caught tuberculous infection very quickly.

The treatment of these patients were on similar lines of tuberculosis of involved joint, except strict vigilance was necessary to avoid the precipitation of Sickle cell crisis, and to reduce the morbidity and mortality.

DISCUSSION

The incidence of osteoarticular tuberculosis is high in Sickle cell haemoglobinopathy patients. The major defects in the host defence mechanism acts in these group of sicklers. These are functional asplenia, a deficiency of serum opsonins and a defect in alternative pathway of complement activation. Local pathology in bones, exhaustion of reticuloendothelial system due to chronic haemolysis and hepatic dysfunction predispose for increased incidence of tubercular infection (Figs. 15.7-15.10).

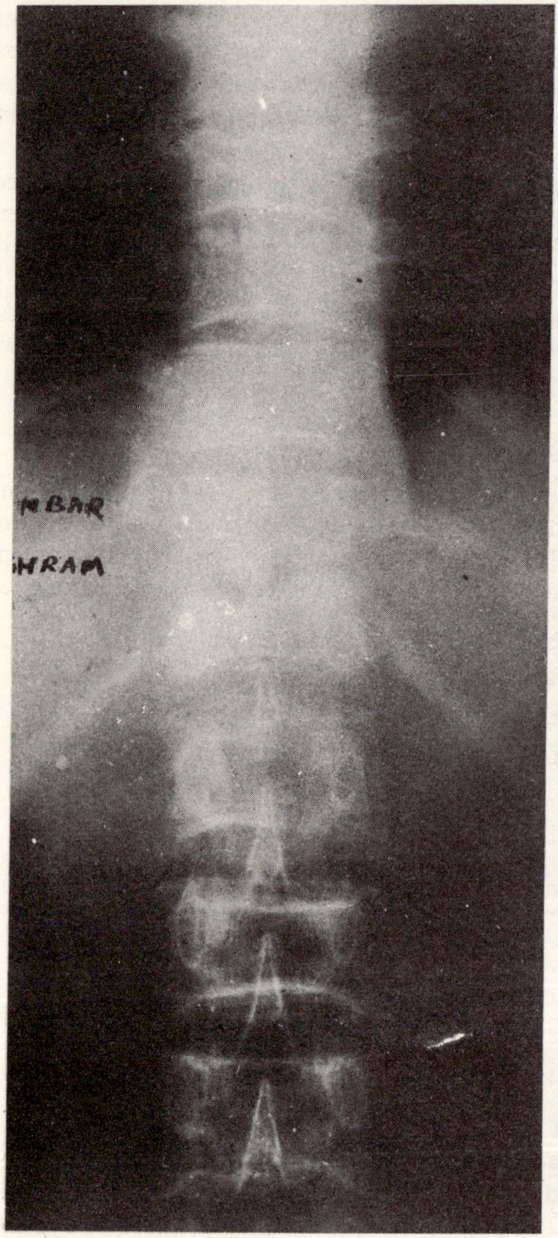

Fig. 15.7

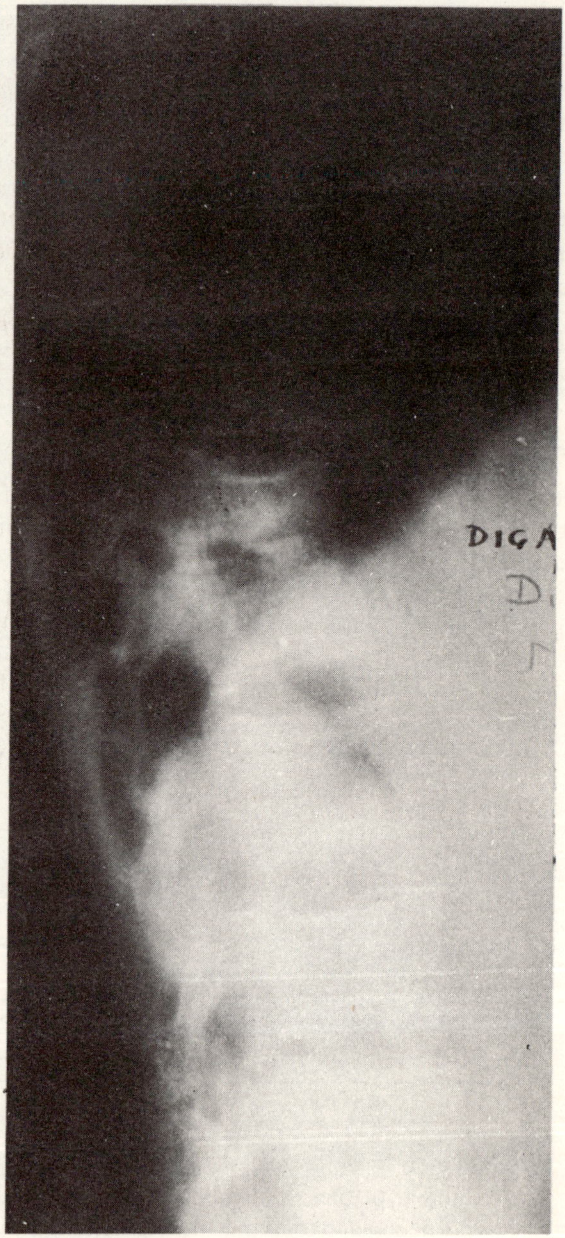

Fig. 15.8

Fig. 15.7 and 15.8. X-ray of thoracolumbar spine showing classical changes of Pott's spine with destruction of adjoining surfaces of vertebral body with complete loss of intervertebral disc space. The same X-rays are showing typical radiological sign of vertebral involvement of sickle cell haemoglobinopathy including "step- sign".

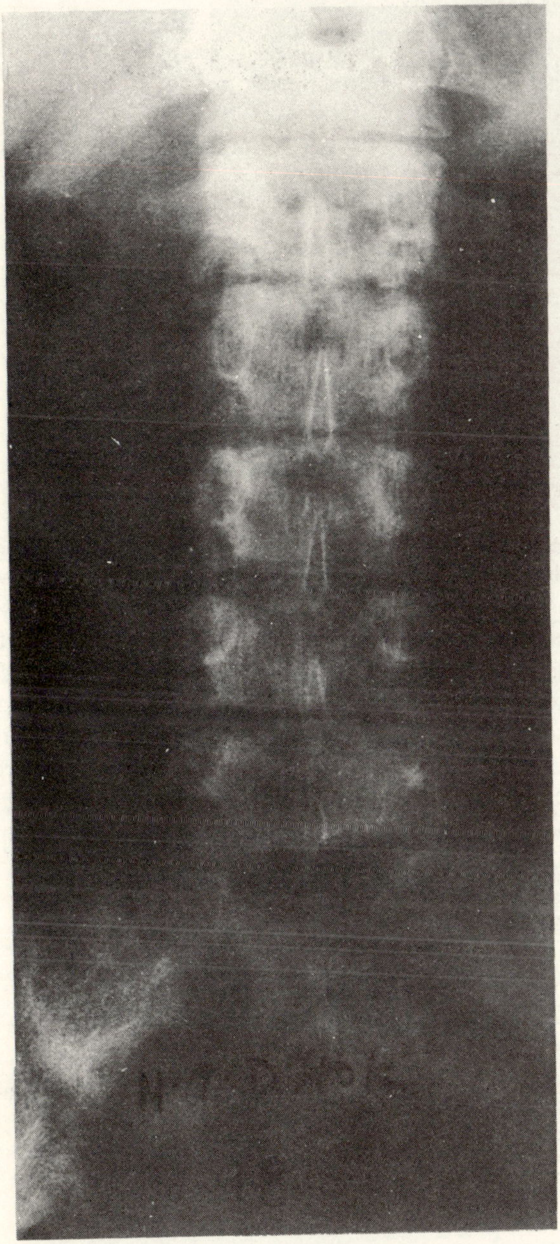

Fig. 15.9

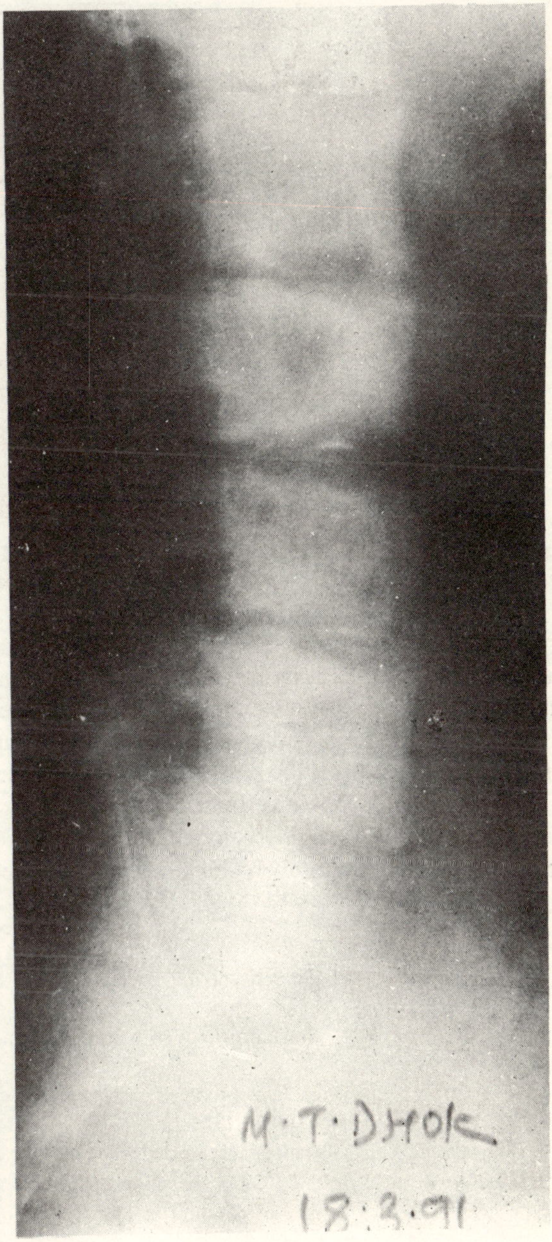

Fig. 15.10

Fig. 15.9 and 15.10. X-ray of young sickler who had multifocal tuberculosis. Entire lumbar spine was affected with mainly involvement of adjoining surfaces of vertebral body. The tubercular nature was confirmed by histopathology.

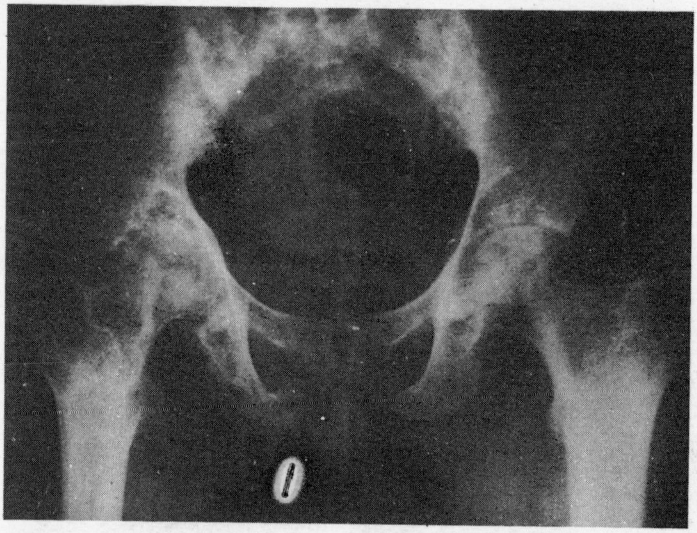

Fig. 15.11. X-ray pelvis showing marked destruction of articular surfaces of right hip with complete loss of joint space suggesting of tuberculosis of hip joint with typical generalised changes of sickle cell haemoglobinopathy.

Initially there is enlargement of spleen, which becomes progressively reduced with increasing age to a siderofibrotic segment by repetitive episodes of vaso-occlusion and infarction - a phenomenon termed "autosplenectomy". The spleen has a dual role in bacterial infection - biological filtering and phagocytosis of blood-borne bacteria, and production of specific antibody, IgM and tufsin. Repeated marrow thrombosis, infarction and necrosis would make the bone a favoured site of localisation and lodgement of microbacteria in these patients of Sickle cell haemoglobinopathy. Incidence of osteoarticular tuberculosis is very high in these sicklers who largely belong to poor socioeconomic strata of the society. Active steps and prompt treatment including antitubercular drugs is necessary to reduce the morbidity.

REFERENCES

1. Alleyne S., Went E. and Serjeant G. : Social effects of leg ulceration in Sickle cell anaemia. South. Med. J. 70(2);213, 1977.
2. Camilla Noel, R.N., Nursing Clinics of North America, Complications of Sickle cell disease, Leg Ulcers, Mar 1983; 155-59.
3. Chernoff A., Shapleigh J. & Moore C. : Therapy of chronic ulceration of legs associated with Sickle cell anaemia J.A.M.A., 155 : 1487-1491, 1954.
4. Serjeant G. Leg ulcerations in Sickle cell anaemia. Arch. Intern. Med. 133; 690-694, 1974.
5. Wolfort F. & Kriget T.: Skin ulcerations in Sickle cell anaemia. Plast. Reconstr. Surg., 43(1); 71. 1969.

16

Clinical & Anthropometric Studies in Patients of Sickle Cell Haemoglobinopathies (Body Shape, Growth and Development)

INTRODUCTION

The patients of Sickle cell haemoglobinopathies are rampant and are frequently seen in this region, around the vicinity of Nagpur, Central India. The disease is not commonly seen everywhere, but it has some topographical distribution. Sickle cell haemoglobinopathy, though infrequently observed, is of great pathological significance since it can be diagnosed in the early years of life. Different disorders in Sickle cell haemoglobinopathy may differ and vary in severity, symptoms and signs.

There are various orthopaedic manifestations of this haematological disorder. Sickle cell haemoglobinopathy was observed frequently in a specific community of scheduled castes and scheduled tribes belonging to backward classes and the surveys were conducted especially in the areas where this specific community is thickly populated. The anthropometric studies were carried out in the identical sicklers and normal individuals in children, adolescents and adults. Sickling was done in all patients by sealed moist preparation described by Daland and Castle (1948). The haemoglobin electrophoresis was done by paper electrophoresis.

PURPOSE OF THE STUDY

The main aim of this project was to study the group of proved Sickle cell haemoglobinopathy patients especially with skeletal affection and compare them with identical normal individuals to establish certain visual impressions. The study was designed to establish physical abnormalities so that even the trait can be diagnosed much earlier (in advance) than their expected time of reporting to the hospital or earlier than clinical presentation.

Bony changes are commonly seen in Sickle cell haemoglobinopathy and there are different causes and presentations depending upon the site, time and pattern of involvement. In this disorder, apart from the genetic factors, growth and development to a large extent is influenced by socio-cultural, economic, nutritional, hormonal and environmental factors. Physical dimensions of the body are largely influenced by nutritional factors especially in the rapidly growing period of early childhood. During the growth period of these sicklers it produces few changes which lead to different presentations of their faces and physique. Anthropometry is concerned with the measurements of variations of physical dimensions and the gross composition of human body at different age levels. It is one of the important parameters for assessment of growth and development of human body.

Apart from physical anthropometry, the faces were studied by clinical photographs and X-rays of skull to study the radiological changes and anthropometric measurements (Figs. 16.1-16.6). The X-rays of the other parts were taken if any suspicion of skeletal involvement was noticed during the physical examination. There is hyperplasia of bone marrow and other pathological changes which affect the growth and shape of the bones. Skeleton is the basic structure on which presentation of individuals' size, shape, figure depends which gives the look of physical personality.

Since the skeleton is affected by this dreaded disease it produces certain changes in physical look (including faces) of individual. Hence skeletal survey was considered as an important factor in early detection. Accordingly, apart from facial anthropometry (face photograph) skull X-ray, X-rays of suspected parts and other growth measurements were considered as important landmarks in producing definite results of diagnosing sicklers at the earliest amongst the community at large.

Material and Methods

The patients who were detected during various camps were directed to "Sickle cell centre" at Sushrut Hospital, Research Centre and Post Graduate Institute of Orthopaedics and Indira Gandhi Medical College Nagpur for detailed study and follow up. A total of 7380 patients of Sickle cell haemoglobinopathy were detected during this period and followed up regularly with an average follow up of 12 years. Among these 7380 sicklers only 944 patients had skeletal affection though in many patients multiple bones were involved. Besides these 944 patients 124 proved sicklers without any obvious skeletal affection were chosen for anthropometric studies. In these 124 patients 62 patients had SS pattern and 62 had AS pattern on electrophoresis.

The subjects (children, adolescents and adults) were measured wearing light clothing, without any footwear. Height was measured by using Anthropometer with the subject standing erect and heels touching together and against the vertical bar of height scale. Weight was measured by the same weighing machine for all the subjects by the same person.

The photographs of the subjects were taken by the same camera and the same photographer from a distance of 3 feet.

The X-Ray skull of the subjects were taken from the fixed distance between the X-Ray tube and the subject.

The precautions were taken to minimise the errors in measurements as much as possible.

PILOT STUDY OF ANTHROPOMETRY

Apart from detailed clinical examination, these 124 patients (fifty percent SS and fifty percent AS) were selected for Physical Anthropometry, Facial Anthropometry, and Radiographic Anthropometry (X-ray of Skull) in the age group of 05-20 years, since the growth period is maximally affected during this age group. Radiological survey was done even at minimal suspicion. The patients were divided in the following groups according to the age and sex in this anthropometric study.

Table 16.1. Age and sex distribution

Age group	*Age*	*S/C*	*Male*	*Female*
A	00-05	S	26	09
		C	23	09
B	06-10	S	18	10
		C	18	09
C	11-15	S	23	11
		C	23	11
D	16-above	S	20	07
		C	19	07

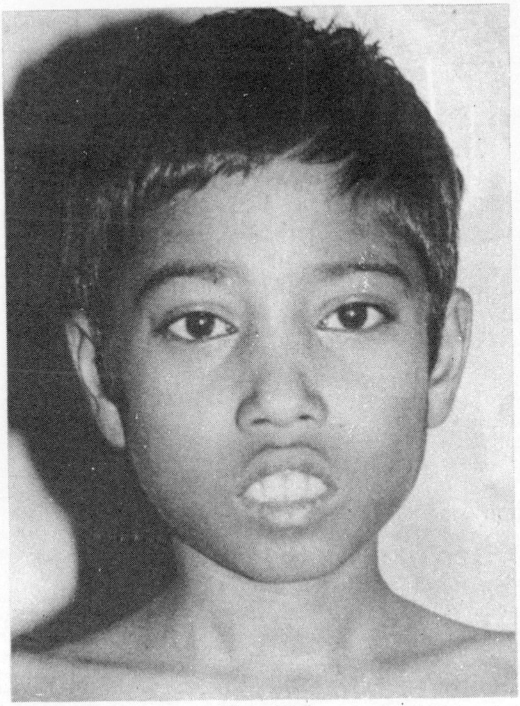

Fig. 16.1

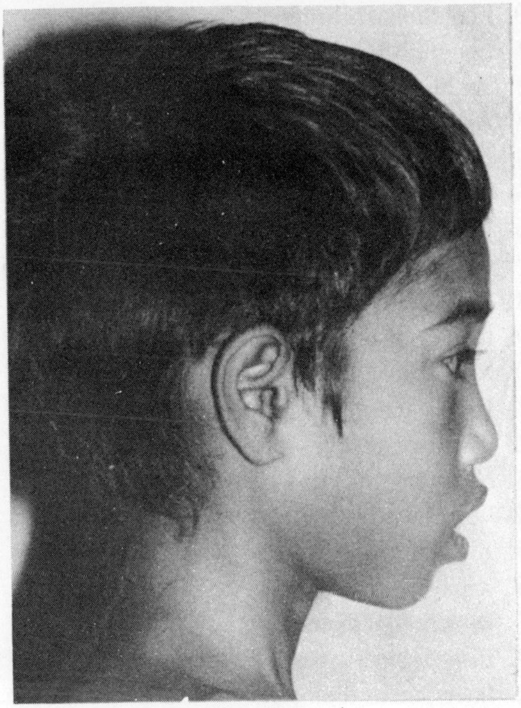

Fig. 16.2

Fig. 16.1 & 16.2. Clinical photograph of face from front and side of a classical Sickle cell disease patient showing typical "Sicklers face"

All these Sickle Cell haemoglobinopathy patients were compared with normal individuals of the group of same age and sex. As mentioned earlier, in this project 243 patients were studied amongst which 124 were sicklers and 119 controlled individuals. The normal/controlled individuals were selected from 5 to 15 years of age from Somalwar High School, Ramdaspeth, Nagpur and 16 to 20 years from Medical students from Indira Gandhi Medical College and the rest of the patients from outdoor of General Hospital.

Table 16.2. Frequencies according to categories

Patients	*Physical anthropometry*	*Facial anthropometry*	*Radiological anthropometry*
Sickle cell	124	88	84
Control	119	119	119

PHYSICAL ANTHROPOMETRY

1. Weight.
2. Height.
3. Circumference of head.
4. Distance between Inion and Nasion.
5. Distance between Hair line - Chin.
6. Distance between Nasion - tip of the nose.
7. Distance between preauricular - preauricular.
8. Width of the Lips. (both)

9. Width of the Nose.
10. Length of Philtrum.
11. Length of Chin.
12. Width of the Oral Fissure.
13. Angle of Mandible to angle of Mandible.
14. Bi-Mastoid diameter.
15. Bi-Temporal diameter.
16. Bi-Frontal diameter.
17. Distance between Nasion to preauricular point.
18. Bi-Zygomatic distance.
19. Length of palpebral fissure.
20. Nasion to Zygomatic distance.
21. Inter Canthal distance (inner)
22. Circumference of Neck at Thyroid prominence.
23. Neck length - in front.
24. Length of the sternum to centre of pubic symphysis.
25. Xiphysternum to pubic symphysis.
26. Xiphysternum to suprasternal border.
27. Bi-acromial diameter.
28. Bi-trochanteric diameter.
29. Interspinous diameter.
30. Length of the superior limb. (both)
31. Length of the Hand.
32. Length of the Arm.
33. Length of Forearm.
34. Length of Thigh.
35. Length of ASIS to greater trochanter.
36. Length of Leg.

FACIAL ANTHROPOMETRY BY PHOTOGRAPHS

1. Distance between Inion & Nasion (Lat.)
2. Distance between Hairline to chin (AP)
3. Distance between Nasion-tip of the nose (AP)
4. Distance between Preauricular to preauricular (AP)
5. Width of the lower lip (AP)
6. Width of the nose (AP)
7. Length of the oral fissure (AP) :
8. Angle of mandible to angle of mandible (AP)
9. Bi-Frontal distance (AP)
10. Distance between Nasion to preauricular (Lat.)
11. Bi-Zygomatic dist. (Intermaxillary) (AP)
12. Nasion to Zygomatic distance (AP)
13. Inter-inner canthal distance (AP)

14. Inter-outer canthal distance (AP)
15. Length of Ear (Lat.)
16. Width of Ear (Lat.)
17. Length of Hair line to Nasion (AP)
18. Chin to angle of mandible (Lat.)

ANTHROPOMETRY BY SKULL X-RAYS

1. Bi-Frontal distance (AP)
2. Bi-Zygomatic distance (AP)
3. Nasion to Zygomatic distance (AP)
4. Nasion to Chin distance (AP)
5. Distance between Medial border of orbit (AP)
6. Distance between Lateral border of orbit (AP)
7. Distance between Nasion to top of the skull (AP)
8. Bi-Maxilla distance (AP)
9. Angle of Mandible to angle of Mandible. (AP)
10. Distance between Inion and Nasion. (Lat)
11. Distance between Nasion to Anterior Border of pituitary fossa (Lat)
12. Distance between posterior border of pituitary fossa to Inion (Lat)
13. X-ray findings
    X-ray skull (AP & Lat)
    Other X-rays

ANTHROPOMETRIC STUDY

I. Statistical Analysis

Means and standard deviation for the groups of "Sicklers" are compared with those of the group of "controlled" or normal children. Student's t-tests are calculated to establish the statistical reliability of the mean differences for each individual measure. Percentage changes - growth or retardation in the mean values of the each indicator values for the two groups are also presented.

Statistical analyses, given in the present study, relate to:

A. Physical Anthropometric data.
B. Facial Anthropometric data.
C. Skull X-ray Anthropometric data.
D. Indices.
E. Observations.
F. Statistical Analyses according to Sex.

II. Results

A. Physical Anthropometry

The statistical calculations for the 36 indicators, physical anthropometric measurements (Fig. 16.3, 16.4), according to the three age groups, are presented in the Table 16.3.

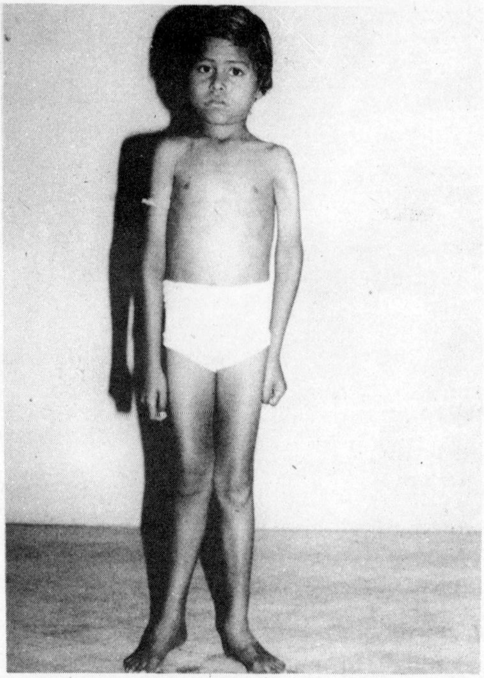

Fig. 16.3

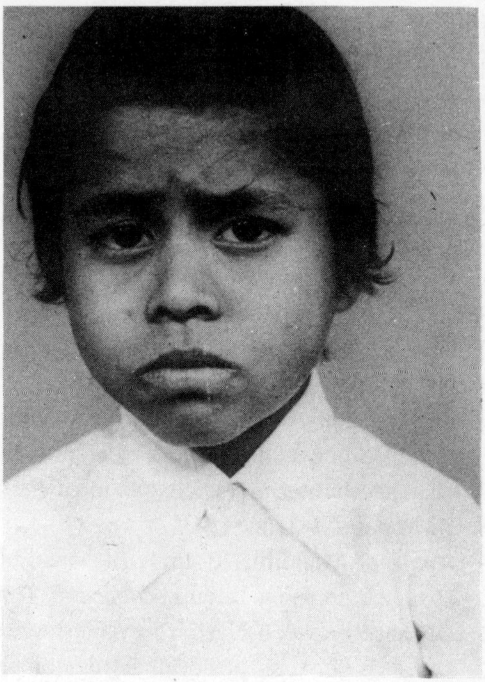

Fig. 16.4

Fig. 16.3 & 16.4. Complete body photograph and front view of face of a SS pattern child showing multiple deformities—Genu valgum, angular deformity in left arm with shortening with a typical "Sickler face".

Table 16.3. Calculations for physical anthropometric data

Ind. No.	*Name*	*Age group Group*	*Controlled*		*Sickler*		*t value*	*% change*	*Remark*
			Mean	*SD*	*Mean*	*SD*			
1.	Weight	05-09	20.96	5.51	15.53	3.71	4.60	-25.91	
		10-15	35.96	7.92	28.38	6.60	4.17	-20.64	
		16-20	45.64	4.61	42.40	4.61	2.62	-7.10	
2.	Height	05-09	120.58	10.18	117.50	0.42	2.18	-2.55	
		10-15	147.97	10.12	133.00	1.42	11.65	-10.12	
		16-20	160.85	4.84	157.40	1.24	5.00	-2.14	
3.	Circumference of Head	05-09	51.85	3.51	46.68	7.41	2.70	-9.97	
		10-15	52.15	6.60	50.18	3.47	1.56	-3.78	
		16-20	52.30	2.17	51.29	3.56	1.07	-1.93	
4.	Distance Between Inion & Nasion	05-09	18.09	0.70	18.06	3.34	0.04	-0.16	
		10-15	19.76	4.27	18.38	4.50	1.22	-6.98	
		16-20	22.63	2.70	19.06	0.77	8.44	-15.77	
5.	Distance between hair-line & Chin	05-09	16.21	1.46	14.02	2.85	3.04	-13.51	
		10-15	16.30	1.29	15.33	1.31	2.91	-5.95	
		16-20	16.69	0.73	16.37	1.25	1.03	-1.92	
6.	Distance between Nasion & Tip of Nose	05-09	4.15	0.46	3.71	1.18	1.50	-10.60	
		10-15	4.55	0.52	4.71	0.70	0.95	3.52	
		16-20	4.78	0.47	4.86	0.42	0.69	1.67	

(Contd.)

Ind. No.	*Name*	*Age group Group*	*Controlled Mean*	*Controlled SD*	*Sickler Mean*	*Sickler SD*	*t value*	*% change*	*Remark*
7.	Distance between Pre-auricular to Pre-auricular	05-09	11.84	0.71	11.06	2.10	0.68	-6.59	
		10-15	13.47	3.44	11.37	1.36	4.03	-15.59	
		16-20	19.44	1.50	12.44	0.66	26.36	-36.01	
8.	Width of Lips (Both)	05-09	0.87	0.37	1.33	0.42	3.94	52.87	
		10-15	0.90	0.12	1.46	0.97	2.58	62.22	
		16-20	0.92	0.19	1.60	1.14	2.38	73.94	
9.	Width of Nose	05-09	2.97	0.23	2.75	0.69	3.28	-7.41	
		10-15	3.07	0.21	3.09	0.55	-1.58	0.00	
		16-20	3.30	0.10	3.17	0.51	0.16	-3.94	
10.	Length of Philtrum	05-09	1.38	0.29	1.24	0.49	1.12	-10.14	
		10-15	2.37	0.24	1.24	0.33	14.22	-47.68	
		16-20	2.45	0.40	1.75	0.34	7.34	-28.57	
11.	Length of Chin	05-09	2.69	0.46	2.44	0.55	1.69	-9.29	
		10-15	2.75	0.54	3.02	0.38	-0.04	9.10	
		16-20	3.15	0.67	3.05	0.78	0.49	-3.17	
12.	Width of Oral Fissures	05-09	4.27	0.44	4.01	1.09	0.96	-6.09	
		10-15	4.42	0.78	4.07	0.74	1.20	-7.92	
		16-20	4.44	1.18	4.14	0.43	1.53	-6.33	
13.	Angle of Mandible to Angle of Mandible	05-09	7.87	0.48	9.61	1.19	-5.87	22.11	
		10-15	9.42	1.13	9.56	1.14	-0.48	1.49	
		16-20	9.85	1.05	10.48	1.56	-1.61	6.40	
14.	Bi-Mastoid Diameter	05-09	13.49	0.63	11.62	1.51	15.33	-13.86	
		10-15	13.85	2.11	12.12	0.95	5.16	-12.49	
		16-20	17.33	0.49	12.72	0.89	3.42	-26.60	
15.	Bi-Temporal Diameter	05-09	9.60	2.59	13.22	0.83	-9.11	39.06	
		10-15	12.73	2.55	13.35	0.94	-1.30	3.85	
		16-20	14.37	2.58	13.93	0.74	1.17	-3.06	
16.	Bi-Frontal Diameter	05-09	5.10	0.45	8.89	0.83	-17.89	74.31	
		10-15	5.17	1.46	8.31	2.54	-5.27	60.74	
		16-20	5.54	1.53	7.09	0.69	-6.06	27.98	
17.	Distance between Nasion to Pre-auricular point	05-09	10.76	1.82	8.97	2.12	3.46	-18.08	
		10-15	10.95	0.99	10.06	0.88	3.02	-6.51	
		16-20	11.25	0.26	11.04	0.28	2.84	-1.87	
18.	Bi-Zygomatic Distance	05-09	7.62	0.69	10.11	1.07	-9.00	32.68	
		10-15	9.63	1.28	10.45	1.41	-2.33	8.52	
		16-20	11.06	0.64	11.78	0.75	-3.69	6.51	
19.	Length of Palpebral Fissure	05-09	2.54	0.55	3.34	0.63	-4.68	31.50	
		10-15	2.93	0.42	3.76	2.08	-1.77	28.33	
		16-20	2.96	0.33	3.86	0.39	-8.88	30.41	
20	Nasion to Zygomatic Distance	05-09	5.75	0.43	6.00	1.38	-0.74	4.35	
		10-15	6.10	0.50	6.47	1.61	-1.01	6.07	
		16-20	7.34	2.17	7.16	1.83	0.35	-2.45	
21	Inter-Canthal Distance Inner	05-09	2.28	0.39	2.55	0.56	-1.85	11.84	
		10-15	2.49	0.62	2.69	0.16	-2.37	8.03	
		16-20	2.56	0.50	2.79	0.66	-1.37	8.98	
22.	Circumference of Neck at Thyroid prominence	05-09	26.75	1.45	28.41	1.87	-3.35	6.21	
		10-15	28.18	2.37	28.54	3.37	-0.45	1.28	
		16-20	28.98	3.28	29.01	5.12	-0.02	0.10	
23.	Neck Length - In front	05-09	5.88	0.61	5.42	1.19	1.53	-7.82	
		10-15	8.18	1.27	7.93	2.57	0.42	-3.06	
		16-20	9.24	2.27	8.76	4.54	0.43	-5.19	

(Contd.)

Ind. No.	Name	Age group Group	Controlled Mean	Controlled SD	Sickler Mean	Sickler SD	value	% change	Remark
24.	Length of Sternum to centre of pubic Symphysis	05-09	36.37	4.82	34.80	3.88	1.36	-4.32	
		10-15	42.26	3.63	40.78	8.43	0.76	-3.50	
		16-20	46.17	1.47	46.55	1.62	-0.89	0.82	
25.	Xiphy-sternum to Pubic Symphysis	05-09	30.17	2.63	29.11	4.22	0.98	-3.51	
		10-15	30.24	5.37	30.54	2.52	-0.35	0.99	
		16-20	31.81	3.65	38.29	2.57	-8.44	20.37	
26.	Xiphy-Sternum to Suprasternal border	05-09	12.52	1.20	11.68	3.10	1.09	-6.71	
		10-15	14.92	2.15	13.79	2.31	1.95	-7.57	
		16-20	19.93	2.63	16.00	2.52	5.74	-19.72	
27.	Biacromial Diameter	05-09	20.21	2.51	24.08	2.68	-5.25	19.15	
		10-15	29.08	5.37	28.39	4.19	0.60	-2.37	
		16-20	31.37	2.40	31.11	2.52	0.39	-0.83	
28	Bi-trochanteric Diameter	05-09	28.00	2.75	19.25	5.02	6.86	-31.25	
		10-15	28.95	6.14	22.54	4.56	5.05	-22.14	
		16-20	34.00	5.02	30.11	8.67	1.81	-11.44	
29.	Interspinous Diameter	05-09	21.52	5.03	18.41	3.40	2.88	-14.45	
		10-15	22.09	4.05	20.41	4.71	1.44	-7.61	
		16-20	26.54	3.77	21.56	3.71	4.92	-18.76	
30.	Length of the Superior Limb (Both)	05-09	39.44	12.52	47.83	3.40	-4.37	21.27	
		10-15	65.39	5.88	62.35	2.93	0.42	28.33	
		16-20	72.53	2.35	69.72	1.90	5.19	-3.87	
31.	Length of Hand	05-09	13.56	1.32	12.59	2.83	1.37	-7.15	
		10-15	16.67	1.26	15.63	1.98	2.22	-6.24	
		16-20	18.80	1.95	17.40	1.70	2.96	-7.45	
32.	Length of Arm	05-09	20.69	2.39	19.54	2.72	1.56	-5.56	
		10-15	26.50	3.42	24.86	3.62	1.80	-6.19	
		16-20	29.18	2.92	27.93	2.22	1.94	-4.28	
33.	Length of Forearm	05-09	20.83	2.24	16.78	2.70	5.59	-19.44	
		10-15	24.20	2.11	28.81	3.49	4.12	-14.01	
		16-20	24.52	2.85	24.18	2.73	0.46	-1.39	
34.	Length of Thigh	05-09	27.10	3.86	31.50	7.77	-2.25	16.24	
		10-15	42.48	5.92	41.34	6.03	0.75	-2.68	
		16-20	47.92	2.16	45.70	2.71	3.19	-1.63	
35.	Length of ASIS to greater trochanter	05-09	9.44	1.05	8.01	1.64	3.38	-15.15	
		10-15	11.37	2.12	9.89	2.07	2.79	-13.02	
		16-20	11.87	2.17	10.45	2.09	2.51	-11.96	
36.	Length of Leg	05-09	30.75	2.99	26.53	4.12	3.90	-13.72	
		10-15	36.83	3.26	33.79	4.62	2.82	-8.47	
		16-20	39.72	2.84	36.67	2.72	4.13	-7.68	

The results are as follows:

1. Out of the 36 indicators, it is observed that in case of 19 indicators, the Sickle cell disease has led to growth- retardation in all the age groups;
2. In case of the six indicators, the Sickle cell disease has led to abnormal growth irrespective of age; and
3. In respect of the remaining 11 indicators the results are mixed, i.e., there is abnormal growth in some age groups and growth-retardation in respect of the others.

The results relating to the individual indicators of physical anthropometric measurements are presented in the following paragraphs.

1. Weight : It may be observed that the Sickle cell disease has led to growth-retardation of weight in the children of all the age groups. The difference between the mean weights of the two catagories of children are observed to be statistically significant at 5 percent level of significance. The percentages of growth-retardation of weight, it is observed, decrease with the advancement of age.

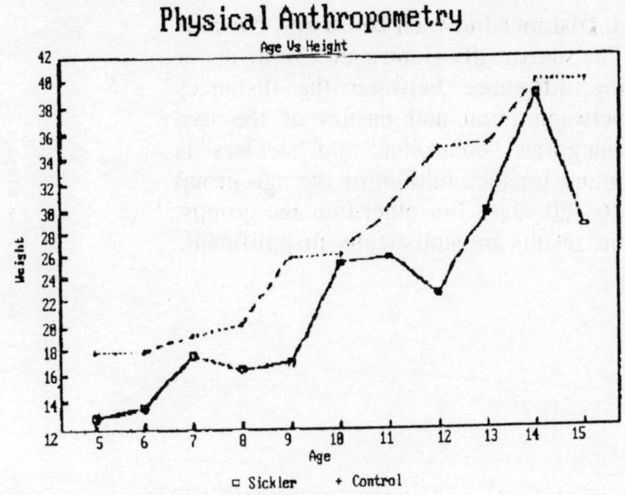

2. Height : It has been hypothesized by the earlier researchers that the sicklers are generally shorter than the normal children. Statistical calculations of the anthropometric measurements confirm the hypothesis for the children of all the three age groups. The differences in the heights of the two categories of children for all the three age groups are found to be statistically significant. The differ- ence between the mean heights of the children of two categories is more pronounced in the age group, 10-15 years.

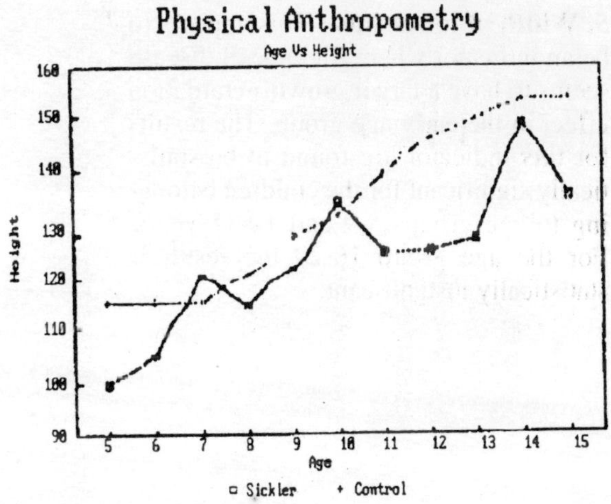

3. Circumference of the head : This is another indicator where the Sickle cell disease has not only arrested the growth but also led to growth retardation in the circumference of the head of the sickle cell disease affected children of all the three age groups. The difference between the mean circumference of the head of the "controlled" children and the mean circumference of the head of the "sicklers" is found to be statistically significant for the children of age group 5 - 9 years. For the other two age groups, the results are statistically insignificant. The foregoing analysis implies that the Sickle cell disease affects more seriously in the early years of life as far as this indicator is concerned.

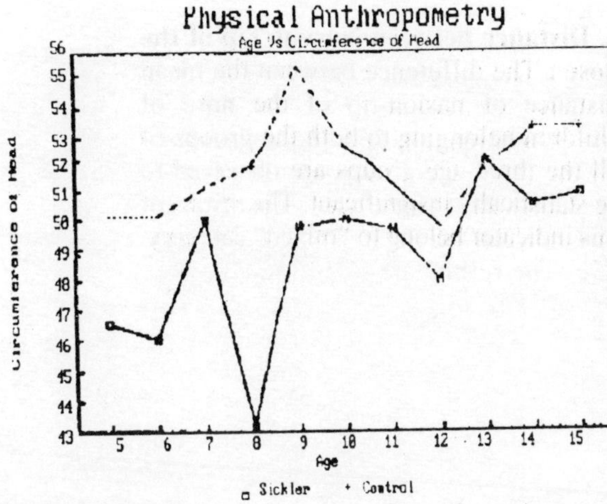

4. Distance between Inion and Nasion: The statistically significant results about the difference between the distances between inion and nasion of the two categories; "controlled" and "sicklers" is found for the children of the age group 16 - 20 years. For other two age groups, the results are statistically insignificant.

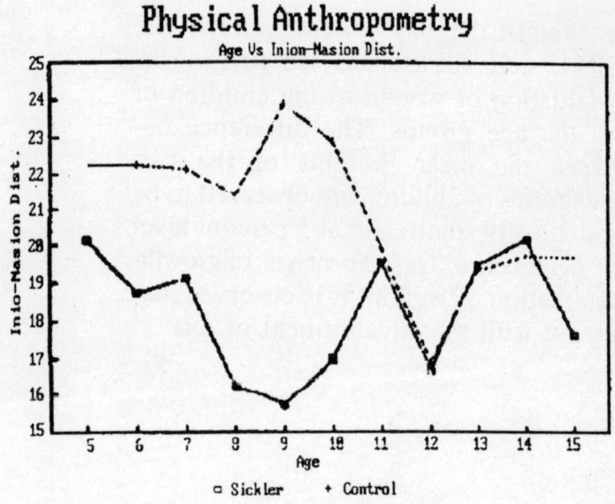

5. Width of lower lips : This appears to be an indicator where Sickle cell disease seems to have a larger growth-retardation effect in the early age group. The results for this indicator are found to be statistically significant for the children belonging to age groups 5-9 and 10-15 years. For the age group 16-20 the result is statistically insignificant.

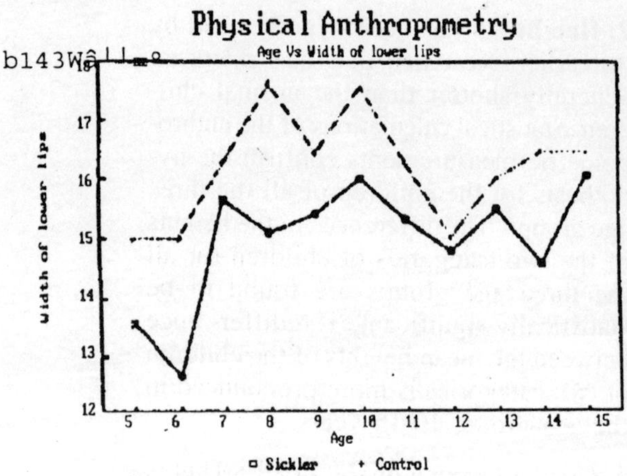

6. Distance between Nasion-Tip of the nose : The difference between the mean distance of nasion-tip of the nose of children belonging to both the groups of all the three age groups are observed to be statistically insignificant. The results of this indicator belong to "mixed" category.

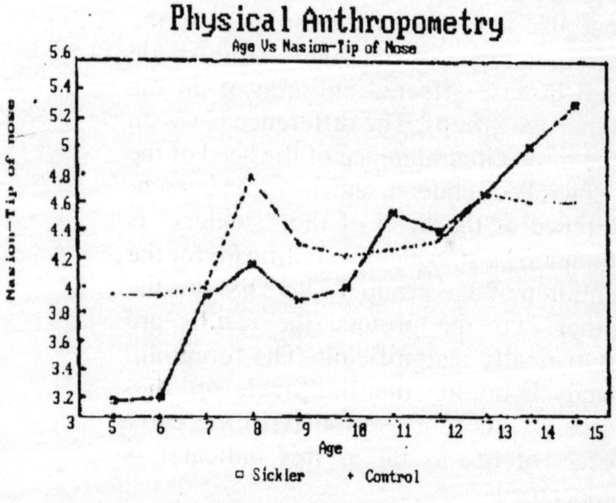

7. Distance between preauricular - perauricular : The Sickle cell disease appears to have been responsible for growth retardation as far as this indicator is concerned. The results are statistically significant. Another distinguishing feature of the statistical calculations is that the degree of growth retardation increases with the advancement of age.

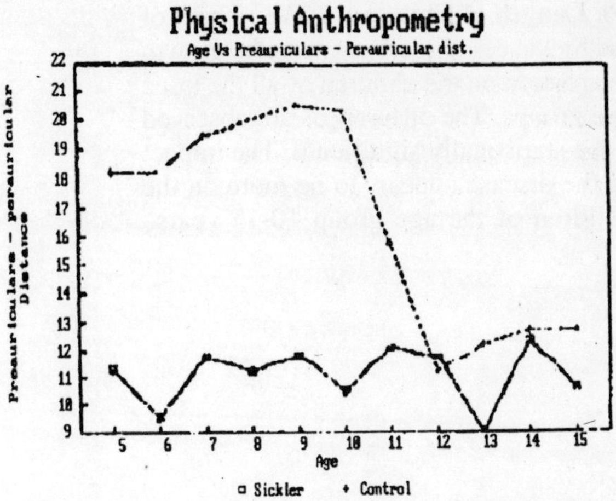

8. Width of lips : The Sickle cell disease, it seems, has led to abnormal growth in this indicator. The difference between the mean widths of lips are found to be statistically significant. It is also observed that widths of lips increases more with the advancement of age.

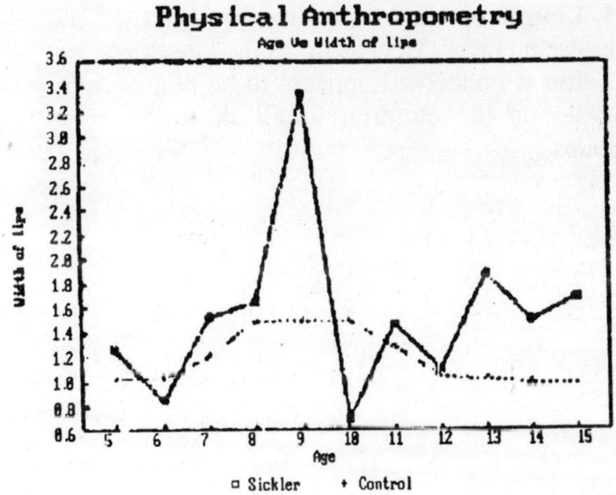

9. Width of Nose : The children belonging to the group of "sicklers" appears to have growth-retardation due to the sickle cell disease. The result is statistically significant for the children belong to the age group 5 - 9 years. For the other two age groups the results are found to be statistically insignificant. This implies that the impact of the Sickle cell disease is more pronounced in the early age group.

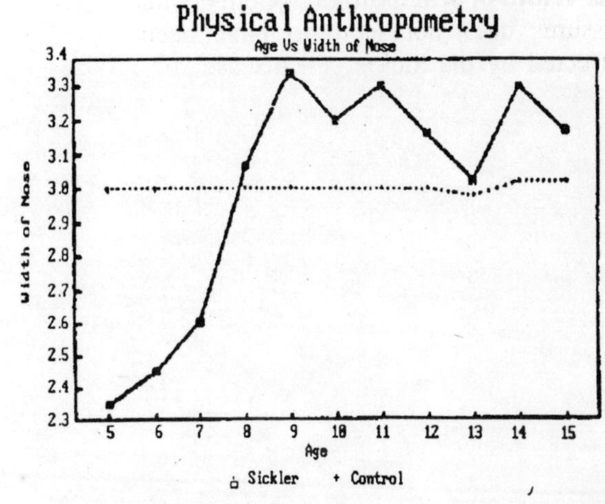

10. Length of Philtrum : The impact of the Sickle cell disease seems to be growth retardation on the children of all the three age groups. The differences are observed to be statistically significant. The impact of the disease appears to be more on the children of the age group 10-15 years.

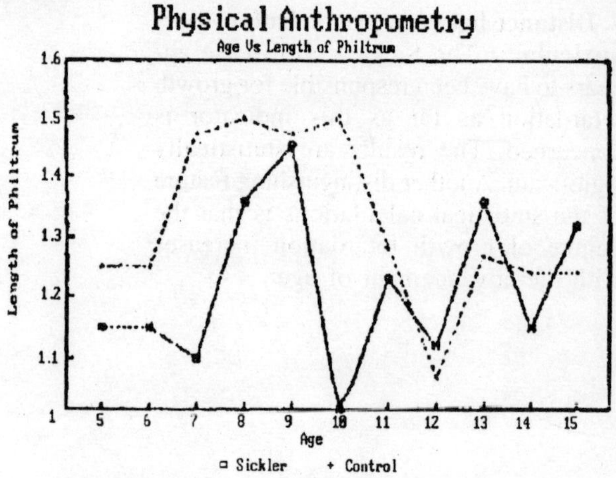

11. Length of Chin : The impact of the disease on the sicklers as far as the length of chin is concerned appears to be negligible on the children of all the age groups.

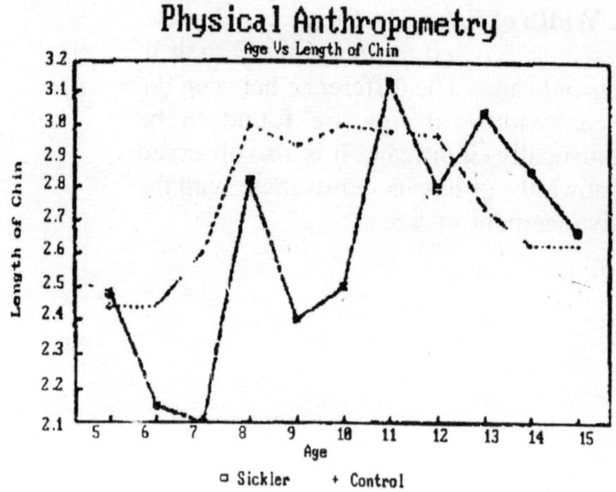

12. Width of oral fissures : Width of oral fissures does not seem to have been affected by the Sickle cell disease.

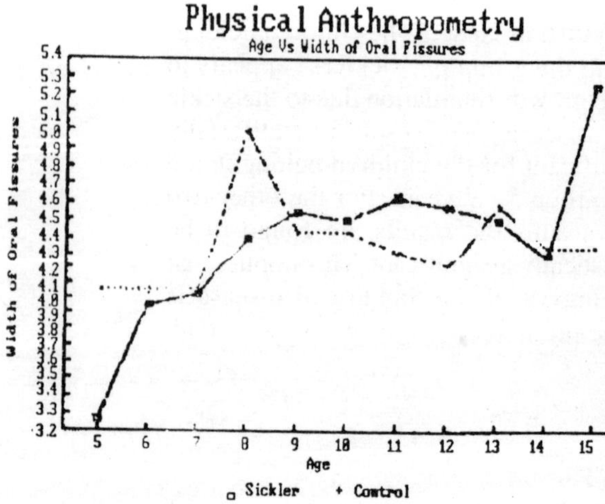

13. Angle of mandible to angle of mandible : This is one of those indicators where abnormal growth is observed due to the disease in the children of all the age groups. The abnormal growth is more visible during the early age group as is evident from the statistically significant results for the children of the age group 5-9. For the children of other two age groups, the results are statistically insignificant. The statistically significant results for the children of the age group 5-9 years may be able to identify the "sicklers" in the early age and for early medical treatment.

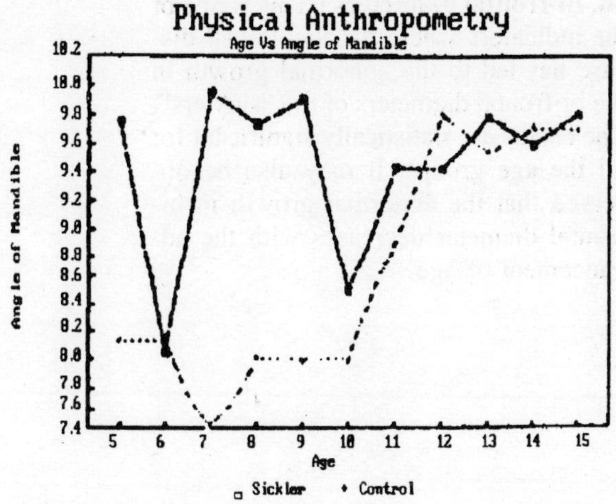

14. Bi-Mastoid diameter : The sickle cell disease seem to have led to growth-retardation of the sicklers of all the age groups. But the result is prominent in the age group 16-20 years.

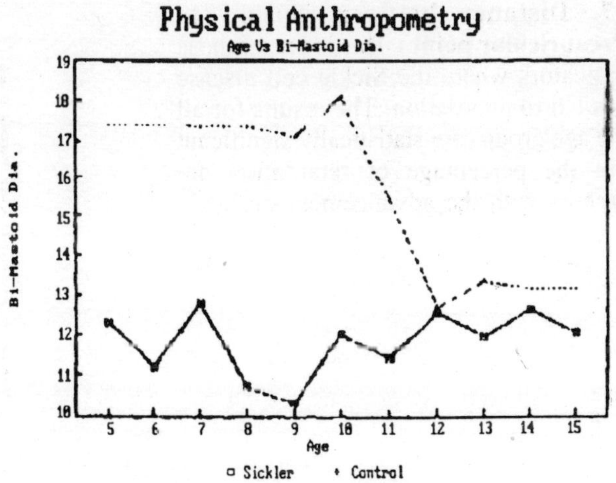

15. Bi-Temporal diameter : Bi-temporal diameter is one of those indicators where it appears, the Sickle cell disease has led to abnormal growth, to the extent of 39 percent, in the early age group. This is also evident from the student's T-test which is significant for the children of age group 5-9 years. The student's T-tests for the other two age groups are observed to be statistically insignificant implying that the difference between the bitemporal diameters of the children of the two age groups, "controlled" and "sicklers" are almost negligible.

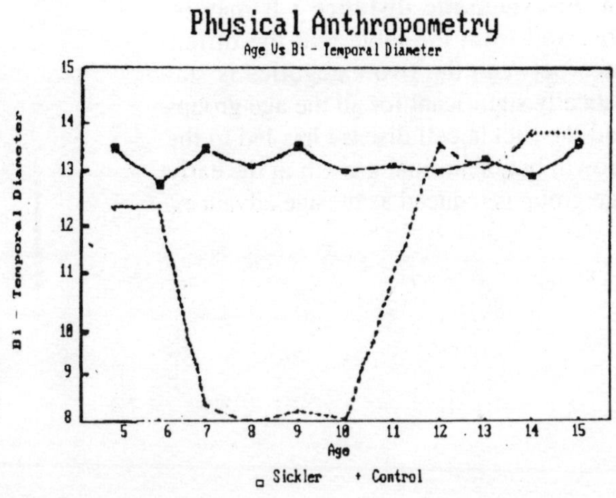

16. Bi-frontal diameters : This is one of the indicators where the Sickle cell disease has led to the abnormal growth in the bi-frontal diameters of the "sicklers". The results are statistically significant for all the age groups. It may also be observed that the abnormal growth in bi-frontal diameter decreases with the advancement of age.

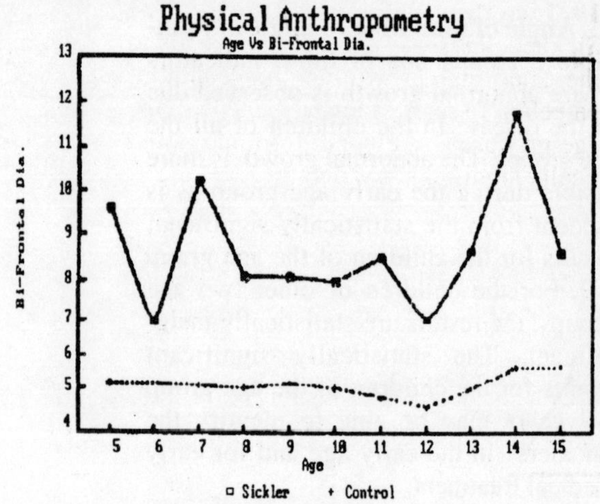

17. Distance between Nasion to Preauricular point : This is one of those indicators where the Sickle cell disease has led to retardation. The results for all the age groups are statistically significant but the percentage of retardation decreases with the advancement of age.

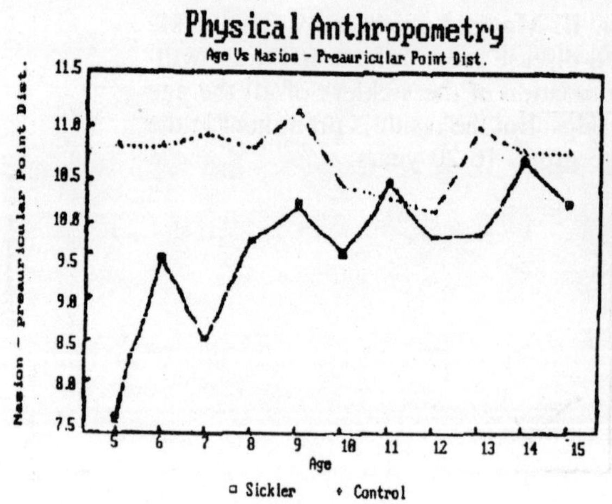

18. Bi-zygomatic distance : It may be observed from the table that the difference between the two categories is statistically significant for all the age groups and the Sickle cell disease has led to the growth but, abnormal growth in the early age group is reduced as the age advances.

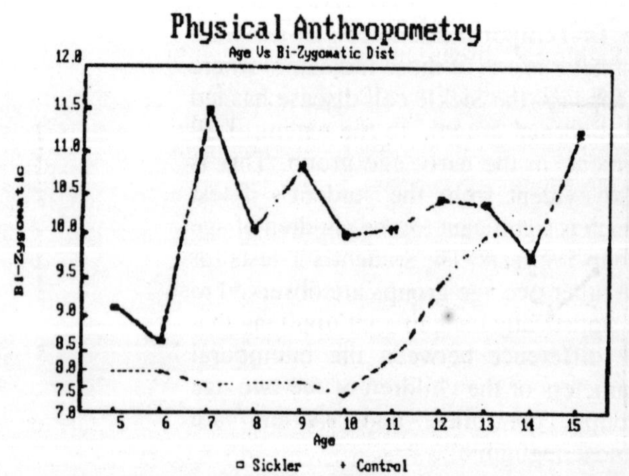

19. Length of Palpebral fissures : The Sickle cell disease appears to have led to the abnormal growth in the length of palpebral fissures of the sicklers of all the age groups, as is evident from the statistically significant results.

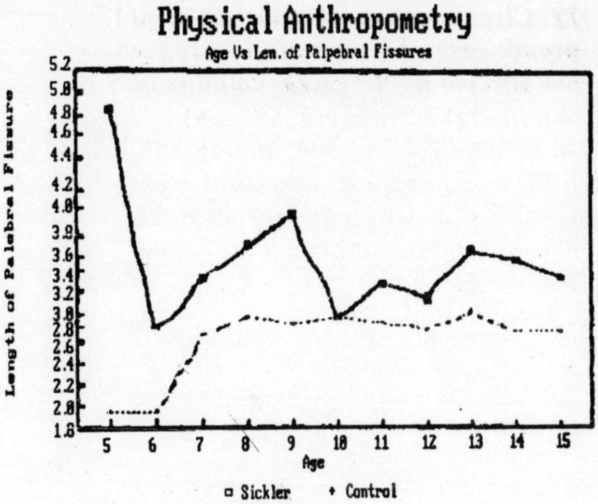

20. Nasion to Zygomatic distance : Nasion to zygomatic distance of the "sicklers" does not seem to have been affected by the sickle cell disease.

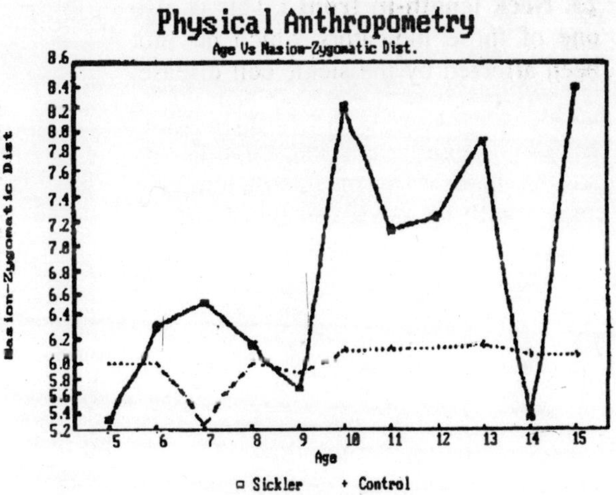

21. Inter-canthal distance inner : The Sickle cell disease appears to have led to the abnormal growth in the inter-canthal distance-inner of the "sicklers". The effect is more visible in the children of the age group 10-15 years.

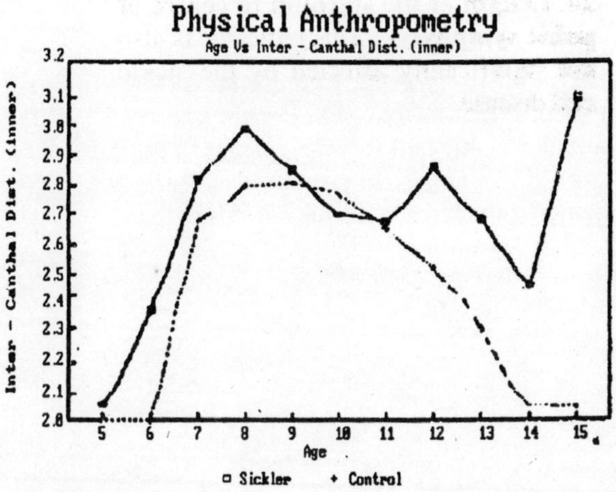

22. Circumference of neck at thyroid prominence : This appears to have been not affected by the Sickle cell disease.

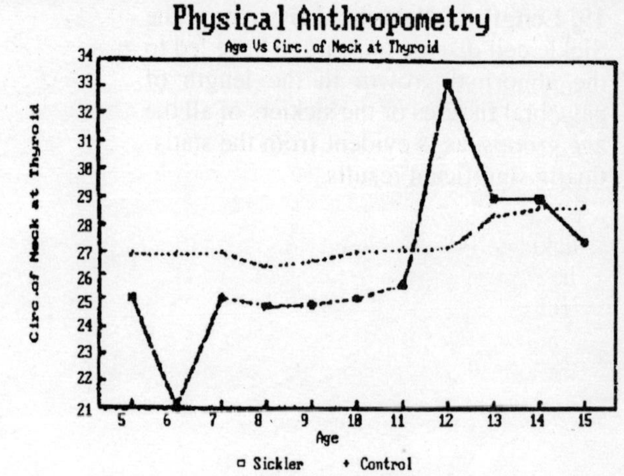

23. Neck length-in front : This is also one of those indicators which has not been affected by the sickle cell disease.

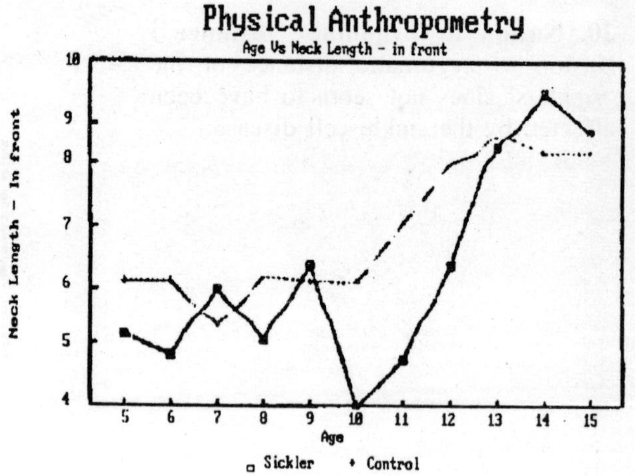

24. Length of the sternum to centre of pubic symphysis : This indicator is also not significantly affected by the sickle cell disease.

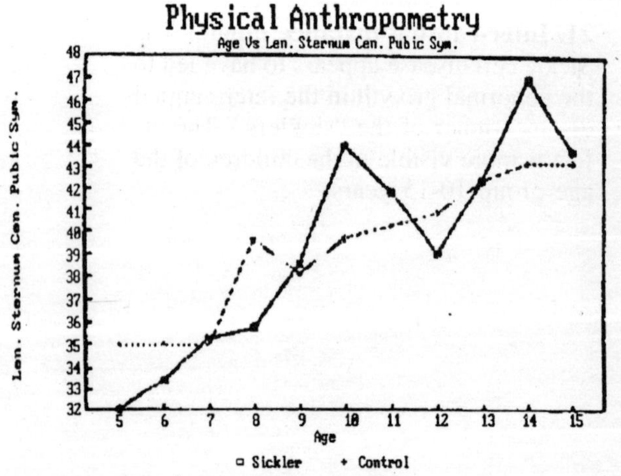

25. Xiphysternum to pubic symphysis: A somewhat curious result has been observed for this indicator. In the early age group, the disease has led to growth retardation as is evident from the statistically significant results for the children of the age group 5-9 years. After this, the sickle cell disease appears to have led to the abnormal growth in the other two age groups. The effect appears to be more pronounced in the age group 10-15 years and almost negligible in the age group 16-20 years.

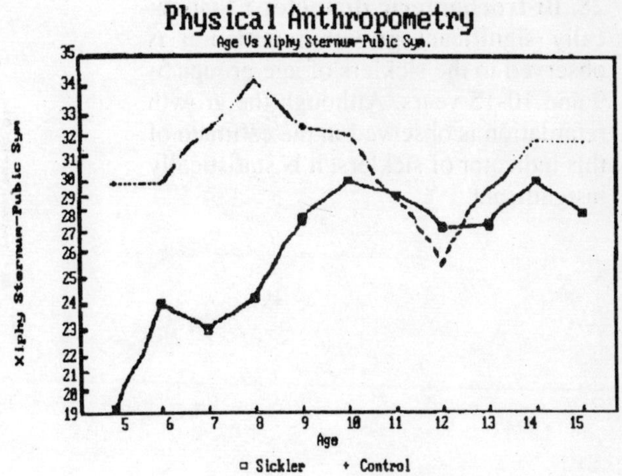

26. Xiphysternum to suprasternal border : As far as this indicator is concerned, there is growth retardation in all the age groups but the statistically significant growth retardation is observed in the sicklers of age group 16-20 years.

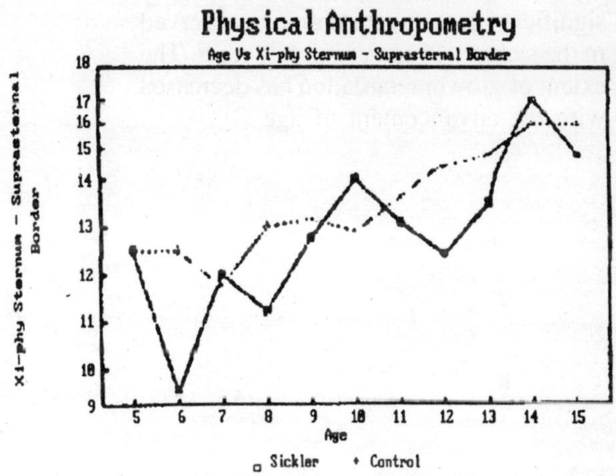

27. Bi-acromial diameter : Abnormal growth statistically significant is observed in the sicklers of age group 5-9 years. But this abnormal growth has not only reduced, but also there was a growth retardation with the advancement of age.

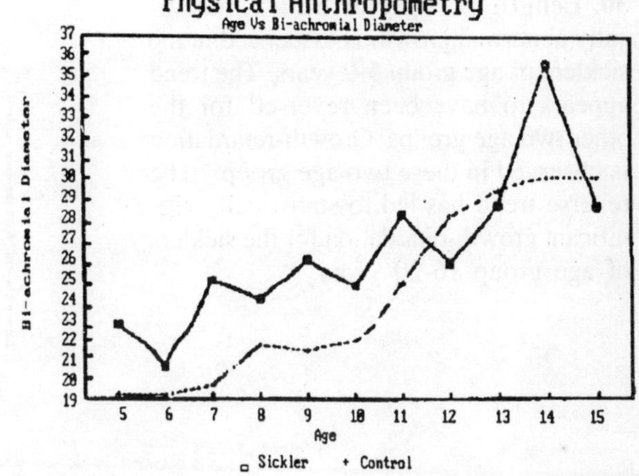

28. Bi-trochanteric diameter : Statistically significant growth retardation is observed in the sicklers of age groups 5-9 and 10-15 years. Although the growth retardation is observed in the estimate of this indicator of sicklers, it is statistically insignificant.

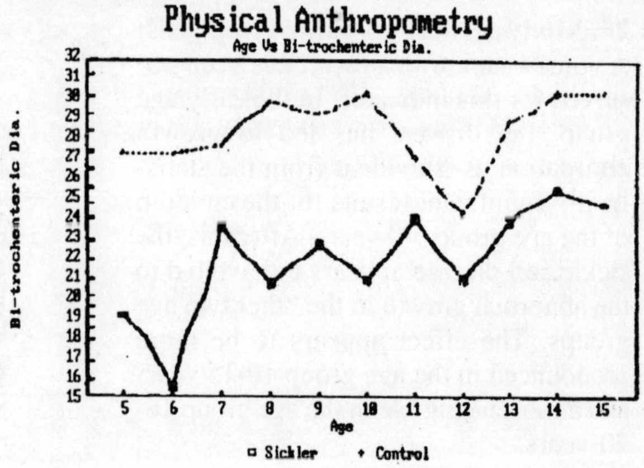

29. Interspinous diameter : Statistically significant growth retardation is observed in the sicklers of age group 5-9 years. The extent of growth retardation has decreased with the advancement of age.

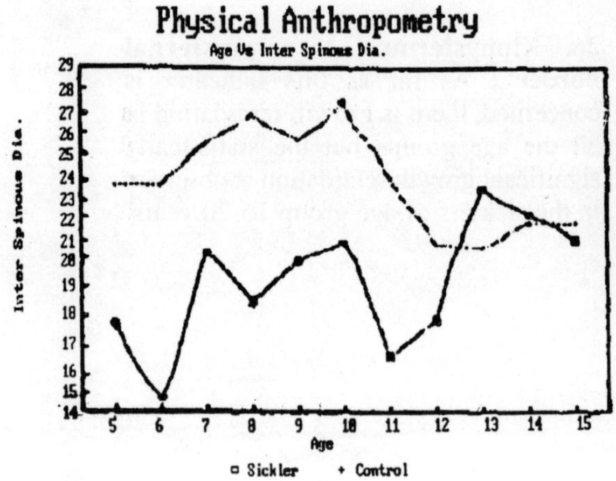

30. Length of superior limb : Statistically abnormal growth is evidenced in the sicklers of age group 5-9 years. The trend appears to have been reversed for the other two age groups. Growth-retardation is observed in these two age groups. The reverse trend has led to statistically significant growth-retardation for the sicklers of age group 16-20 years.

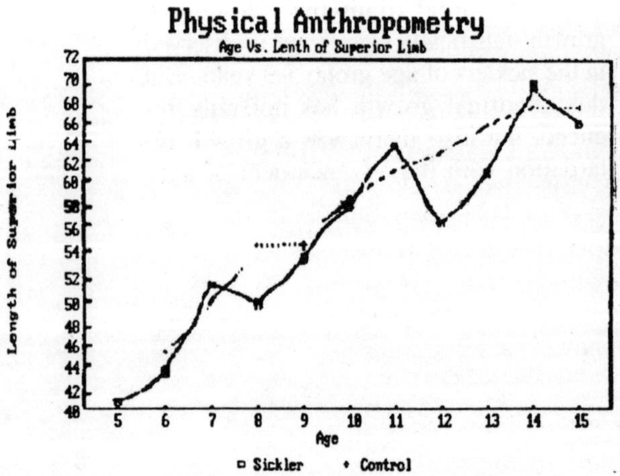

31. Length of Hand : Sicklers appear to have shorter hands as compared to the "Controlled" children. The results are statistically significant for sicklers of all the three age groups.

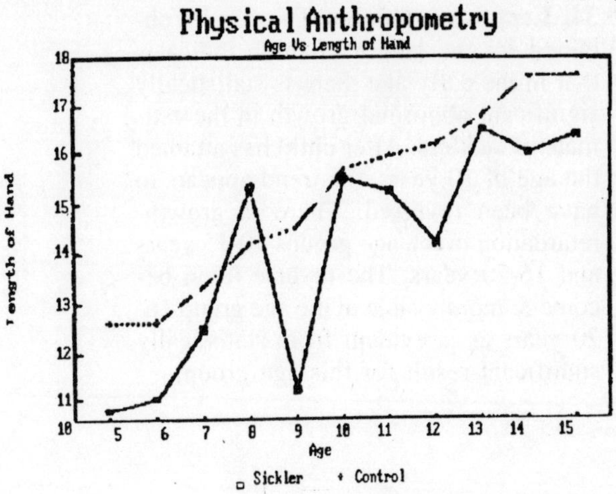

32. Length of Arm : Length of arm of the sicklers does not appear to have been significantly affected by the sickle cell disease. However, there is growth retardation in the length of arms of sicklers of all the three age groups.

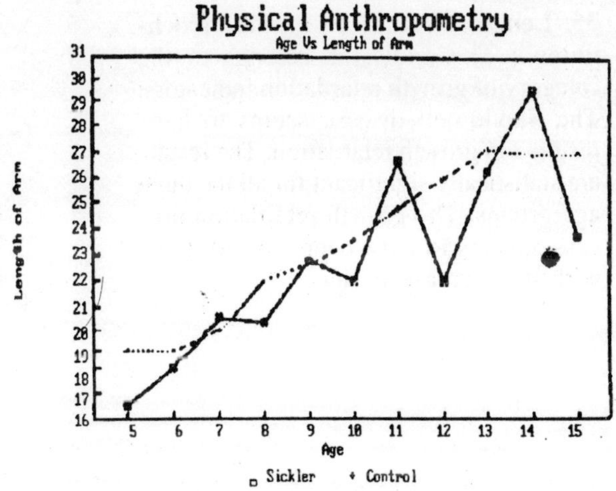

33. Length of Forearm : The Sickle-cell disease has led to growth-retardation in the length of forearm of the sicklers of all the three age groups. But the results are more pronounced in the age groups, 5-9 years and 10-15 years as may be evident from the statistically significant results for these two age groups. The growth-retardation is observed to be declining with the advancement of age.

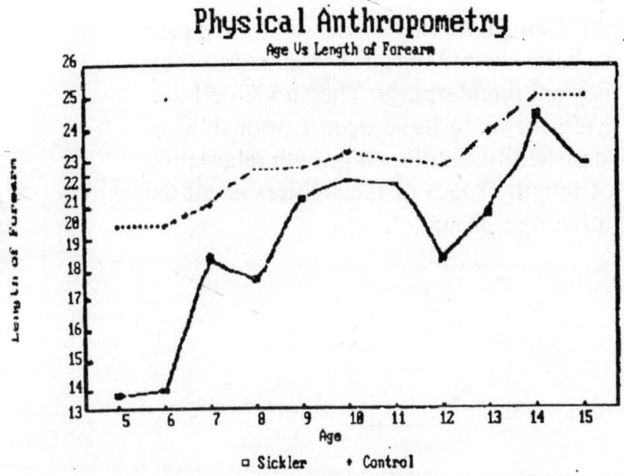

34. Length of Thigh : The results obtained for the length of thigh indicates that in the early age there is statistically significant abnormal growth in the estimate of sicklers. After child has attained the age of 10 years, the trend appears to have been reversed. There is growth-retardation in the age groups 10-15 years and 16-20 years. The reverse trend become & more visible in the age group 16-20 years as is evident from statistically significant result for this age group.

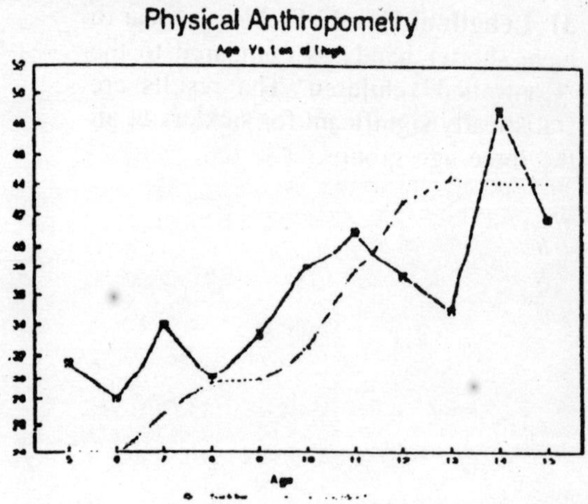

35. Length of ASIS to greater trochanter : This indicator belongs to the category of growth retardation indicators. The Sickle cell disease seems to have resulted in growth retardation. The results are statistically significant for all the three age groups. The growth retardation process appears to have been slowed down with the increase in age.

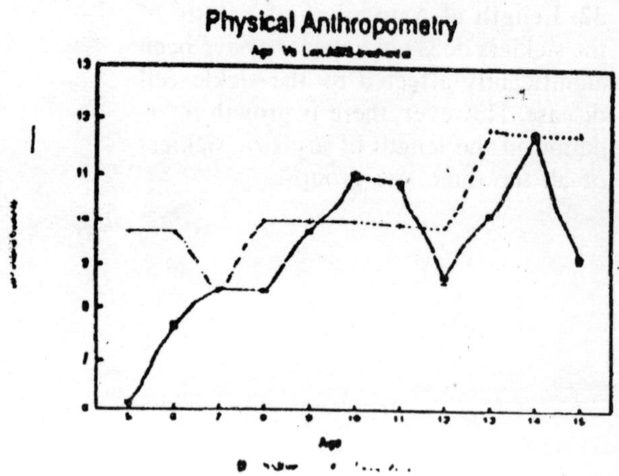

36. Length of Leg : The sicklers appear to have shorter legs as compared to their normal counterparts. The sickle cell disease seems to have been responsible of statistically significant growth retardation of length of legs of the sicklers of all the three age groups.

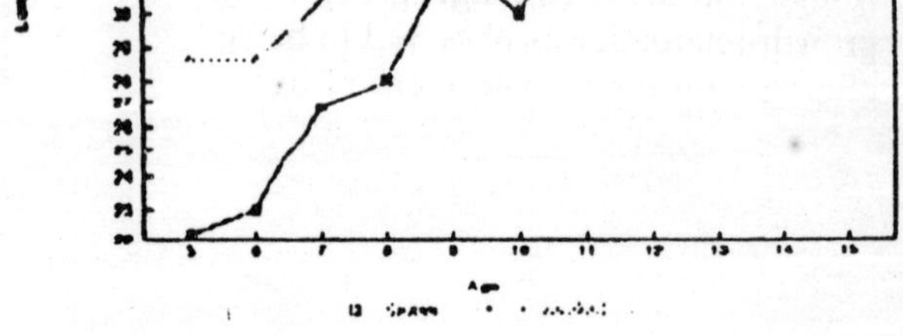

B. Facial Anthropometry

Facial Anthropometry (Fig. 16.1 and 16.2) plays an important role in the diagnosis of sicklers. The results of the quantitative measuresments, comparison between the sicklers and normal children are presented in the Table 16.2.

Table 16.4. Calculations for facial anthropometric data

Ind. No.	Name	Age group Group	Controlled Mean	Controlled SD	Sickler Mean	Sickler SD	t vdlue	% change	Remark
1	Distance between Inion and Nasion (Lat.)	05-09	2.91	.21	2.96	.34	-.51	1.72	
		10-15	2.97	.26	3.14	.44	-1.48	5.72	
2	Distance between Hairline to Chin	05-09	2.44	.25	2.85	.56	-2.58	16.80	
		10-15	2.55	.20	3.08	.33	-6.16	20.78	
3	Distance between Nasion-tip of the Nose (AP)	05-09	.77	.11	.82	.10	-1.58	6.49	
		10-15	.83	.09	.93	.11	-3.37	12.05	
4	Distance between Preauricular to Preauricular (AP)	05-09	.60	.15	2.14	.20	-26.00	256.67	
		10-15	1.75	.29	2.24	.28	-6.24	28.00	
5	Width of lower lips (AP)	05-09	.13	.08	.24	.05	-6.19	84.62	
		10-15	.18	.04	.29	.03	-12.26	61.11	
6	Width of Nose (AP)	05-09	.55	.07	.55	.07	00.00	00.00	
		10-15	.60	.05	.60	.10	00.00	00.00	
7	Length of Oral Fissure (AP)	05-09	.76	.09	.83	.12	-1.97	9.21	
		10-15	.82	.06	.97	.14	-4.19	18.29	
8	Angle of Mandible to angle of Mandible (AP)	05-09	1.27	.25	1.66	.23	-5.37	30.71	
		10-15	1.44	.13	1.76	.18	-6.70	22.22	
9	Bi-Frontal distance (AP)	05-09	1.77	.17	1.62	.25	2.05	-8.47	
		10-15	1.85	.12	1.76	.22	1.58	-4.86	
10	Distance between Nasion to Pre-auricular (Lat)	05-09	1.41	.18	1.32	.17	1.69	-6.38	
		10-15	1.38	.14	1.23	.15	3.63	-10.87	
11	Bi-Zygomatic distance (Intermaxillary AP)	05-09	1.20	.16	1.71	.19	-8.92	42.50	
		10-15	1.33	.12	1.74	.22	-7.20	30.83	
12	Nasion to Zygomatic distance (AP)	05-09	.63	.06	1.02	.07	-18.46	61.90	
		10-15	.78	.07	1.05	.17	-6.23	34.62	
13	Inter Inner Canthal distance (AP)	05-09	.44	.06	.58	.08	-5.91	31.82	
		10-15	.49	.05	.58	.08	-4.30	18.37	
14	Inter Outer Canthal distance (AP)	05-09	1.47	.18	1.83	.16	-7.07	24.49	
		10-15	1.52	.08	1.90	.19	-7.83	25.00	
15	Length of Ear (Lat.)	05-09	.91	.10	.97	.11	-1.79	6.59	
		10-15	.99	.06	1.06	.21	-1.32	7.07	
16	Width of Ear (Lat.)	05-09	.50	.07	.51	.07	-.46	2.00	
		10-15	.51	.04	.52	.06	-.63	1.96	
17	Length of Hair line to Nasion (AP)	05-09	.90	.17	1.14	.21	-3.82	26.67	
		10-15	.81	.10	1.09	.19	-5.71	34.57	
18	Chin to angle of Mandible (Lat.)	05-09	1.01	.06	1.02	.10	-.35	.99	
		10-15	1.05	.10	1.08	.14	-.81	2.86	

1. Distance between Inion and Nasion (lat.) : The Sickle-cell disease does not seem to have affected the "Sicklers" as is evident from the statistically insignificant results for both the age-groups.

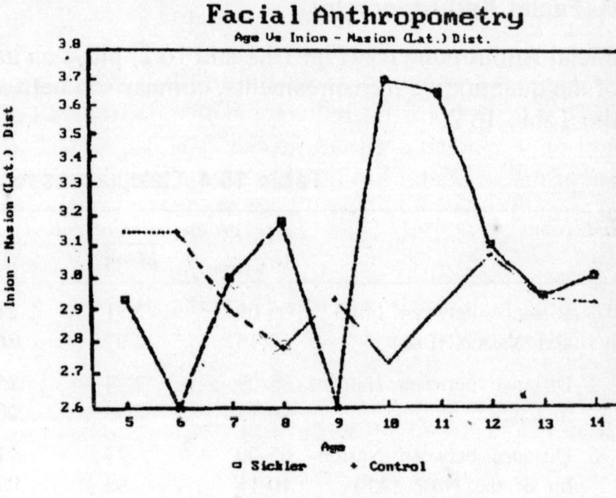

2. Distance Between Hair-line to chin: The Sickle cell disease appears to have affected the sicklers in both the age groups. This is obvious from the statistically significant results. The disease appears to have led to the abnormal growth.

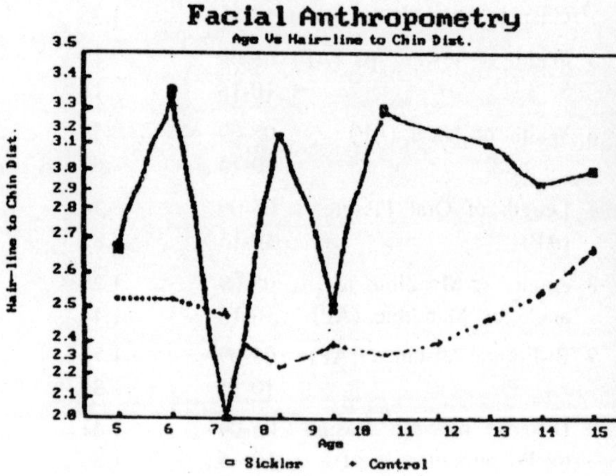

3. Distance Between the Nasion-tip of the Nose (AP) : The sicklers seem to have been led to abnormal growth in the estimates of this indicator in the later age group. This is evident from the statistically significant result for both the age-groups. The abnormal growth in the mean value of the indicator is observed to increase with the advancement of age.

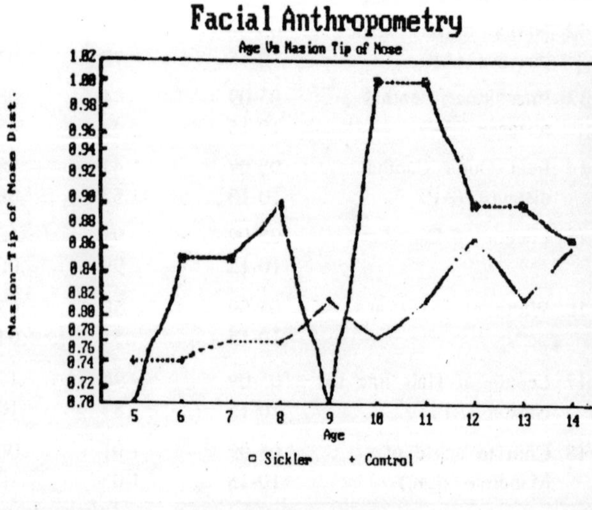

4. Distance Between Preauricular to preauricular (AP) : The Sickle-cell disease appears to have to made the most significant impact on this indicator. There is not only abnormal growth in the estimate of this indicator but also the abnormal growth is highly significant (upto 273.33 percent) in the age group of 10-15 years. This results is in time with the corresponding result observed in the physical Anthropometry.

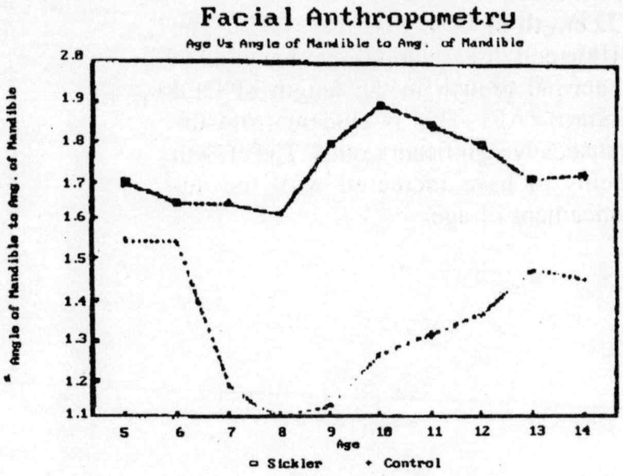

5. Width of Lower Lips (AP) : Width of Lower Lips of the sicklers seems to have grown abnormally. The abnormal growth in the width of the sicklers is found to be statistically significant.

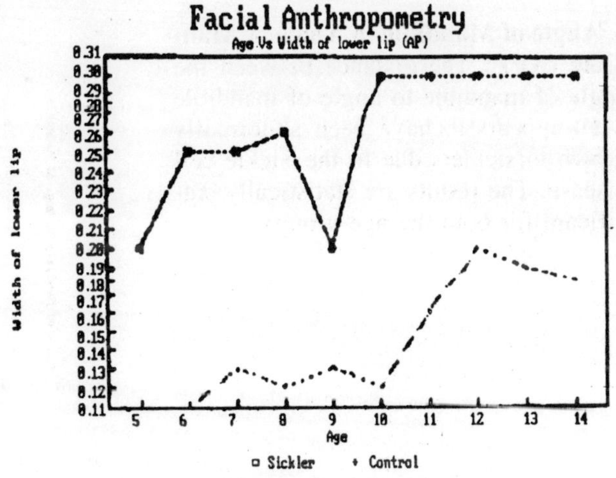

6. Width of Nose (AP) : Width of Nose (AP) does not seem to have affected by the disease as may be seen from the Table 16.4 and the Figs. 16.1, 16.2.

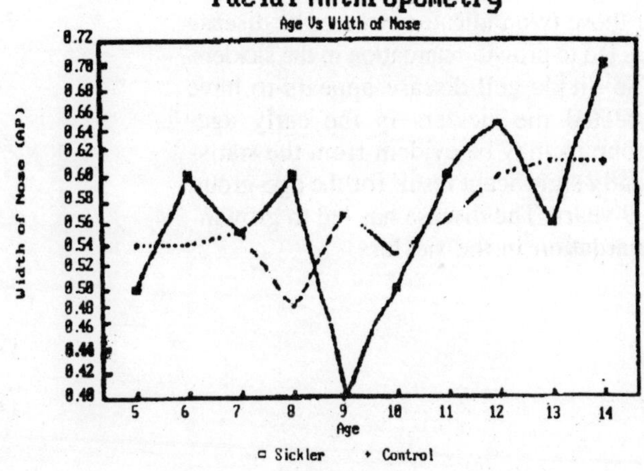

7. Length of Oral Fissures (AP) : The Sickle cell disease appears to have led to abnormal growth in the length of Oral fissures (AP). This is evident from the statistically significant results. The growth seems to have increased with the advancement of age.

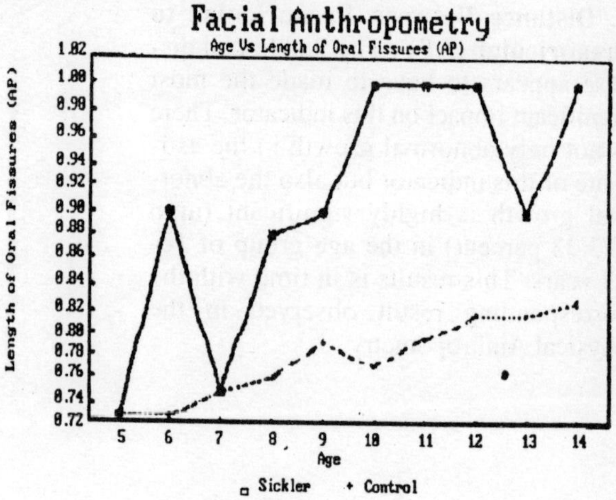

8. Angle of Mandible to Angle of Mandible (AP) : The distance between the angle of mandible to angle of mandible (AP) appears to have been abnormally grown in sicklers due to the Sickle cell disease. The results are statistically significant for both the age-groups.

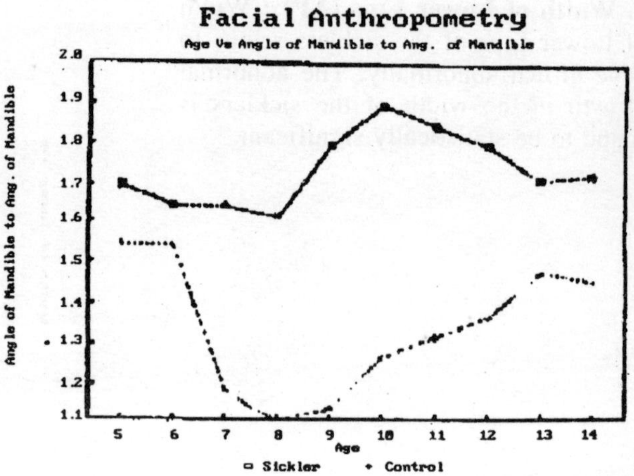

9. Bifrontal distance (AP) : This is one of those two indicators where the disease has led to growth-retardation in the sicklers. The Sickle cell disease appears to have affected the sicklers in the early age-group as may be evident from the statistically significant result for the age-group 5-9 years. The disease has led to growth-retardation in the sicklers.

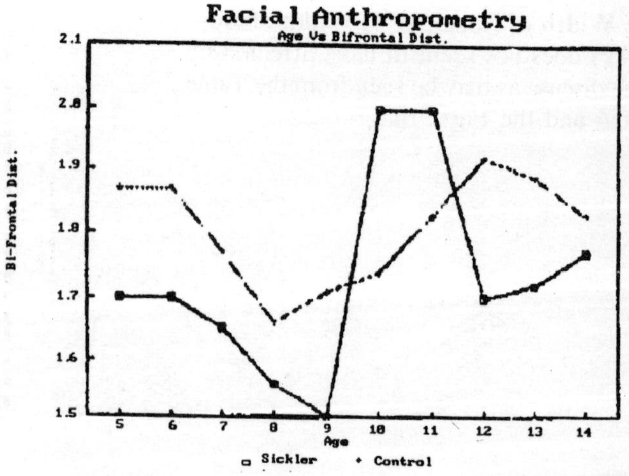

10. Distance Between Nasion to Pre-auricular (Lat.) : This is another indicator where the Sickle cell disease has led to growth retardation in the early age group of the sicklers.

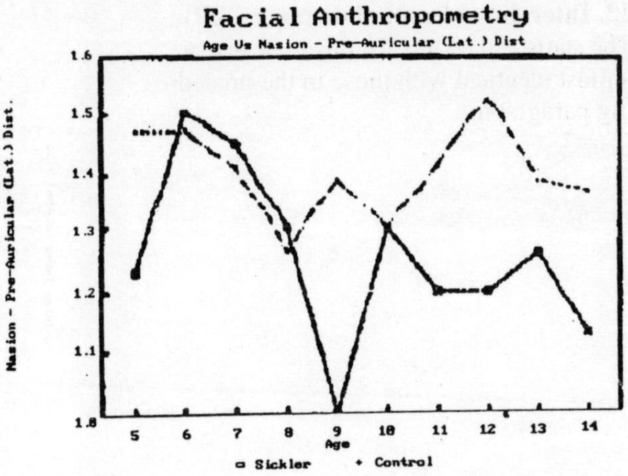

11. Bi-Zygomatic distance (Inter-maxillary AP) : The Sickle-cell disease appears to have led to the statistically significant abnormal growth in both the age groups,

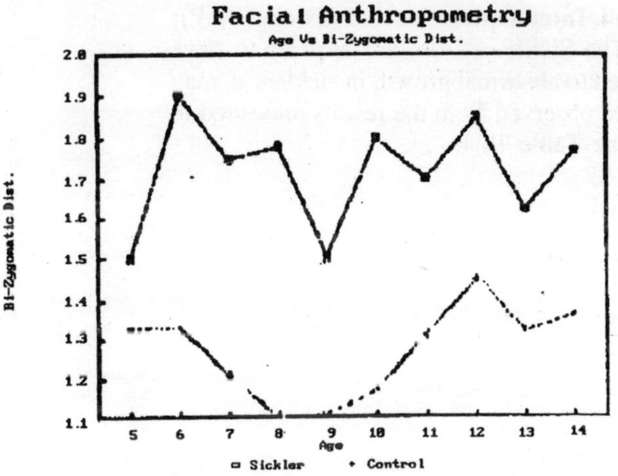

12. Nasion to Zygomatic distance (AP): The abnormal growth in Nasion to Zygomatic distance (AP), due to Sickle cell disease, appears to be statistically significant for both age-groups but more so in the early age-group.

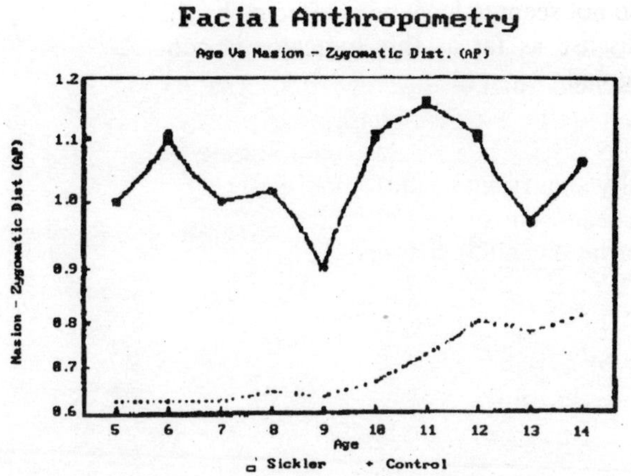

13. Inter-Inner canthal distance (AP) : The statistical results for this indicator are almost identical with those in the preceding paragraph.

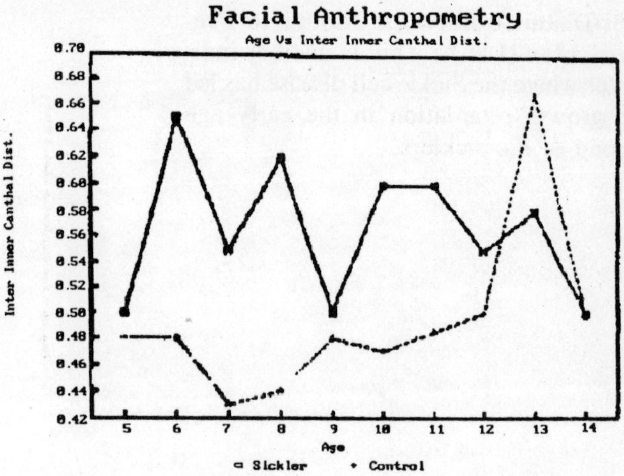

14. Inter-Outer Canthal distance (AP): The Sickle-cell disease appears to have led to abnormal growth in sicklers as may be observed from the results presented in the Table 16.4.

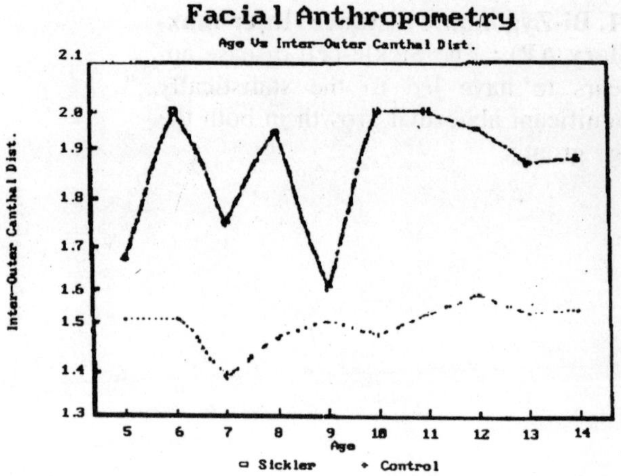

15. Length of Ear (Lat.) : The sicklers do not seem to have been affected by the disease as far as this indicator is concerned.

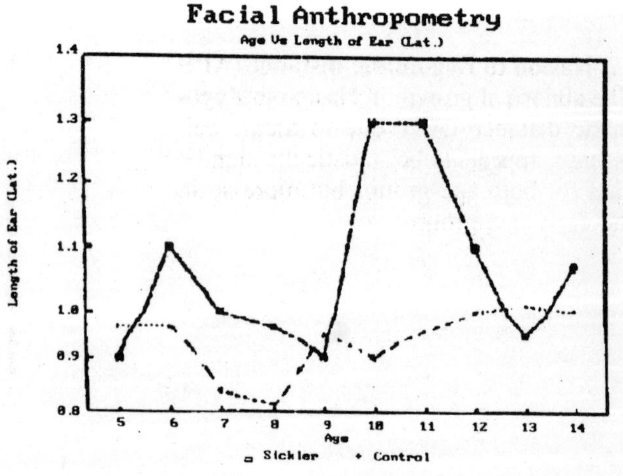

16. Width of Ear (Lat.) : Like the length of Ear (Lat.), the width of Ear (Lat.) is also not affected by the Sickle-cell disease.

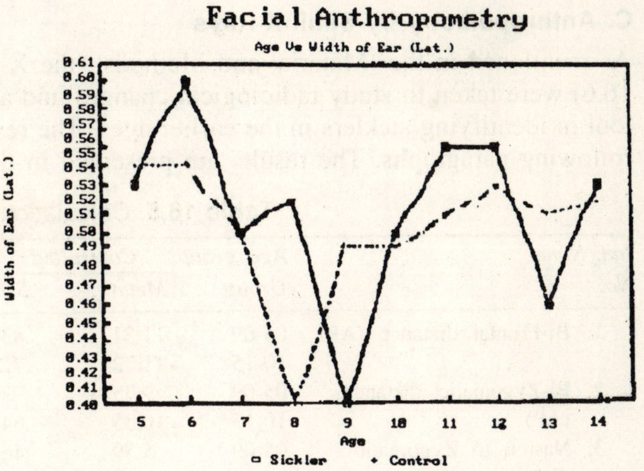

17. Length of Hair-line to Nasion (AP) : The Sickle cell disease, it appears has to led abnormal growth in the value of this indicator for sicklers irrespective of age.

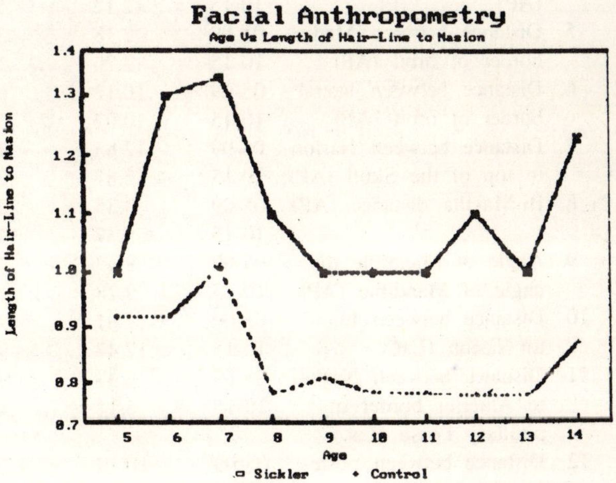

18. Chin to Angle of Mandible : The distance from Chin to angle of mandible does not seem to be affected by the Sickle-cell disease.

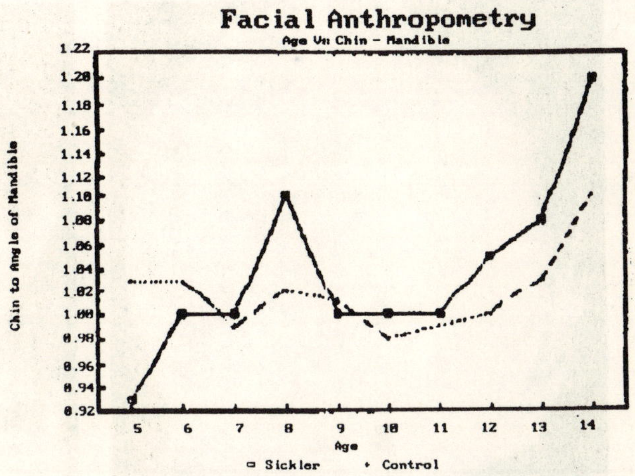

C. Anthropometry by Skull X-Rays

As mentioned in the 'Material and Methods', the X-rays of skull (AP & Lateral views, Figs. 16.5 and 16.6) were taken to study radiological changes and anthropometric measurements. This is an important tool in identifying sicklers in the earlier ages. The results based on the skull X-rays are presented in the following paragraphs. The results are presented in the Table 16.5.

Table 16.5. Calculations for skull X-ray data

Ind. No.	*Name*	*Age group Group*	*Controlled Mean*	*Controlled SD*	*Sickler Mean*	*Sickler SD*	*t value*	*% change*	*Remark*
1.	Bi-Frontal distance (AP)	05-09	11.31	.83	14.00	1.29	-5.72	23.78	
		10-15	11.72	.72	14.72	.81	-13.57	25.60	
2.	Bi-Zygomatic distance	05-09	9.75	.72	9.17	.53	2.73	-5.95	
	(AP)	10-15	10.35	.64	9.53	.89	3.47	-7.92	
3.	Nasion to Zygomatic	05-09	5.59	.46	5.39	.57	.95	-3.58	
	distance (AP)	10-15	6.31	.53	5.34	.61	5.85	-15.37	
4.	Nasion to Chin distance	05-09	10.20	.51	11.00	.88	-2.51	7.84	
	(AP)	10-15	12.12	.58	12.28	1.12	-.55	1.32	
5.	Distance between Medial	05-09	2.18	.32	2.67	.41	-3.23	22.48	
	border of orbit (AP)	10-15	2.76	.52	3.16	.42	-3.25	14.49	
6.	Distance between lateral	05-09	10.12	.64	10.00	.44	.67	-1.19	
	border of orbit (AP)	10-15	10.92	.89	11.00	.87	-.33	.73	
7.	Distance between Nasion	05-09	12.85	.71	11.72	1.16	2.68	-8.79	
	to top of the Skull (AP)	10-15	12.87	.78	12.25	1.29	1.84	-4.82	
8.	Bi-Maxilla distance (AP)	05-09	3.35	.23	3.56	.44	-1.32	6.27	
		10-15	3.37	.42	3.14	.43	1.93	-6.82	
9.	Angle of Mandible to	05-09	8.43	.71	8.22	.63	.86	-2.49	
	angle of Mandible (AP)	10-15	9.28	1.11	9.34	1.70	-.13	.65	
10.	Distance between Inion	05-09	17.81	.95	16.72	1.60	1.88	-6.12	
	to Nasion (Lat.)	10-15	17.47	.96	17.69	.93	-.84	1.26	
11.	Distance between Nasion	05-09	6.37	.94	5.67	.41	3.59	10.99	
	to Anterior border of pituitary Fossa (Lat.)	10-15	6.11	.49	5.97	.48	1.04	-2.29	
12.	Distance between posterior border of pituitary	05-09	10.19	1.10	9.78	.95	1.11	-4.02	
	Fossa to Inion (Lat.)	10-15	10.28	.91	10.34	.78	-.27	.58	

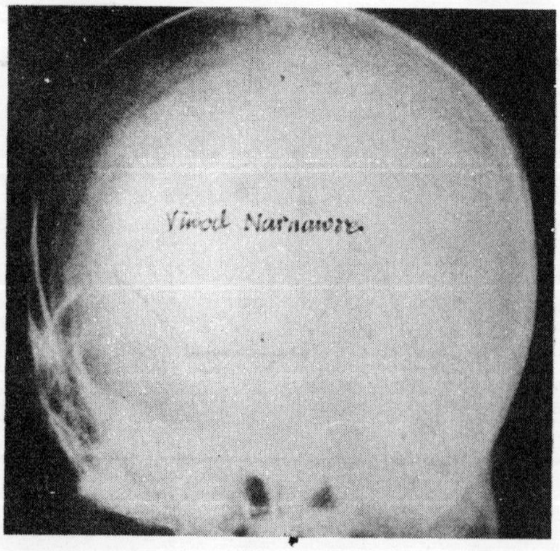

Fig. 16.5

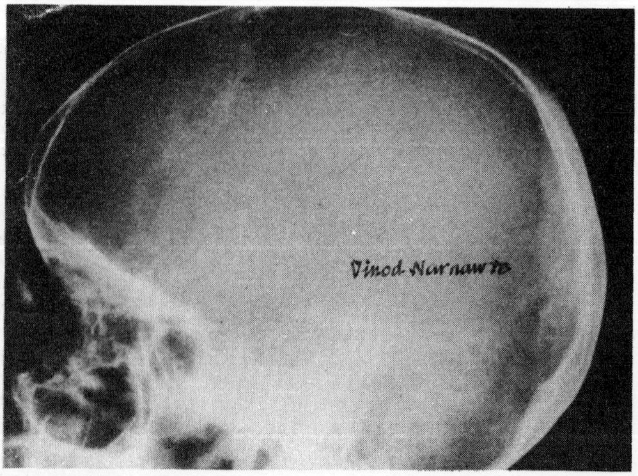

Fig. 16.6

Fig.16.5 & 16.6. X-ray skull Anteroposterior and lateral views of a young sickler child showing widening of diploe for different measurements of Anthropometry.

1. Bi-frontal distance (AP) : The sicklers seem to have been led to abnormal growth in the estimate of this indicator. The statistical results are significant for both the age groups.

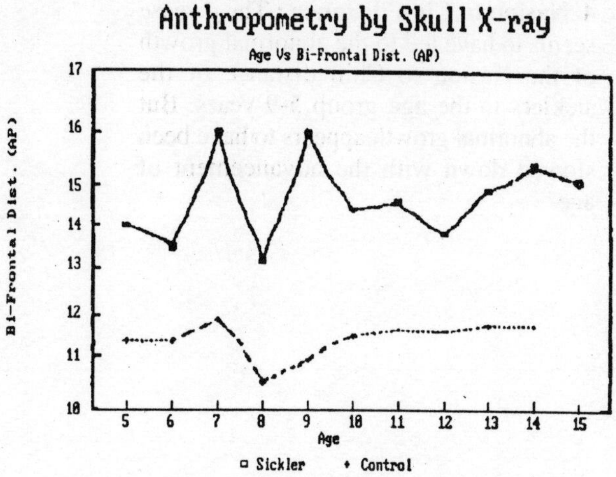

2. Bi-Zygomatic distance (AP) : The student's t-tests applied to test the reliability of the statistical results reveal that the difference between the Bi-Zygomatic distance (AP) of "Controlled" group children and the Bi-Zygomatic distance (AP) of the "Sicklers" are found to be statistically significant for both the age groups. This implies that the disease has led to growth retardation in the sicklers.

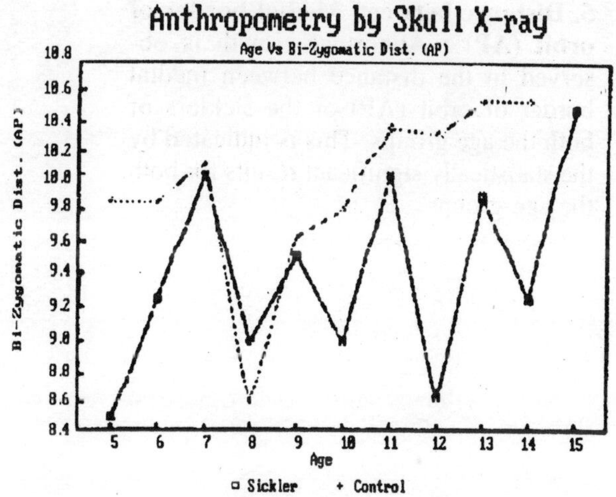

3. Nasion to Zygomatic distance (AP): The Sickle-cell disease seems to have led to growth-retardation of sicklers for this indicator, more so in the age group 10-15 years.

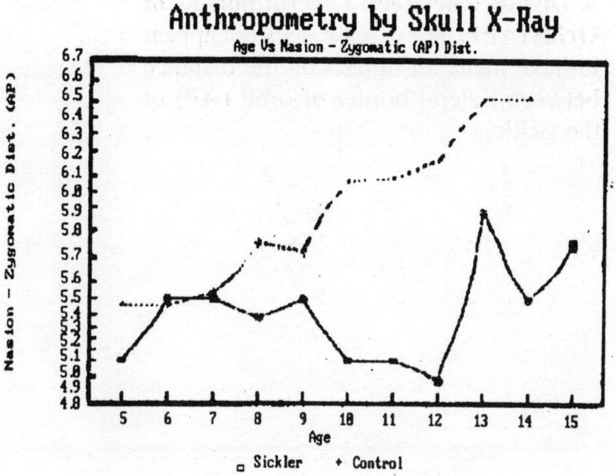

4. Nasion to Chin distance : The disease seems to have led to the abnormal growth of the Nasion to Chin distance of the sicklers in the age group 5-9 years. But the abnormal growth appears to have been slowed down with the advancement of age.

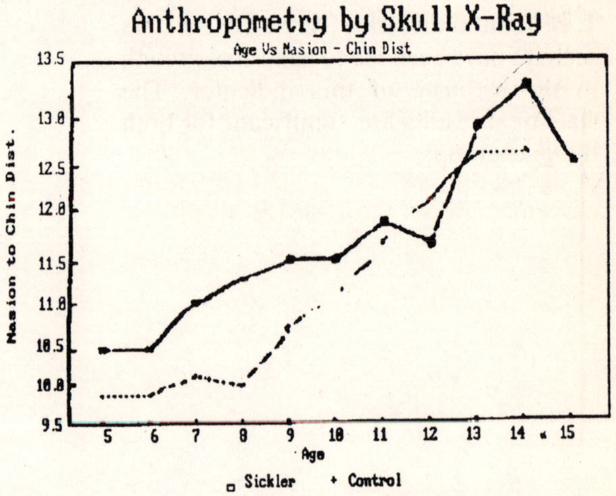

5. Distance between Medial border of orbit (AP) : Abnormal growth is observed in the distance between medial border of orbit (AP) of the sicklers of both the age groups. This is indicated by the statistically significant results for both the age-groups.

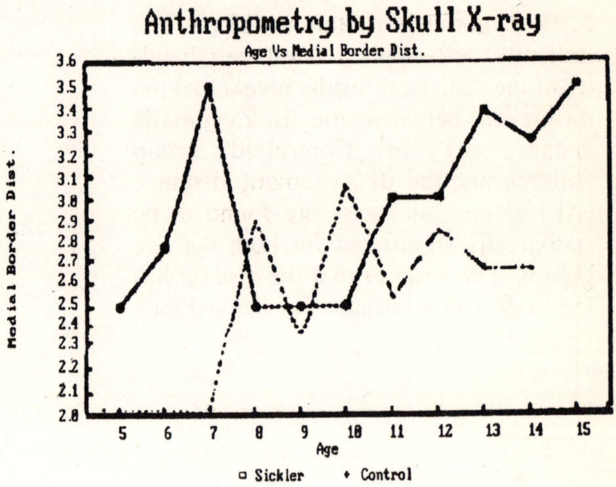

6. Distance between Lateral border of Orbit (AP) : The disease does not appear to have made an impact on the distance between Lateral border of orbit (AP) of the sicklers.

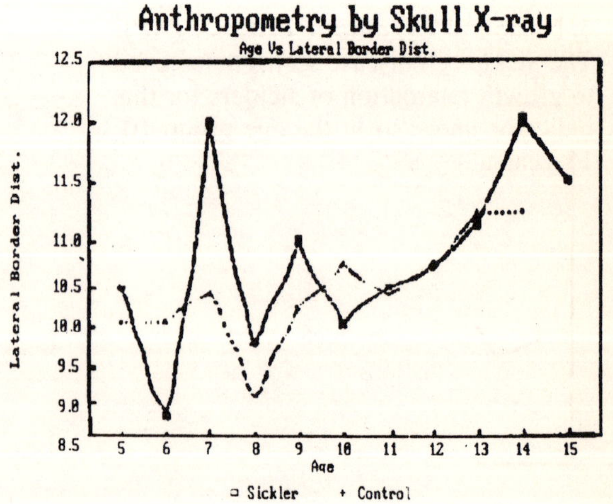

7. Distance between Nasion to the Top of Skull : The Sickle-cell disease appears to name resulted in the growth- retardation of the sicklers as far as this indicator is concerned. The statistically significant results has been observed for the sicklers of age-group 5-9 years. Afterwards, the movement of growth-retardation appears to be slowed down.

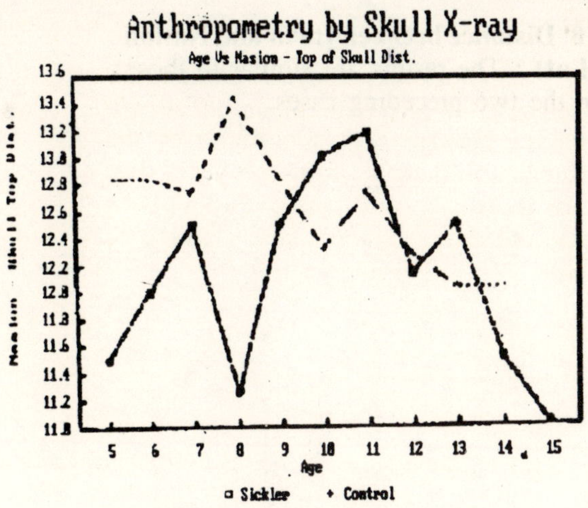

8. Bi-Maxilla distance (AP) : This does not appear to have been affected by the distance.

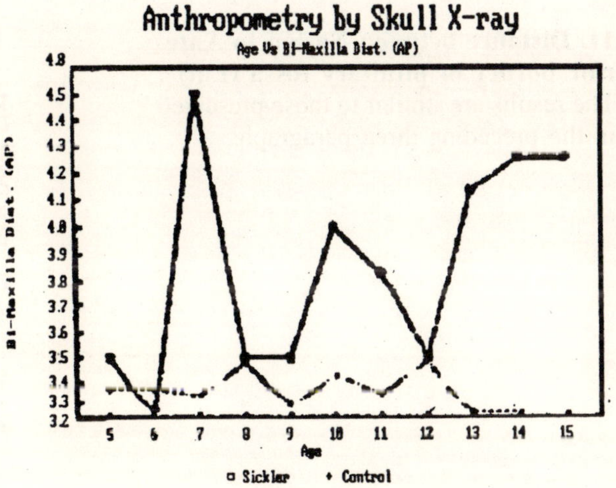

9. Angle of Mandible to Angle of Madible (AP) : The statistical results for this indicator are similar to those in case of Bi-Maxilla distance (AP).

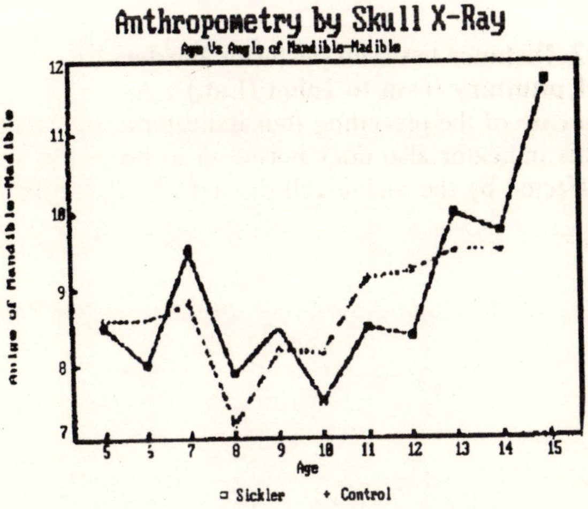

10. Distance between Inion and Nasion (Lat) : The results are similar to those in the two preceding cases.

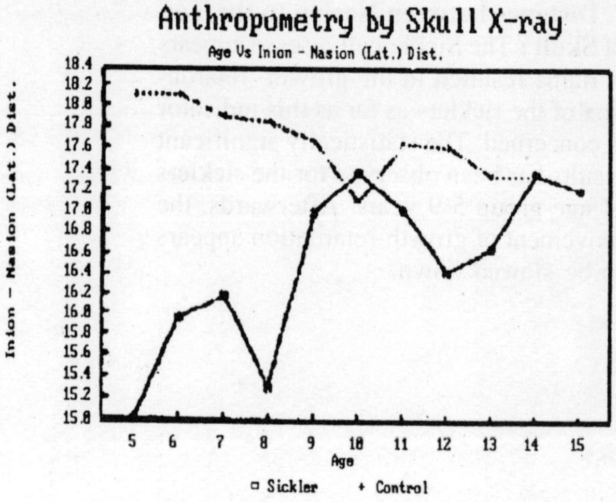

11. Distance between Nasion to Anterior border of pituitary fossa (Lat) : The results are similar to those presented in the preceding three paragraphs.

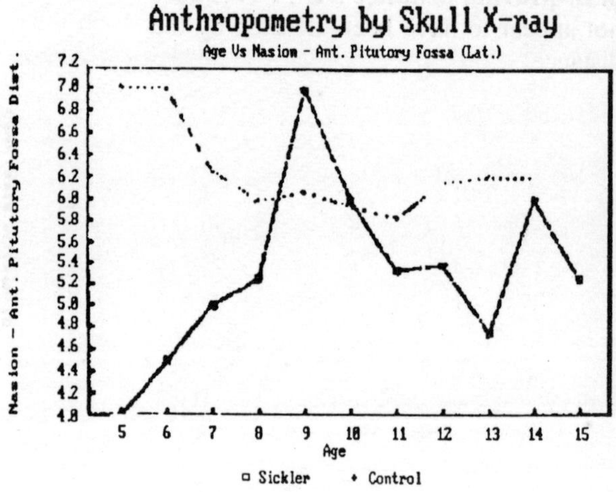

12. Distance between posterior border of pituitary fossa to Inion (Lat.) : As in case of the preceding four indicators, this indicator also does not seem to be affected by the Sickle-cell disease.

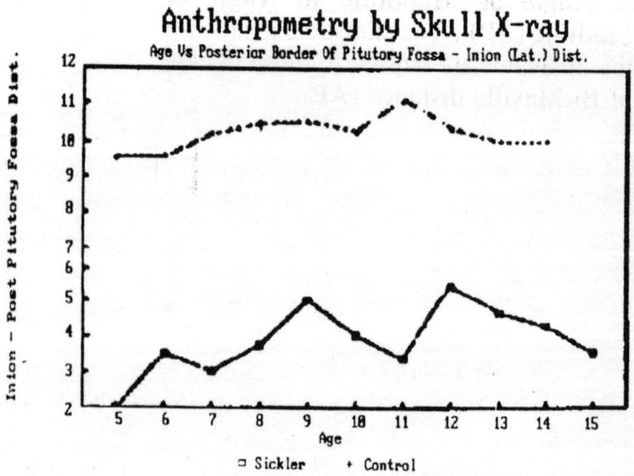

D. Indices

Various indices are calculated for the children of "Controlled" and "Sicklers" groups and compared. The results are presented in Table 16.6.

Table 16.6. Indices of indicators

Age Group	*Controlled*	*Sickler*
1. 100 × Weight/Height		
05-09	17.40	13.28
10-15	24.17	21.34
16-20	28.37	26.94
2. 100 × Bi-Mastoid diameter/Circumference of the Head		
05-09	26.02	24.89
10-15	26.56	24.15
16-20	33.14	24.80
3. 100 × Bi-Temporal diameter/Circumference of the Head		
05-09	18.51	28.32
10-15	24.41	26.60
16-20	27.48	27.16
4. 100 × Bi-Frontal diameter/Circumference of the Head		
05-09	9.84	19.04
10-15	9.91	16.56
16-20	10.59	13.82
5. 100 × Length of Leg/Length of Superior Limb		
05-09	77.97	55.47
10-15	56.32	54.07
16-20	54.76	52.60
6. 100 × Length of Arm/Length of Thigh		
05-09	76.35	62.03
10-15	62.38	60.13
16-20	60.89	61.12
7. 100 × Length of Forearm/Length of Leg		
05-09	67.74	63.25
10-15	65.71	61.73
16-20	61.73	60.94
8. 100 × (Length of Thigh + length of Leg)/Length of Superior Limb (both)		
05-09	146.68	121.36
10-15	121.29	120.37
16-20	120.83	118.14

These indices may be considered as the supporting evidence for the statistical results furnished in the earlier paragraphs.

For the first index, the ratio of weight to height multiplied by 100, it may be noted that the indices for sicklers of all the three age-groups are less than the corresponding indices for the children of "Controlled" age-groups.

For the second index, the ratio of Bi-mastoid diameter to Circumference of the head multiplied by 100, the results are similar to those in the preceding paragraphs.

For the third index, the ratio of Bi-temporal diameter to Circumference of the head multiplied by 100, the indices for the sicklers are greater than the corresponding indices for the children of "Controlled" groups. This is obvious from the fact that the Sickle-cell disease has led to abnormal growth of Bi-temporal diameter but in case of circumference of the head, there is growth retardation.

The results for the fourth index, the ratio of Bi-frontal diameter to Circumference of head multiplied by 100, are similar to those in the preceding paragraph.

The ratio of length of leg to length of superior limb multiplied by 100, the fifth index, is observed to be less for the sicklers as compared to the corresponding index for the "Controlled" group children.

The indices for the sicklers are observed to be less for the sicklers than the corresponding indices of the "Controlled" group children in respect of the following indices also

(i) 100 × length of arm / length of thigh ;
(ii) 100 × length of forearm / length of leg ; and
(iii) 100 × (length of thigh + length of leg)/length of superior limb (both)

E. Observations

From the foregoing statistical analyses for the various indicators of Physical Anthropometry, Facial Anthropometry and Anthropometry by Skull X-Rays, it is possible to identify the indicators where either growth-retardation or abnormal growth takes place in the parameter values of the indicators. The identification of statistically significant indicators may be of help in the diagnosis of the sicklers.

It has already been noted that the Sickle-cell disease has two types of effects

1. Growth - Retardation; and
2. Abnormal Growth.

1. Growth-Retardation

The statistical analysis, presented earlier for the Physical Anthropometric measurements, reveals that there are 18 indicators where statistically significant growth-retardation is the result of the Sickle-cell disease. These are presented, age-group wise, in the Table 16.7, where a * (star) denotes that the disease has a significant impact in an age-group and a dash (-) indicates that the impact is negligible.

Similar results for Facial Anthropometry and Anthropometry by Skull X-Rays are furnished in Table 16.8 and Table 16.9 respectively.

Table 16.7. Physical anthropometry indicators : Statistically significant growth-retardation

S. No.	*Name of the Indicator*	*Age Group*		
		5-9	*10-15*	*16-20*
1.	Weight	*	*	-
2.	Height	*	*	-
3.	Circumference of head	*	*	-
4.	Distance between Inion and Nasion	-	-	*
5.	Distance between Hair line — Chin	*	*	-
6.	Distance between Preauricular — Preauricular	-	*	*
7.	Width of the Nose	*	-	-
8.	Length of Philtrum	-	*	*
9.	Angle of Mandible to Angle of Mandible	*	-	-
10.	Bi-Mastoid diameter	*	-	-

(Contd.)

S. No.	Name of the Indicator	Age Group		
		5-9	10-15	16-20
11.	Distance between Nasion to Preauricular point	-	-	-
12.	Xiphy-sternum to Suprasternal		-	-
13.	Bi-trochanteric diameter	*	*	-
14.	Inter spinous diameter	*	-	*
15.	Length of the Hand	-	*	*
16.	Length of Forearm	*	*	-
17.	Length of ASIS to greater trochanter	*	*	*
18.	Length of Leg	*	*	*

Table 16.8. Facial anthropometry indicators : Statistically significant growth retardation

S. No.	Name of the Indicator	Age Group	
		5-9	10-15
1.	Bi-Frontal Distance (AP)	*	-
2.	Distance Between Nasion to Pre-auricular (Lat.)	-	*

Table 16.9. Anthropometry by skull X-rays

S. No.	Name of the Indicator	Age Group	
		5-9	10-15
1.	Bi-Zygomatic Distance (AP)	*	*
2.	Nasion to Zygomatic Distance (AP)	-	*
3.	Distance between Nasion to Top of the Skull (AP)	-	-
4.	Distance between Nasion to Anterior border of pituitary fossa (Lat.)	*	-

2. Abnormal Growth

Statistical Analysis also evinced the abnormal growth in the indicator measurements of Physical Anthropometry, Facial Anthropometry and Anthropometry by Skull X-Rays. There are 7 indicators of Physical Anthropometry, 11 of Facial Anthropometry and only 3 of Anthropometry by Skull X-Rays which are observed to be the ones where the Sickle-cell disease has led to the abnormal growth.

The indicators where statistically significant abnormal growth is observed are depicted in the Table 16.10 for Physical Anthropometry, in the Table 16.11 for Facial Anthropometry and in the Table 16.12 for Anthropometry by Skull X-Rays.

Table 16.10. Physical anthropometry indicators : Statistically significant abnormal growth

S. No.	Name of the Indicator	Age Group		
		5-9	10-15	16-20
1.	Width of Lips both	*	*	*
2.	Angle of Mandible to angle of Mandible	*	-	-
3.	Bi-Temporal Diameter	*	-	-
4.	Bi-Frontal Diameter	*	*	*
5.	Bi-Zygomatic Distance	*	*	*
6.	Length of Palpebral Fissure	*	-	*
7.	Inter Canthal distance Inner	-	*	-

Table 16.11. Facial anthropometry indicators : Statistically abnormal growth

S. No.	*Name of the Indicator*	*Age Group* 5-9	10-15
1.	Distance between Hair line to Chin	*	*
2.	Distance between Nasion - Tip of Nose (AP)	-	*
3.	Distance between Pre-auricular to Pre-auricular (AP)	*	*
4.	Width of lower Lips (AP)	*	*
5.	Length of oral Fissure (AP)	-	*
6.	Angle of Mandible to angle of Mandible (AP)	*	*
7.	Bi-Zygomatic Distance Intermaxillary (AP)	*	*
8.	Nasion to Zygomatic Distance (AP)	*	*
9.	Inter-Inner Canthal Distance (AP)	*	*
10.	Inter-Outer Canthal Distance (AP)	*	*
11.	Length of Hair line to Nasion (AP)	*	*

Table 16.12. Anthropometry by skull X-rays : Statistically significant abnormal growth

S. No.	*Name of the Indicator*	*Age Group* 5-9	10-15
1.	Bi-Frontal Distance (AP)	*	*
2.	Nasion to Chin Distance (AP)	*	-
3.	Distance between Medial border of orbit (AP)	*	*

F. Statistical Analysis according to Sex

In the preceding paragraphs the statistical analysis of the combined sample (both males and females) are presented. With the objective to find out whether the Sickle cell disease affects the males and females in a similar way or in a different way, the statistical exercise has been repeated for the disaggregate samples of males and females. Tables 19.1 to 19.6 are given in the Annexure.

The results relate to:

1. Physical anthropometry;
2. Facial anthropometry; and
3. Skull X-ray anthropometric data.

1. Physical anthropometry

The results of the statistical calculations for the physical anthropometric data for males are presented in Table 19.1 and for the females in the Table 19.2.

A. Growth-Retardation

It may be observed from the tables that the statistically significant growth-retardation in the estimates of the following indicators of both the males and females, in all the three age-groups, is seen.

(i) Weight
(ii) Height
(iii) Distance between Pre-auricular to Pre-auricular
(iv) Length of Philtrum

(v) Distance between Nasion to Pre-auricular point
(vi) Length of ASIS to greater trochanter.

B. Abnormal Growth

This is observed in case of the following indicators for both the sexes and all the three age-groups.
(i) Width of Lips
(ii) Bi-Frontal diameter
(iii) Bi-Zygomatic distance

2. Facial anthropometry

The statistical results relating to the facial anthropometric data of males are depicted in the table 19.3 and of females in Table 19.4.

A. Growth-retardation

It may be observed from the statistical results presented in Table 19.3 for males that the Sickle cell disease has led to the growth retardation of the following indicators irrespective of age:
(i) Bi-frontal distance (AP); and
(ii) Distance between Nasion to Pre-auricular (Lat).

It may be observed from the Table 19.4 for females that the Sickle cell disease has led to growth retardation of the following indicator in all the age groups.

Distance between Nasion to Preauricular (Lat.)

In addition to the above inferences, it may also be noted that although the Sickle cell disease has led to growth retardation of the estimates of the indicators mentioned above, the results are statistically insignificant. Thus, it may be inferred that the growth retardation in the indicators of both males and females are negligible.

B. Abnormal Growth

Males: Abnormal growth in the following indicators of males can be observed from the Table 19.3.
(i) Distance between Inion and Nasion (Lat.);
(ii) Distance between hair-line to chin;
(iii) Distance Between Nasion-tip of the nose;
(iv) Distance between Pre-auricular to Pre-auricular (AP)
(v) Width of lower lips (AP);
(vi) Length of Oral Fissures (AP);
(vii) Angle of mandible to Angle of Mandible (AP);
(viii) Bi-Zygomatic Distance (Intermaxillary AP);
(ix) Nasion to Zygomatic distance (AP);
(x) Inter-inner Canthal distance (AP);
(xi) Inter-outer Canthal distance (AP);
(xii) Length of Hair-line to Nasion (AP); and
(xiii) Chin to Angle of Mandible.

Out of the above indicators, the Sickle-cell disease has led to statistically significant abnormal growth of males in respect of the following indicators :
(i) Width of Lower Lips (AP) (age groups 5-9, 10-15 years) and
(ii) Nasion to Zygomatic distance (AP) (Age groups 5-9 years)

Females: The abnormal growth in the following indicators in respect of females may be observed from Table 19.4.

(i) Distance Between hair-line to chin
(ii) Distance between the Nasion-Tip of the Nose(AP);
(iii) Distance between Pre-auricular to Pre-auricular(AP);
(iv) Width of lower Lips(AP);
(v) Width of Nose(AP);
(vi) Length of Oral Fissure (AP);
(vii) Angle of Mandible to Angle of Mandible (AP);
(viii) By Zygomatic distance
(ix) Nasion to Zygomatic distance (AP);
(x) Inter-outer Canthal distance (AP);
(xi) Length of Ear (Lat.)
(xii) Width of Ear (Lat.); and
(xiii) Length of Hair-line to Nasion (AP).

Out of the above indicators for females, statistically significant abnormal growth is observed in respect of the following indicators :

(i) Width of lower Lips (AP) (age groups 5-9, 10-15);
(ii) Nasion to Zygomatic distance (AP) (age group 5-9 years); and
(iii) Length of Hairline to Nasion (AP).

3. Anthropometry by Skull X-rays

The statistical results for anthropometry by skull X-rays for male are presented in Table 19.5 and those for females in Table 19.6.

A. Growth retardation

Males: It may be observed from the Table 19.5 that the Sickle cell disease, has led to the growth-retardation in respect of the following indicators of males:

(i) Bi-Zygomatic distance (AP);
(ii) Nasion to Zygomatic distance (AP);
(iii) Distance between Lateral border of Orbit (AP);
(iv) Distance between Nasion to the top of Skull;
(v) Angle of Mandible to Angle of Mandible (AP);
(vi) Distance between Inion and Nasion (Lat);
(vii) Distance between Nasion to Anterior border of pituitary fossa (Lat);
(viii) Distance between posterior border of pituitary fossa to Inion (Lat).

It may also be observed from the Table 19.5 that the Sickle cell disease has significantly reduced the distance between posterior border of pituitary fossa to Inion (Lat.) of male children of all the age-groups.

Females: Growth-retardation in the following indicators of the female children may also be observed from Table 19.6:

(i) Bi-Zygomatic distance (AP);
(ii) Distance between Nasion to the top of Skull;
(iii) Distance between Inion and Nasion (Lat);

(iv) Distance between Nasion to Anterior border of pituitary fossa (Lat);

(v) Distance between posterior border of pituitary fossa to Inion (Lat).

As in the case of males, it may be observed that the Sickle cell disease has also led to statistically significant growth-retardation of distance between posterior border of pituitary fossa to Inion (Lat)of female children of all the age-groups.

B. Abnormal Growth

Males: It may be observed from Table 19.5 that the Sickle cell disease has led to the abnormal growth in the following indicators of the male children:

(i) Bi-frontal distance (AP);

(ii) Nasion to Chin distance;

(iii) Distance between Medial border of Orbit (AP);and

(iv) Bi-Maxilla distance (AP)

Out of the above indicators, the Sickle cell disease appears to have significantly affected the Bi-frontal distance (AP) of the male children of age-group 5-9 years.

Females: In respect of the female children, the Sickle cell disease has led to the abnormal growth in the following indicators:

(i) Bi-frontal distance (AP):

(ii) Distance between Medial border of Orbit (AP):

(iii) Distance between Lateral border of Orbit (AP);

(iv) Bi-Maxilla distance (AP); and

(v) Angle of Mandible to Angle of Mandible (AP).

Bi-frontal distance (AP) of the female children of age-group 5-9 years seems to have been significantly affected by the Sickle cell disease

AN IMPORTANT CONCLUSION

The foregoing results for all the three anthropometric data indicate that the Sickle cell disease affect the children irrespective of sex. This implies that the Sickle cell disease leads to almost similar bony changes in both males and females

The Sickle cell trait is usually considered to be a clinically benign condition and may produce medical problems only under certain relatively rare circumstances. Our research was designed to examine the growth of a large group of patients which were representing an "Entire - at Risk Population" in and around Nagpur, Central India and correlate the observed growth and development with identical normal controlled persons.

According to our anthropometric study we are convinced that these patients weigh less and there is retardation in many physical developments as compared to normal individual children & adults. These children were light in weight at greater heights than normal controlled children.

Multiple assessments and physical developments were made. Thirty six measures of physical anthropometry were studied. Means and standard deviations for the group of sicklers (Children, Adolescents & Adults) were compared with those of normal controlled children, Adolescents & Adults. Student's t-tests were calculated to establish the statistical reliability of mean differences for each individual measurement.

An important distinction can be made, however, between measures of linear growth and measures related to muscular development and body weight. Sickle cell children showed decreased weight and height or many other physical measures.

Although Sickle cell trait is benign condition it was observed in our study that it affects the physical growth and development and these patients are susceptible to patho physiological changes as seen in Sickle cell disease which was noticed in our clinical study. Amongst 944 patients who had skeletal manifestations in sicklers, more than 50 per cent of patients had "AS" Haemoglobin pattern (Sickle cell trait). The spectrum of skeletal manifestations in number of Sickle cell trait cases, combined with subtle differences seen in growth and development of Sickle cell carrier (sickle cell trait) raises doubt regarding the common opinion that Sickle cell trait is a totally benign condition.

Our study is in general agreement with Whitten's study (1961) & M.K. McCormack et al (1976) that as a group, children with Sickle cell anaemia weigh less, are shorter, and of thinner body built than comparable normal controlled individuals. This is nicely demonstrated in graphic representation for all measures in anthropometric study.

The reasons for low height of Sickle cell patients are obscure. Growth is affected by many factors and it is not, perhaps, surprising that clear cut relationship with any one factor are difficult to demonstrate.

The study of L.A. Altemus & C.W. Epps (1960) by taking lateral cephalometric radiographs demonstrated that the sickle cell group to be slightly more convex in the lower facial region. This increase in convexity seems to be due primarily to mandibular retrusion which is accompanied by steepening of mandibular plane.

The pathophysiology of low weight is exactly not known but there are two hypotheses. The patients with more sickling have more acute or chronic vaso occlusion which may lead to poor nutritional intake. Patients with more haemolysis have lower haematocrit, more marrow and cardiovascular compensation and large caloric requirements. Probably combination of these factors can explain the observations that patients treated by transfusion show an increase in weight gain.

This genetic disorder has a high prevalence rate in this region of Central India. From the observations it is established that Sickle cell haemoglobinopathy patients are prone to repeated attacks of vosoocclusive crisis, thrombosis, infarction, & infection. All the possible bony changes and complications should be kept in mind when such patients are diagnosed and are under follow-up. To reduce the morbidity and mortality of this disease, need was felt to diagnose this disorder very early, before it manifest clinically, and prevent the sickler community from above mentioned complications and its sequelae. Observations on anthropometric studies in this series is in general agreement with most of the previous researchers regarding the retardation of physical growth and development. However, our keen observation during the anthropometric study detected few abnormal findings in Facial, Physical Anthropometry. **"Face is the index of mind"**. It gave a suspicion regarding the look of the patient and one could formulate and roughly imagine the typical face, these patients are likely to have. **"Your face doth testifie what you are inwardly" L. Evas**. The so called "Sickler's Face" which is basically because of osseous manifestation of the disease is much different than normal individuals and hence they could be detected amongst the population in a large crowd (Figs. 16.1, 16.2). It will be worthwhile to quote, **"From a man's face I can read his character; if I can see him walk I know his thoughts."** Petronious.

The sicklers are plagued throughout their life with attacks of "Pains", which might be ischaemic - voscoocclusive in origin, and are frequently in great agony and seriously ill. Pain is usually very severe, agonising and intolerable. Patients are very sickly, ill with frequent and recurrent infections, usually respiratory tract. The pain is excruciating during the period of crisis. The exact precipitating factors for the crisis are not yet determined, however infection appears to be one of the commonest cause, which compels the patients for repeated hospitalisation, which in turn increases the morbidity and percentage of mortality.

To avoid these possible sequelae, our anthropometric study has proved worth in detecting the sickler community at the earliest possible time of life, much before these persons present with any symptoms and clinical features. If all the possible care of these children is taken and they are prevented from precipitating factors like hypoxia, anoxia, high altitude and infection (to avoid crisis) and prompt timely treatment by protecting the involved bone or joint along with antibiotics, will certainly reduce the morbidity and will improve the life span and quality of the life they live.

17

Anaesthesia Care in Surgical Treatment for Patients of Sickle Cell Haemoglobinopathy

Every possible anaesthetic and operative complication has been reported in patients with Sickle cell disease, like splenic infarction, atelectasis, pulmonary embolisation, lung infection, jaundice, renal failure etc.

The exact incidence of excess of anaesthetic and surgical complications are difficult to estimate. The incidence of morbidity and mortality is definitely high in Sickle cell disease patients than in normals.

The most common type of complications were postoperative fever of unknown origin, painful crisis, wound infections and transfusion related problems. Complications in general were multiple and generally unpredictable.

Few patients of Sickle cell disease were managed with preoperative transfusion, the combination of preoperative transfusion with intravenous hydration 2-3 times, maintenance of fluid requirement reduces the chances of morbidity. The measures for the prevention and treatment of complications of Sickle cell disease, arising as a result of surgery and anaesthesia should be considered together. The treatment of established complications is quite unsatisfactory and consists mainly of supportive measures, hence emphasis should be placed more on prevention.

No definitive guidelines are given for preoperative preparation or conduction of anaesthesia. Each procedure in every case should be treated individually as the management depends upon the condition of the patient, type of surgical procedure, type of anaesthesia and the degree of emergency.

Recognition of patient with Sickle cell disease is necessarily first step in management. Elective procedures should be scheduled when the patient is in the best of health, free from symptoms of pain or infection. Premedication should not produce respiratory or circulatory depression.

PREOPERATIVE PREPARATION

In Sickle cell trait patient management should consist of basic measures of preoxygenation prior to induction. Surplus maintenence of adequate oxygenation during anaesthesia, careful monitoring including arterial blood gases, avoidance of acidosis and hypotension and post-anaesthetic oxygenation.

In patients of Sickle cell disease lot of precaution is necessary since in these group of patients complications are very high with lot of morbidity and mortality.

Preoperative transfusion with packed red cells is not without any risk. A transfusion should not routinely be employed only for haemoglobin values less than 5-7 gm%. The efficacy of preoperative blood transfusion is not very certain. The rationale for preoperative transfusion is reduction of the level of HbS by diluting or partial exchange with HbA blood. By this way it limits the maximum increase in viscosity resulting from the condition of lowered pH and decreased oxygen tension. In a case of planned surgery packed cell transfusion should be administered 2-3 weeks prior to surgery, which will raise the haemoglobin level to normal or higher side, which suppresses endogenous erythropoiesis. Whenever emergency procedure is required partial exchange transfusion may be carried out, which dilutes the sickled cells with normal cells and increases the blood oxygen carrying capacity without increasing the blood volume and producing circulatory overload. The regimen of blood transfusion consisted of monthly transfusion with leucocyte poor, packed erythrocytes till the desired level of haemoglobin is achieved.

BONE MARROW TRANSPLANTATION

The ability to predict who will not do well with their Sickle cell disease is critical because for some, bone marrow transplantation may be curative. More than 60 such transplants have been performed so far in patients with Sickle cell anemia, based on successful use of this treatment approach in beta-thalassemia major. The most frequent indication for bone marrow transplantation in children with Sickle cell anemia in the United States is a prior cerebrovascular accident, which is one of the few events complicating Sickle cell disease that clearly defines a subsequent course characterised by serious morbidity and early mortality.

The real cure for Sickle cell disease probably resides with gene therapy. Until that therapy becomes available, we will have to muddle along. Fortunately, as this study shows, the majority of patients are living long enough to still benefit from innovative therapies.

Other methods which reduce and prevent sickling are necessary. This includes alkalization, hydration, prophylactic folic acid, magnesium sulphate, zinc sulphate, heparinisation and low molecular weight dextran. Alkalization is frequently required for management of patients requiring surgery. Soda bicarb should be given orally 1 g/kg/hour in divided doses or I.V. 3.3 mEq/kg/hour with recommendation to use it before, during and after surgery. It is essential to avoid acidosis to prevent vaso-occlusive crisis. Good hydration is also essential.

MANAGEMENT OF THE ANAESTHETIC

Amongst the wide variety of agents and technique of anaesthesia none has been found to have deleterious effect in patients of Sickle cell disease. Hence no particular anaesthesia drug or technique is contraindicated. However whenever possible local anaesthesia, nerve block, regional anaesthesia, epidural block or spinal anaesthesia is preferred over general anaesthesia.

Excessive cold in operation theatre should be avoided; use of tourniquet should be avoided though it can be employed with apparent safety. Monitoring of cardiopulmonary functions, acid base status and renal functions is essential. Arterial blood gas analysis should be carried out intraoperatively for all major operations. Maintenence of adequate oxygen is absolutely essential. Administration of hundred percent oxygen prior to induction is recommended and maintained throughout the surgical procedure. During surgery inspired oxygen should be adjusted in such a way that pO_2 of at least 80 to 100 tarr is achieved. Administration of hundred percent oxygen prior to extubation and supplemental oxygen postoperatively until full recovery is necessary.

Premedication is usually effected with atropine and promethazine. Promethazine provides sedation without respiratory depression. Drugs which cause respiratory depression should be avoided. After premedication oxygenation of at least 5 minutes is necessary. Induction is achieved with small doses of thiopentone and short muscle relaxants are used for intubation. Anaesthesia is maintained with halothane with 50% nitrous oxide & oxygen. The patient is allowed to breathe spontaneously or ventillation is controlled depending upon the time for surgical procedure.

Early recovery of consciousness and upper respiratory tract reflexes is important. Postoperatively oxygen is given through nasal catheters for 24 hours. The hypoxia is avoided and blood gases should be monitored postoperatively.

The detailed schedule of Anaesthesia is as given below:

1. Keep the patient in equable temperature in O.T. (Cold encourages vasoconstriction and warm causes sweating and dehydration.)
2. Set up I.V. infusion to maintain hydration and alkalization, (low molecular weight dextran or partial exchange blood transfusion may be required.)
3. I.V. alkalization is reasonable if preoperative oral regimes was omitted or discarded. Administer 3.3 mEq/kg/hour of soda bicarbonate over 90 minutes.
4. Pre-oxygenate with 100% oxygen for at least 5 minutes.
5. After induction, ventilate or hyperventilate with nitrous oxide and 50% oxygen to promote respiratory alkolosis.
6. A judicious concentration of volatile agents (Halothane) which will minimise hypocapnic vasoconstriction and promote good tissue perfusion.
7. Avoid cardiac depression, peripheral vasodilatation and vasoconstriction and decreased blood volume. (All this will result in impairment of tissue blood flow.)
8. Give hundred percent oxygenation prior to extubation.
9. Continue oxygenation for 12-24 hrs. after operation.
10. Maintain adequate hydration postoperatively.
11. Early mobilisation of patient to promote optimal tissue concentration.
12. Prophylactic antibiotics.

In short, simple anaesthesia technique, with adequate oxygenation, ventilation and maintenence of circulatory volume and efficient postoperative management is essential to minimise complications in these patients of Sickle cell haemoglobinopathy.

18

Recommendations

Based on the conclusions of the present research work, we offer the following suggestions and recommendations.

1. Early Detection and Mass Education

Morbidity and mortality associated with Sickle cell disease is as a result of its complications and their hazardous sequelae. Hence it is advisable to detect this genetic disorder at the earliest much before it presents with clinical manifestations. This can be achieved by mass education especially of the susceptible community. Doctors, paramedical staff and medical social workers should be updated with knowledge regarding early diagnosis of the disease as well as they should take up the task of propogating the awareness of this disease in the community. Population surveys, screening tests through frequent camps especially in the susceptible community should be carried out. Sickling test (early and late) and haemoglobin solubility test should be performed wherever indicated to confirm the diagnosis.

2. Sickler's Face

From the experience of this clinical and anthropometric study, it has been concluded that most of these patients have common facial presentation, a little different than normal individuals. This is called as **"Sickler's Face"** (as explained in Chapter 16). If the visual impression of these facies is kept in mind, which obviously comes by experience, it is extremely easy.to suspect the sicklers. Such suspected people from the large population should be further screened by a simple outdoor test of sickling or solubility test which will confirm the diagnosis of Sickle cell haemoglobinopathy. Once the person who is diagnosed as Sickle cell patient, he should be provided with "Identity Card" of a "Sickler" and should be referred to Sickle cell centre of a neighbouring medical centre for further investigations like haemoglobin electrophoresis, Skeletal survey etc. and should be followed up for their life-time. All these sicklers must be educated regarding the disease, its various complications and sequelae.

3. Genetic and Marriage Counselling

Genetic counselling is a very important factor in those patients (who are labelled as Sicklers) and the welfare of the sicklers' community at large. Investigations of their parents, siblings and children are mandatory. Haemoglobin electrophoresis is necessary to help them in detecting whether they are carriers (SA Sickle cell trait), or whether they have disease (SS) or they are normal. If one detects Sickle cell trait patients who are likely to have normal life, one can guide them to avoid unphysiological conditions, avoid hypoxia and anoxia. Preferably they should avoid air travel (only compressed air travel) and higher altitude.

One must encourage "Marriage Counselling" which will certainly help them in dilution of the disease by advising them and discouraging them for consanguineous marriage to another Sickler.

4. Prevention of Sequelae and Complications

The Sickle cell disease has a variety of sequelae and its complications. Many times Orthopaedist might be the first doctor where patient presents with osseous manifestations and complications. He/she should be made aware and familiar about the complications of disease and variety of osseous manifestations. The children might present in acute phase like, Sickle cell crisis, "Hand-Foot Syndrome", acute osteotomyelitis, Sickle cell arthralgia, arthritis, pathological fracture or chronic stage with any of the osseous presentation as discussed in various chapters. If treating Physician and Surgeon is aware of these complications the prognosis of the disease is fairly good.

5. Prompt Treatment

Your eyes don't see what your mind does not know. If one is not aware about the sequelae, he is likely to miss such disabling complications. All these complications can be prevented as well as effectively managed.

Even if these persons get these complications, prompt treatment is essential to avoid permanent damage. To take care of such Sicklers throughout their life time, they should be identified like diabetic patients by providing "Identification Card" - "Sickler".

19

Anthropometric Data for Males and Females

Table 19.1. Physical anthropometry for males

S. No.	Age Group	Controlled Mean	Controlled SD	Sicklers Mean	Sicklers SD	t Value	% Change
1	05-09	20.69	4.72	15.44	4.14	3.16	-25.36
1	10-15	36.03	8.28	28.46	19.33	2.01	-22.24
1	16-20	50.40	4.18	46.20	13.06	1.19	-8.33
2	05-09	121.77	10.82	117.50	0.42	2.18	-3.51
2	10-15	148.87	9.36	133.29	15.62	3.01	-11.24
2	16-20	139.67	6.97	165.00	9.64	0.76	-2.75
3	05-09	51.46	1.34	55.17	3.61	2.89	-12.23
3	10-15	52.42	1.64	49.96	3.69	2.65	-8.08
3	16-20	54.67	1.23	53.80	2.54	1.19	-1.59
4	05-09	18.25	0.70	18.06	2.54	0.80	-1.04
4	10-15	20.06	4.24	18.44	4.57	1.22	-6.94
4	16-20	22.81	1.39	17.20	13.84	2.06	-2.59
5	05-09	16.38	1.82	14.82	2.85	2.96	13.70
5	10-15	16.42	1.39	15.47	1.14	2.91	-5.77
5	16-20	17.57	0.77	17.38	1.16	1.01	-1.08
6	05-09	4.15	0.46	3.89	3.08	0.43	-6.38
6	10-15	4.65	0.51	4.31	3.45	0.11	-1.49
6	16-20	4.82	0.31	4.58	0.40	1.84	-4.97
7	05-09	13.59	3.85	9.69	8.64	2.37	-4.05
7	10-15	13.70	3.56	10.98	2.11	2.41	-1.98
7	16-20	19.67	1.58	12.67	0.66	28.18	-35.90
8	05-09	1.23	0.25	2.00	1.45	-2.66	62.50
8	10-15	1.10	0.11	1.66	0.96	-2.57	51.00
8	16-20	0.90	0.38	1.36	0.40	-4.18	50.10
9	05-09	3.60	0.11	2.85	0.67	3.27	-20.83

(Contd.)

S. No.	Age Group	Controlled Mean	Controlled SD	Sicklers Mean	Sicklers SD	t Value	% Change
9	10-15	3.27	0.22	3.20	0.51	1.12	-2.14
9	16-20	3.09	0.21	3.11	0.49	-0.20	0.63
10	05-09	1.40	0.28	1.26	0.50	1.12	-10.04
10	10-15	2.40	0.25	1.57	0.33	10.31	-34.58
10	16-20	2.51	0.39	1.82	0.33	7.34	-27.49
11	05-09	2.71	0.47	2.46	0.53	1.70	-9.26
11	10-15	2.77	0.53	3.34	0.39	-5.28	20.54
11	16-20	3.17	0.66	3.07	0.77	0.51	-3.15
12	05-09	4.13	0.42	4.04	1.11	0.95	-6.07
12	10-15	4.46	0.75	4.70	0.77	-1.22	5.14
12	16-20	4.48	1.18	4.16	0.43	1.53	-7.12
13	05-09	7.89	0.46	9.58	1.12	-6.01	20.04
13	10-15	9.46	1.10	9.63	1.19	-0.70	2.43
13	16-20	9.87	1.03	10.50	1.58	-1.61	6.20
14	05-09	13.51	0.62	11.64	1.49	4.97	-13.56
14	10-15	13.87	2.09	12.14	0.19	5.09	-12.17
14	16-20	14.39	2.56	13.95	0.73	1.19	-3.04
15	05-09	5.12	0.43	7.11	0.67	-11.37	38.93
15	10-15	5.20	1.44	8.34	2.56	-5.27	60.24
15	16-20	5.58	1.52	8.92	0.82	-12.06	60.21
16	05-09	9.62	2.57	13.24	0.96	-8.49	37.52
16	10-15	12.75	2.54	13.77	0.84	-1.28	8.00
16	16-20	14.56	2.57	14.12	0.74	-1.17	-3.02
17	05-09	10.97	1.18	8.99	2.10	3.48	-17.99
17	10-15	10.79	0.99	10.09	0.89	3.02	-6.47
17	16-20	11.28	0.27	11.06	0.29	2.82	-1.84
18	05-09	7.64	0.70	10.13	1.08	9.02	32.65
18	10-15	9.64	1.27	10.46	1.40	-2.34	8.45
18	16-20	11.08	0.65	11.81	0.77	-3.70	6.47
19	05-09	2.57	0.53	3.35	0.64	-4.66	31.38
19	10-15	2.95	0.47	3.78	2.04	-1.73	28.03
19	16-20	2.98	0.33	3.88	0.37	-8.92	30.22
20	05-09	5.75	0.44	6.00	1.37	-0.74	4.35
20	10-15	6.12	0.48	6.49	1.63	-1.02	6.03
20	16-20	7.36	2.15	7.18	1.85	0.33	-2.35
21	05-09	2.30	0.37	2.57	0.58	-1.87	11.34
21	10-15	2.50	0.62	2.71	0.16	-2.36	7.98
21	16-20	2.58	0.48	2.81	0.64	-1.41	8.36
22	05-09	26.77	1.43	28.43	1.85	-3.51	6.17
22	10-15	28.20	2.32	28.56	3.39	0.44	1.18
22	16-20	29.00	3.25	29.02	5.13	-0.02	1.25

(Contd.)

S. No.	Age Group	Controlled		Sicklers		t Value	% Change
		Mean	SD	Mean	SD		
23	05-09	5.90	0.60	5.44	1.21	1.50	-7.76
23	10-15	8.20	1.30	7.95	2.60	0.38	-3.02
23	16-20	9.25	2.25	8.77	4.56	0.42	-5.08
24	05-09	38.40	4.84	34.83	3.86	1.34	4.23
24	10-15	42.30	3.64	40.82	8.42	0.78	-3.45
24	16-20	46.20	1.45	46.58	1.65	-0.87	0.79
25	05-09	30.20	2.61	29.13	4.22	0.99	-3.49
25	10-15	30.25	5.35	30.55	2.52	-0.34	0.98
25	16-20	31.83	3.65	38.31	2.56	-8.42	20.27
26	05-09	12.55	1.21	11.71	3.09	1.08	-6.57
26	10-15	14.95	2.17	13.81	2.32	1.92	-7.42
26	16-20	19.95	2.65	16.02	2.50	5.71	-19.53
27	05-09	20.24	2.52	24.11	2.70	5.18	-19.64
27	10-15	29.10	5.35	28.41	4.20	0.61	-2.34
27	16-20	31.39	2.41	31.13	2.51	0.38	-0.80
28	05-09	28.02	2.77	19.27	5.00	6.83	-30.97
28	10-15	28.97	6.11	22.56	4.58	5.01	-22.01
28	16-20	34.02	5.03	30.13	8.65	1.79	-11.24
29	05-09	21.54	5.01	18.43	3.41	2.89	-14.27
29	10-15	22.11	4.07	20.43	4.71	1.43	-7.29
29	16-20	26.57	3.69	21.59	3.85	4.89	-18.67
30	05-09	39.48	12.15	47.87	3.42	-4.35	21.90
30	10-15	65.41	5.90	62.37	8.31	1.49	-4.58
30	16-20	72.55	2.36	69.74	1.87	5.20	-3.78
31	05-09	13.58	1.30	12.61	2.85	1.37	-7.08
31	10-15	16.68	1.25	15.64	1.97	2.20	-6.17
31	16-20	18.83	1.92	17.47	1.73	2.98	-7.39
32	05-09	20.71	2.40	19.56	2.70	1.59	-5.38
32	10-15	26.53	3.39	24.89	2.72	1.58	-5.39
32	16-20	29.20	2.91	27.95	2.23	1.93	-4.19
33	05-09	20.85	2.22	16.80	2.70	5.61	-19.24
33	10-15	24.22	2.01	20.83	3.59	4.82	-13.93
33	16-20	24.54	2.83	24.20	2.70	0.50	-1.22
34	05-09	27.12	3.84	31.52	7.75	-2.26	16.09
34	10-15	42.50	5.89	41.36	6.00	0.75	-1.21
34	16-20	47.94	2.11	45.72	2.69	3.21	-4.58
35	05-09	9.46	1.03	8.03	1.61	3.42	-15.02
35	10-15	11.39	2.10	9.91	2.05	2.81	-12.98
35	16-20	11.89	2.15	10.47	2.06	2.62	-11.87
36	05-09	30.77	3.00	26.55	4.09	3.87	-13.65
36	10-15	36.85	3.26	33.73	4.61	2.84	-8.33
36	16-20	39.75	2.82	36.69	2.70	4.15	-7.59

Table 19.2. Physical anthropometry for females

S. No.	*Age Group*	*Controlled*		*Sicklers*		*t*	*%*
		Mean	*SD*	*Mean*	*SD*	*Value*	*Change*
1	05-09	20.65	4.02	15.40	3.94	4.21	-25.40
1	10-15	34.03	8.28	27.94	19.33	2.01	-17.86
1	16-20	42.47	4.59	39.23	4.54	2.65	-7.61
2	05-09	118.70	10.08	115.62	0.40	2.20	-2.51
2	10-15	147.07	10.12	132.10	1.56	11.45	-9.49
2	16-20	152.85	4.75	145.40	1.20	5.04	-4.87
3	05-09	51.42	1.34	45.12	3.59	2.89	-12.21
3	10-15	52.37	1.52	49.91	3.29	3.04	-8.03
3	16-20	54.17	1.10	53.20	2.24	3.01	-1.78
4	05-09	18.21	0.52	18.02	2.34	0.92	-1.03
4	10-15	20.02	4.14	18.00	4.34	1.34	-10.09
4	16-20	22.79	1.35	17.16	13.80	2.11	-25.57
5	05-09	16.32	1.71	14.76	2.81	3.02	-9.56
5	10-15	16.35	1.20	15.42	1.22	2.91	-5.67
5	16-20	17.07	0.72	17.88	1.16	1.07	-1.11
6	05-09	4.10	0.44	3.83	3.06	0.61	-7.05
6	10-15	4.55	0.48	4.21	3.44	0.13	-7.47
6	16-20	4.78	0.31	4.54	0.40	1.84	-4.93
7	05-09	13.50	3.75	9.58	8.50	2.17	-29.04
7	10-15	13.65	3.54	10.93	2.01	2.53	-19.93
7	16-20	19.62	1.55	12.61	0.64	28.31	-35.73
8	05-09	1.20	0.24	1.97	1.44	-2.67	64.17
8	10-15	1.06	0.10	1.62	0.92	-2.62	52.83
8	16-20	0.86	0.35	1.32	0.40	-4.23	53.49
9	05-09	3.55	0.12	2.80	0.62	3.31	-21.13
9	10-15	3.20	0.23	3.13	0.50	1.13	-2.19
9	16-20	3.05	0.20	3.07	0.48	-0.21	-0.66
10	05-09	1.35	0.26	1.22	0.48	1.15	-9.63
10	10-15	2.36	0.24	1.53	0.31	10.52	-35.17
10	16-20	2.47	0.37	1.78	0.32	7.38	-27.93
11	05-09	2.65	0.50	2.40	0.55	1.67	-9.43
11	10-15	2.75	0.52	3.32	0.42	-5.08	20.73
11	16-20	3.15	0.62	3.05	0.75	0.61	-3.17
12	05-09	4.25	0.44	4.00	1.12	0.91	-5.88

(Contd.)

S. No.	Age Group	Controlled		Sicklers		t Value	% Change
		Mean	SD	Mean	SD		
12	10-15	4.42	0.76	4.65	0.79	-1.20	5.20
12	16-20	4.46	1.19	4.14	0.42	1.53	-7.17
13	05-09	7.85	0.45	9.53	1.14	-6.01	-21.40
13	10-15	9.43	1.11	9.60	1.17	-0.72	1.80
13	16-20	9.85	1.02	10.46	1.46	-1.62	6.19
14	05-09	13.45	0.59	11.57	1.45	5.01	-13.98
14	10-15	13.85	2.07	12.12	0.88	5.12	-12.49
14	16-20	14.35	2.55	13.90	0.70	1.31	-3.14
15	05-09	9.60	2.59	13.22	0.98	-8.31	37.71
15	10-15	12.70	2.57	13.71	0.86	-1.67	7.95
15	16-20	14.53	2.59	14.10	0.80	-1.20	-2.96
16	05-09	5.09	0.49	7.08	0.70	-10.92	39.10
16	10-15	5.15	1.43	8.30	2.55	-5.30	61.17
16	16-20	5.55	1.51	8.89	0.81	-12.10	60.18
17	05-09	10.92	1.68	8.93	2.05	3.61	-18.22
17	10-15	10.75	0.98	10.05	0.90	3.01	-6.51
17	16-20	11.25	0.25	11.03	0.25	3.01	-1.96
18	05-09	7.60	0.69	10.09	1.06	-9.04	32.76
18	10-15	9.62	1.25	10.44	1.39	-2.42	8.52
18	16-20	11.04	0.60	11.77	0.72	-3.81	6.52
19	05-09	2.51	0.53	3.31	0.63	-4.67	31.87
19	10-15	2.91	0.46	3.74	2.14	-1.69	28.53
19	16-20	2.94	0.31	3.84	0.35	-8.93	30.62
20	05-09	5.17	0.48	6.00	1.40	-0.72	5.26
20	10-15	6.10	0.50	6.47	1.61	-1.03	6.06
20	16-20	7.31	2.15	7.13	1.84	0.34	-2.46
21	05-09	2.26	0.36	2.53	0.57	-1.88	11.95
21	10-15	2.47	0.61	2.68	0.15	-2.40	8.50
21	16-20	2.55	0.45	2.78	0.75	-1.37	9.01
22	05-09	26.75	1.44	28.41	1.81	-3.57	6.21
22	10-15	28.00	2.30	28.36	3.35	-0.51	1.29
22	16-20	28.75	3.21	28.77	5.14	-0.02	1.21
23	05-09	5.70	0.61	5.24	1.20	1.48	-8.07
23	10-15	8.00	1.40	7.76	2.61	0.36	-3.00
23	16-20	9.10	2.15	8.61	4.52	0.45	-5.38
24	05-09	37.40	4.80	33.33	3.85	1.46	-9.54
24	10-15	41.30	3.70	39.72	8.42	0.75	-3.85

(Contd.)

S. No.	Age Group	Controlled Mean	Controlled SD	Sicklers Mean	Sicklers SD	t Value	% Change
24	16-20	45.30	1.50	45.48	1.64	-0.85	0.40
25	05-09	29.10	2.51	28.03	4.12	1.02	-3.68
25	10-15	29.25	5.15	29.55	2.25	-0.61	1.01
25	16-20	30.85	3.62	37.33	2.55	-8.51	20.91
26	05-09	12.15	1.12	11.31	3.09	1.08	-6.54
26	10-15	13.95	2.15	13.81	2.36	1.91	-8.17
26	16-20	18.85	2.64	15.02	2.48	5.74	-20.32
27	05-09	19.25	2.51	23.12	2.71	5.16	20.10
27	10-15	28.20	5.40	27.51	4.40	0.51	-2.45
27	16-20	30.40	2.70	30.33	2.61	0.35	-0.23
28	05-09	27.20	2.77	18.47	4.96	6.78	-32.09
28	10-15	27.95	6.10	21.55	4.56	5.03	-22.50
28	16-20	33.20	5.06	29.31	8.64	1.76	-11.72
29	05-09	20.55	5.01	17.44	3.39	2.90	-15.13
29	10-15	21.21	4.10	19.53	4.90	1.42	-7.92
29	16-20	25.56	3.65	20.58	3.84	4.91	-19.48
30	05-09	38.58	12.47	46.89	3.39	-4.51	21.79
30	10-15	64.42	5.95	61.39	8.35	1.45	4.70
30	16-20	71.75	2.35	68.94	1.85	5.24	-7.92
31	05-09	12.57	1.40	11.60	2.90	1.21	-7.72
31	10-15	16.08	1.24	15.03	1.95	2.24	-6.53
31	16-20	18.33	1.92	16.94	1.71	2.99	-7.58
32	05-09	19.72	2.60	18.58	2.81	1.49	-5.78
32	10-15	26.03	3.50	24.43	2.75	1.54	-6.15
32	16-20	28.20	3.01	26.97	3.32	1.74	-4.36
33	05-09	19.86	2.20	15.82	2.56	5.62	-20.34
33	10-15	23.25	2.01	19.85	3.51	4.02	-14.62
33	16-20	23.55	3.01	23.21	2.75	0.47	-1.44
34	05-09	26.12	3.84	30.52	7.72	-2.27	16.84
34	10-15	41.76	6.01	40.62	6.05	0.71	-2.72
34	16-20	46.96	2.11	44.74	2.65	3.22	-4.73
35	05-09	8.50	1.04	7.07	1.62	3.43	-16.82
35	10-15	10.13	2.08	8.90	2.03	2.82	-14.26
35	16-20	10.90	2.12	9.48	2.05	2.64	-13.03
36	05-09	29.77	2.73	25.60	3.79	3.91	-14.01
36	10-15	16.35	3.16	33.33	4.65	2.81	-8.31
36	16-20	39.25	2.79	36.17	2.68	4.17	-7.85

Table 19.3. Facial anthropometry for males

S. No.	Age Group	Controlled		Sicklers		t Value	% Change
		Mean	SD	Mean	SD		
1	05-09	3.01	0.26	3.05	0.26	-0.40	1.40
1	10-15	2.97	0.18	3.01	2.50	-0.09	1.38
1	16-20	3.01	0.17	3.07	8.71	-0.12	5.17
2	05-09	2.43	0.22	2.96	2.44	-1.09	22.01
2	10-15	2.53	0.20	2.96	2.47	-0.95	16.97
2	16-20	2.60	0.02	3.03	8.64	-0.82	18.08
3	05-09	0.78	0.13	0.83	0.68	-0.36	6.31
3	10-15	0.82	0.10	0.92	0.77	-0.70	12.01
3	16-20	0.83	0.13	0.91	2.61	-0.62	9.87
4	05-09	1.76	0.27	2.13	1.75	-1.04	21.01
4	10-15	1.81	0.15	2.17	1.81	-1.08	19.71
4	16-20	1.89	0.20	2.29	6.50	-0.95	21.16
5	05-09	0.12	0.04	0.24	0.19	-2.86	91.53
5	10-15	0.17	0.04	0.28	0.23	-2.43	60.26
5	16-20	0.18	0.06	0.59	0.24	-3.01	33.33
6	05-09	0.55	0.08	0.56	0.46	-0.11	1.90
6	10-15	0.58	0.05	0.58	0.48	0.06	-0.95
6	16-20	0.58	0.06	0.57	1.61	-0.07	-1.72
7	05-09	0.76	0.11	0.85	0.70	-0.61	11.26
7	10-15	0.80	0.06	0.90	0.75	-0.75	12.97
7	16-20	0.91	0.07	1.01	0.86	-0.75	10.98
8	05-09	1.31	0.24	1.60	1.31	-1.09	22.32
8	10-15	1.42	0.13	1.71	1.43	-1.10	20.22
8	16-20	1.54	0.13	1.80	5.13	-0.92	16.88
9	05-09	1.77	0.15	1.52	1.25	0.98	-13.94
9	10-15	1.86	0.11	1.70	1.42	0.62	-8.60
9	16-20	1.87	0.17	1.79	5.10	0.47	-4.28
10	05-09	1.40	0.18	1.25	1.03	0.74	-10.97
10	10-15	1.37	0.13	1.20	1.00	0.93	-12.41
10	16-20	1.37	0.17	1.36	3.89	0.00	-0.42
11	05-09	1.21	0.16	1.67	1.38	-1.68	38.66
11	10-15	1.29	0.13	1.67	1.39	-1.49	29.53
11	16-20	1.42	0.14	1.80	5.12	-0.97	26.97
12	05-09	0.62	0.05	1.00	0.82	-2.33	62.34

Contd.)

S. No.	*Age Group*	*Controlled*		*Sicklers*		*t Value*	*% Change*
		Mean	*SD*	*Mean*	*SD*		
12	10-15	0.76	0.07	1.02	0.85	-1.66	33.92
12	16-20	0.86	0.08	1.12	3.23	-0.98	30.23
13	05-09	0.48	0.19	0.59	0.48	-1.03	22.40
13	10-15	0.49	0.07	0.59	0.49	-1.13	21.00
13	16-20	0.51	0.08	0.52	1.48	0.00	1.96
14	05-09	1.42	0.16	1.83	1.50	-1.33	28.16
14	10-15	1.52	0.07	1.83	1.52	-1.09	19.88
14	16-20	1.56	0.06	1.87	1.50	-1.08	19.87
15	05-09	0.92	0.10	0.98	0.80	-0.37	6.44
15	10-15	0.98	0.06	0.99	0.80	0.09	-1.36
15	16-20	0.99	0.06	1.00	2.84	0.00	1.00
16	05-09	0.51	0.07	0.47	0.43	-0.15	2.54
16	10-15	0.52	0.04	0.51	0.39	-0.15	1.91
16	16-20	0.53	0.06	0.53	1.46	0.00	0.00
17	05-09	0.79	0.16	1.05	0.87	-1.06	21.53
17	10-15	0.86	0.09	1.00	0.84	-1.37	26.58
17	16-20	0.89	0.12	1.09	3.14	-1.23	23.71
18	05-09	1.02	0.07	1.04	0.85	-0.13	2.12
18	10-15	1.04	0.07	1.04	0.87	-0.03	0.43
18	16-20	1.09	0.10	1.10	3.15	0.00	0.91

Table 19.4. Facial anthropometry for females

S. No.	*Age Group*	*Controlled*		*Sicklers*		*t Value*	*% Change*
		Mean	*SD*	*Mean*	*SD*		
1	05-09	2.94	0.25	2.82	0.40	0.66	-4.16
1	10-15	2.85	0.22	3.31	2.96	-0.92	16.23
1	16-20	2.42	0.27	2.30	0.50	0.62	-4.87
2	05-09	2.47	0.27	2.66	2.36	-0.40	7.56
2	10-15	2.58	0.21	3.23	2.88	-1.33	25.28
2	16-20	2.73	0.29	2.60	2.32	0.42	4.76
3	05-09	0.77	0.09	0.82	0.74	-0.32	6.07
3	10-15	0.84	0.08	0.94	0.84	-0.72	12.24
3	16-20	0.88	0.09	0.98	0.90	-0.69	11.36
4	05-09	1.75	0.31	2.16	1.94	-1.06	23.16
4	10-15	1.81	0.34	2.33	2.08	-1.46	28.75
4	16-20	1.90	0.35	1.90	2.10	-1.20	28.75
5	05-09	0.12	0.04	0.24	0.21	-2.82	101.29
5	10-15	0.18	0.04	0.30	0.27	-2.55	64.06

Contd.)

S. No.	*Age Group*	*Controlled*		*Sicklers*		*t*	*%*
		Mean	*SD*	*Mean*	*SD*	*Value*	*Change*
5	16-20	0.18	0.05	0.32	0.32	-2.47	78.88
6	05-09	0.54	0.06	0.54	0.48	-0.02	0.29
6	10-15	0.61	0.05	0.63	0.56	-0.21	3.29
6	16-20	0.68	0.05	0.70	0.60	-0.20	11.76
7	05-09	0.75	0.07	0.80	0.72	-0.33	6.12
7	10-15	0.83	0.05	0.84	0.94	-0.36	3.61
7	16-20	0.88	0.06	0.89	0.93	-0.36	-3.21
8	05-09	1.25	0.25	1.76	1.58	-1.63	40.80
8	10-15	1.44	0.12	1.81	1.62	-1.35	25.74
8	16-20	1.50	0.13	1.86	1.65	-1.32	24.00
9	05-09	1.78	0.18	1.78	1.60	0.01	-0.26
9	10-15	1.84	0.12	1.84	1.65	-0.01	0.16
9	16-20	1.86	0.14	1.87	1.66	0.00	0.10
10	05-09	1.42	0.19	1.42	1.27	0.01	-0.22
10	10-15	1.39	0.15	1.24	1.11	0.80	-10.86
10	16-20	1.45	0.30	1.60	1.27	-0.75	10.34
11	05-09	1.20	0.16	1.76	1.58	-1.79	46.20
11	10-15	1.36	0.11	1.83	1.63	-1.71	34.74
11	16-20	1.40	0.21	1.87	1.65	-1.56	33.56
12	05-09	0.64	0.06	1.04	0.93	-2.19	62.89
12	10-15	0.79	0.06	1.09	0.97	-1.83	38.18
12	16-20	0.80	0.07	1.10	0.96	-1.82	37.50
13	05-09	0.44	0.06	0.56	0.50	-1.19	26.61
13	10-15	0.61	0.75	0.56	0.50	0.37	-9.30
13	16-20	0.65	0.76	0.60	0.51	0.36	-7.69
14	05-09	1.51	0.19	1.84	1.65	-1.02	22.04
14	10-15	1.52	0.08	2.00	1.79	-1.59	31.58
14	16-20	1.53	0.09	2.00	1.80	-1.58	30.71
15	05-09	0.90	0.10	0.96	0.86	-0.35	6.67
15	10-15	0.99	0.06	1.19	1.06	-1.07	19.25
15	16-20	1.01	0.80	1.20	1.07	-1.03	5.94
16	05-09	0.49	0.08	0.52	0.47	-0.34	6.46
16	10-15	0.51	0.05	0.56	0.50	-0.61	10.17
16	16-20	0.56	0.05	0.58	0.51	-0.21	3.57
17	05-09	0.93	0.17	1.28	1.14	-1.52	36.95
17	10-15	0.83	0.10	1.21	1.08	-2.09	46.05
17	16-20	0.92	0.11	1.30	1.07	-3.10	4.13
18	05-09	1.01	0.05	1.00	0.90	0.07	-1.14
18	10-15	1.05	0.11	1.13	1.01	-0.43	7.05
18	16-20	1.06	0.13	1.14	1.10	-0.41	7.55

Table 19.5. Anthropometry by skull X-rays for males

S. No.	Age Group	Controlled Mean	Controlled SD	Sicklers Mean	Sicklers SD	t Value	% Change
1	05-09	11.37	0.83	13.50	1.38	-3.32	18.68
1	10-15	11.96	0.77	14.63	11.32	-1.29	22.32
1	16-20	12.54	0.82	15.11	12.82	-1.27	20.49
2	05-09	9.82	0.77	9.10	8.09	0.43	-7.30
2	10-15	10.46	0.47	9.54	7.37	0.68	-8.78
2	16-20	10.81	0.44	9.89	8.07	0.69	-8.51
3	05-09	5.67	0.45	5.10	4.53	0.62	-10.13
3	10-15	6.18	0.49	5.25	4.05	1.25	-15.05
3	16-20	6.82	0.50	5.89	6.70	1.15	-13.64
4	05-09	10.14	0.61	11.20	9.95	-0.52	10.44
4	10-15	12.03	0.59	12.42	9.59	-0.22	3.24
4	16-20	13.44	0.60	13.83	9.18	-0.22	2.90
5	05-09	2.23	0.34	2.60	2.31	-0.77	16.42
5	10-15	2.84	0.62	3.13	2.41	-0.64	10.16
5	16-20	3.65	0.63	3.94	2.64	-0.62	7.95
6	05-09	10.18	0.68	9.50	8.44	0.40	-6.71
6	10-15	11.12	0.92	10.92	8.44	0.13	-1.80
6	16-20	12.09	0.93	11.89	8.47	0.13	-1.65
7	05-09	13.01	0.71	11.90	10.57	0.51	-8.52
7	10-15	12.51	0.80	12.46	9.61	0.03	-0.41
7	16-20	11.98	0.81	11.56	9.62	0.02	-3.51
8	05-09	3.38	0.26	3.40	3.02	-0.03	0.49
8	10-15	3.40	0.42	3.83	2.96	-0.79	12.75
8	16-20	3.42	0.43	3.85	2.96	-0.78	12.57
9	05-09	8.54	0.81	7.80	6.94	0.52	-8.68
9	10-15	9.19	0.72	8.88	6.85	0.25	-3.43
9	16-20	10.08	0.74	9.78	7.76	0.23	-2.98
10	05-09	17.90	1.10	15.76	14.01	0.75	-11.98
10	10-15	17.55	1.01	16.87	13.05	0.29	-3.91
10	16-20	17.68	1.01	17.00	18.12	0.19	-3.85
11	05-09	6.48	0.84	5.40	4.78	1.08	-16.60
11	10-15	6.27	0.48	5.25	3.90	1.42	-16.22
11	16-20	6.37	0.50	6.17	3.87	0.00	-3.14
12	05-09	10.13	0.95	3.80	3.36	8.88	-62.50
12	10-15	10.35	0.95	4.50	3.06	10.00	-56.52
12	16-20	10.52	0.96	7.22	3.37	9.58	-31.37

Table 19.6. Anthropometry by skull X-rays for females

S. No.	*Age Group*	*Controlled*		*Sicklers*		*t*	*%*
		Mean	*SD*	*Mean*	*SD*	*Value*	*Change*
1	05-09	11.24	0.83	14.63	0.82	-7.69	30.06
1	10-15	11.52	0.61	15.00	14.14	-1.48	30.21
1	16-20	11.77	0.60	15.25	14.71	-1.42	29.57
2	05-09	9.70	0.67	9.25	8.53	0.27	-4.64
2	10-15	10.27	0.75	9.50	8.90	5.51	-7.47
2	16-20	10.52	0.76	9.75	8.97	0.52	-7.32
3	05-09	5.51	0.46	5.75	5.30	0.23	4.26
3	10-15	6.39	0.56	5.63	5.30	0.86	-11.92
3	16-20	6.40	0.56	5.63	5.85	0.86	-12.03
4	05-09	10.25	0.38	10.75	9.92	-0.26	4.90
4	10-15	12.21	0.56	11.88	11.10	9.18	-2.71
4	16-20	12.33	0.57	13.00	12.57	0.17	5.43
5	05-09	2.14	0.292	0.752	0.53	-1.25	28.68
5	10-15	2.70	0.423	0.25	3.06	-1.07	20.37
5	16-20	3.25	0.52	3.55	3.09	-1.03	9.23
6	05-09	10.07	0.60	10.60	39.80	-0.29	5.51
6	10-15	10.74	0.81	11.25	10.60	-0.29	4.71
6	16-20	10.75	0.81	11.25	10.54	-0.31	4.65
7	05-09	12.70	0.66	11.50	10.61	0.59	-9.48
7	10-15	11.99	0.68	11.63	10.96	0.20	-3.04
7	16-20	12.00	0.69	11.13	10.33	0.20	-7.25
8	05-09	3.31	0.21	3.75	3.46	-0.66	13.26
8	10-15	3.34	0.42	4.25	4.01	-1.36	27.39
8	16-20	3.34	0.70	4.13	4.16	-1.42	23.65
9	05-09	8.32	0.70	8.75	8.07	-0.28	5.17
9	10-15	9.17	0.76	10.75	10.10	-0.93	17.20
9	16-20	9.20	0.73	10.76	10.38	-0.91	16.96
10	05-09	17.88	0.80	15.63	14.42	0.81	-12.60
10	10-15	17.40	0.92	16.98	16.00	0.16	-2.44
10	16-20	17.40	0.94	16.96	17.79	0.21	-2.70
11	05-09	6.36	1.13	4.75	4.38	1.84	-25.26
11	10-15	5.99	0.46	5.50	5.18	0.56	-8.12
11	16-20	6.24	0.56	5.75	5.31	0.55	-7.85
12	05-09	10.12	1.27	3.25	2.98	11.02	-67.89
12	10-15	10.22	0.88	4.00	3.77	9.64	-60.86
12	16-20	10.72	0.89	5.50	3.79	6.72	-48.69

Bibliography

1. Acurio M.T., Richard J. Friedman. Hip arthroplasty in patient with sickle cell haemoglobinopathy. JBJS Vol. 74-B No. 3 May 1992. 367-371.
2. Ali Kalamchi, G. Dean, MacEwen. Avascular necrosis following treatment of congenital dislocation of the hip. JBJS Vol. 62-A No. 6, Sep 1980. 876-888.
3. Altemus L.A., Epps C.W. Cephalofacial characteristics of North American Black Individuals with Sickle Cell Disease. Angle Orthodont-50 : 223-240, 1960.
4. Alavi A., Schumacher R., Dorwart B. and Kuhl D.E. Bone Marrow scan evaluation of Arthropathy in Sickle Cell disorder. Arch Intern Med. Vol. 136, 436, April 1976.
5. Allen B.J. and Andrews B.S. Bilateral aseptic necrosis of calcenai in an adult male with Sickle cell disease treated by a surgical coring procedure. The Journal of Rheumatology. Brief Communication. Vol. 10, No.2: 294-296, Nov. 83.
6. Almklov J.R., Hansen A.E. and Schneider M. Long bone involvement in Sickle cell anaemia. Paediatrics., 5: 204, 1950.
7. Ashcroft M.T., Lovell H.G. Heights and weights of Jamaican primary school children. The Journal of Tropical Paediatrics. 1237-43, Sep. 1966.
8. Ashcroft M.T., Serjeant G.R. and Desai P. Heights, weights and skeletal age of Jamaican adolescents with Sickle cell anaemia. Archives of Disease in Childhood. 47: 519-524, 1972.
9. Aziz I.M. Extensive Bone Involvement in Sickle Cell disease and its Treatment. Southern Medical Journal. Vol. 64, No. 7 : 889-891, July 1971.
10. Babhulkar S.S.; Avascular Necrosis of Femoral Head in Sickle cell haemoglobinopathy. Indian Journal of Orthopaedics; Vol. 15 No. 2 162-165, 1981.
11. Babhulkar S.S., Pande Ketan C., Babhulkar Sushrut; Hand-Foot Syndrome in sickle cell haemoglobinopathy; Journal of Bone & Joint Surgery (Br.) 77B, 310-312, Mar. '95.
12. Bankar M.P., Kate S.L., Ranade S.A., Barnabas R.J., Mokashi G.D.,Phadake M.A., Hegade M.V.,: Prenatal diagnosis of Sickle cell anaemia using polymerase chain reaction. Indian Paediatrics. Nov. 1993, Vol. 30, 1340-43.
13. Barter S.J. and Hennessy O. Actinomycetes as the causative organism of Osteomyelitis in Sickle cell disease. Skeletal Radiology 11: 271-273, 1984.

14. Barton C.J. and Cockshott W.P. Bone Changes in Haemoglobin Sickle cell disease. Amer. J. Roentgen, 88: 523, 1962.
15. Becker J.A. Haemoglobin Sickle cell disease. Amer. J. Roentgenol, 88: 503, 1962.
16. Bentley P.G. and Howard E.R. Surgery in children with homozygous Sickle cell anaemia. Annals of Royal College of Surgeons of England, Vol.61: 55-58, 1979.
17. Blau S. and Hamerman D. Aseptic necrosis of the femoral heads in Sickle-A haemoglobin disease. Arthritis & Rheumatism. Vol. 10, No. 4 : 397-400, Aug '67.
18. Bobechko W.P. and Harris W.R. Radiographic density of avascular Bone. J. Bone Joint surg., 42-B, No. 3: 626-632, 1960.
19. Bohrer S.P. Growth disturbances of the distal femur following Sickle cell bone infarcts and/or Osteomyelitis. Clinical Radiology. Vol. 25 : 221-235, 1974.
20. Bohrer S.P. Fractures complicating bone infarcts and/or Osteomyelitis in Sickle cell disease. Clinical Radiology. 22 : 83-88, 1971.
21. Bohrer S.P. Acute long bone diaphyseal infarcts in Sickle cell disease. British Journal of Radiology. 43: 685-697, Oct'70.
22. Booker C.R., Scott R.B. and Ferguson A.D. Studies in Sickle cell anaemia. XXII. Clinical Manifestations of Sickle cell anaemia during the first two years of life. Clin. Pediat. 3: 111, 1964.
23. Borzell F.F. Erythroblastic anaemia (Cooley's Syndrome). Amer. J. Roentgen., 30: 657, 1933.
24. Buchi E.C. In Anthropologist. Delhi, 2. QB 6: 256, 1955.
25. Buchman J. Sickle cell disease simulating osteomyelitis. Bull. Hosp. Joint Dis., 10: 239, 1949.
26. Burch J.E. Paratyphoid osteomyelitis. A Case Report. Southern Med. J., 42: 138, 1949.
27. Burko H., Watson J. and Robinson H. Unusual bone changes in Sickle cell disease in childhood. Radiology, 80: 457-962, 1963.
28. Ballas S.K., Talacki C.A., Rao V.N., Steiner R.M. The prevalence of avascular necrosis in Sickle cell anaemia, Haemoglobin 1989, 13(7-8);649-55.
29. Bishop A.R., Roberson J.R., Eckman J.R., Fleming L.L. Total hip arthroplasty in patients who have Sickle cell haemoglobinopathy. J.B.J.S. (Am.) 1988 July, 70(A); 853-5.
30. Bordin J.O., Kerbauy J., Lourenco D.M., Sesso R. A level of foetal haemoglobin as an indicator of clinical complications in Sickle cell anaemia. Braz. J. Med. Biol Res. 1989, 22 (11);347-53.
31. Bomelberg D., Ehringhaus C., Zeigler R., von Lengerke H.J., Timm C. Femur head necrosis in Sickle cell anaemia; Monatsschr Kinderheilkd 1986 Apr. 134[4]; 212-5.
32. Brooks C.H., Revell W.J., Heatley F.W. Vascularity of the humeral head after proximal humeral fractures. J.B.J.S. 1993, 75B, No.1, 132-36.
33. Baumgard S.H. and Leach R.E.; Avascular necrosis of the femoral head secondary to Sickle cell disease. Case reports of the two Caucasian sisters. Clin. Orthop., 69 : 207-212, 1970.
34. Brooks B.J. Jr. et al. Erythropoietin therapy for Sickle cell anaemia in Jehovah's witnesses (letter); South Med. Jr. 1991 Nov, 84(11) 1416-7.
35. Caffey J. Skeletal Changes in Chronic haemolytic anaemias. Amer. J. Roetngen., 37: 293, 1937.
36. Carrington H.T., Ferguson A.D. and Scott R.B. Studies In Sickle cell anaemia XI. Bone Involvement simulating aseptic necrosis. Amer. J. Dis. Child, 95: 157, 1958.
37. Carroll D.S. Roentgen Manifestations of Sickle cell disease. Southern Med. J., 50: 1486, 1957.
38. Carroll D.S. and Evans J.W. Roentgen Findings in Sickle cell anaemia. Radiology, 53: 834, 1949.
39. Casey D.F. and Cathcart E.S. Haemarthrosis & Sickle cell trait, Arthritis & Rheumatism. Vol.13, No.6: 882-886, Dec '70.

40. Cassady J.R., Berdon W.E., Baker D.H. The "typical" Spine Changes of Sickle cell anaemia in a patient with Thalassemia major (Cooley's anaemia). Radiology Vol. 89: 1065-1068, Dec'67.

41. Charache S. and Page D.L. Infarction of bone marrow in the Sickle cell disorders. Annals of internal Medicine. Vol. 67, No. 6: 1195-1200, Dec'67.

42. Chung S.M.K., Alavi A. and Russell M.O. Management of Osteonecrosis in Sickle cell anaemia and its genetic Variants. Clinical Orthopaedics and Related Research. No. 130 : 158-174, Jan-Feb'78.

43. Cockshott W.P. Haemoglobin Sickle cell disease. J. Fac. Radiologists, 9 : 211-216, 1958.

44. Cole W.R. Sickle cell Anaemia - Radiological Features. Surg. Prog., 5: 126, 1955.

45. Cook J.E. and Meyer J. Severe anaemia with remarkable elongated and sickle -shaped red blood cells and chronic leg ulcer. Arch. Intern. Med. (Chicago). 16: 644, 1915.

46. Cooley T.B., Witwer E.R. and Lee P. Anaemia in Children with Splenomegaly and peculiar Changes in Bones: Report of Cases. Amer. J. Dis. Child, 34: 347, 1927.

47. Crout J.E., McKenna C.H. and Pettit R.M. Symptomatic joint effusion in Sickle cell B-Thalassemia disease. JAMA. Vol. 235, No. 17: 1878-1879, April 1976.

48. Curtis E.M. Pregnancy in Sickle cell anaemia, Sickle cell haemoglobin C disease and variants thereof. Amer. J. Obstet. & Gynec., 77: 1312, 1959.

49. Chung S.M.K. and Ralston E.L. Necrosis of femoral head in Sickle cell disease. J.B.J.S. 51A, 33-58, 1969.

50. Christian Gerber, Alberto G. Schneeberger, Tho-son Vinh. The arterial vascularisation of the humeral head; J.B.J.S. Dec. 1990; 72A No.10, 1486-1494.

51. Clarke H.J., Jinnah R.H., Brooker A.F. Total replacement of hip for avascular necrosis in Sickle cell disease; JBJS [Br] 1989 May; 71[3]; 465-70

52. Clark Gunderson, Robert D., D'Ambrosia, and Hiromu Shoji. Total hip replacement in patients with Sickle cell disease. JBJS Vol. 59-A, No.6 Sep 1977. Page 760-762.

53. Currarino G. and Marien E. Erlandson. Premature fusion of epiphysis in Cooley's anaemia, Radiology 83,1964; 656-664.

54. Danford E.A., Marr R. and Elsey E.C. Sickle cell anaemia with unusual bone changes. Amer. J. Roentgen., 45: 223, 1941.

55. Daramola J.O. Massive osteomyelitis of the mandible complicating Sickle cell disease report of case. Journal of Oral Surgery. Vol. 39: 144-146, Feb 1981.

56. Das S.R., Bhattacharjee D.P., Shastri D.B. and Mukherji D.P. Sickle cell trait in Koraput Dist. and other parts of India. Bul. Anthr. Survey of India. 11, 3: 145, 1962.

57. Deibert K.R. Roentgen Changes in Sickle cell anaemia. Amer. J. Roentgen,82. 501, 1959.

58. deTorregrosa M.V., Dapena R.B., Harnandez H. and Ortiz A. Association of Salmonella-Caused osteomyelitis and Sickle cell disease. Report of Three Cases. JAMA, 174: 354, 1960.

59. Diggs L.W. Sickle cell crisis. American Journal Clin. Path. 44: 1-19, 1965.

60. Diggs L.W. Bone and Joint lesions in Sickle cell disease. Clinical Orthopaedics and Related Research. No.52: 119-143, May-June'67.

61. Diggs L.W., Pulliam H.N. and King J.C. The bone changes in Sickle cell anaemia. Southern Med. J., 30: 249, 1937.

62. Diggs L.W. and Ching R.E. Pathology of Sickle cell anaemia. Southern Med. J., 27: 839, 1934.

63. Daland G.A. and Castle W.B. A simple and rapid method of demonstrating sickling of red blood cells, the use of reducing agents. J. Lab. Clin. Med. 33: 1082 - 88, 1948.

64. Dunlop K.J. and Mazumdar U.K. The occurrence of Sickle cell anaemia Among a group of Tea Garden Labourers in Upper Assam. India Med. Gaz, 87: 387, 1952.

65. Dunnagan W.A. Roentgen changes in Salmonella osteomyelitis occurring in children with and without Sickle cell anaemia. N. Carolina Med. J., 21: 45, 1960.
66. Datz F.L., Taylor A. Jr., Technical use of radionuclide bone marrow imaging, Semin Nucal. Med.; 1985 July, 15(3), 239-59.
67. Donald G. Mitchell, Herbert Y. Kressel, Peter H. Arger, Murrey Dalinka, Charles E. Spritzer, Marvin E Skinberg; Avascular necrosis of the femoral head ; Radiology 1986, Vol. 161, No.3; 739-742.
68. Donald G. Mitchell, Micheal Fallon, Herbert Y. Kressel, Vijay M. Rao, Murrey K. Dalinka, Charles E. Spritzer, Abbas Alavi and Marvin E. Steinberg: Femoral head avascular necrosis,correlation of MRI, radiographic staging, radionuclide imaging and clinical findings, Radiology 1987, Vol 162, No. 3; 709-715.
69. Danzig Larry A., Richard D. Coults, and Donald Resnick: Avascular necrosis of the femoral head following cardiac transplantation. Clin orthopaedics and related research. No. 117, June 1976, 217-220.
70. Ebong W.W. Avascular necrosis of the femoral head associated with haemoglobinopathy. Tropical & Geographical Medicine. Vol. 29: 19-23, 1977.
71. Ebong W.W. The treatment of chronic osteomyelitis in Sickle cell anaemia. Int. Surgery. 67: 4, 1982.
72. Ehrenpreis B. and Schwinger H. Sickle cell anaemia. Amer. J. Roentgen., 68: 28, 1952.
73. Engh C.A., Huges J.L., Abrams R.C., Bowerman J.W. Osteomyelitis in the patient with Sickle cell disease. Journal of Bone and Joint Surgery. Vol. 53A, No. 1: 1-15, Jan'71.
74. Espinoza L.R., Spilberg I., Osterland C.K. Joint manifestations of Sickle cell disease. Medicine Vol. 53 No. 4: 295-305, 1974.
75. Exarchou E., Politou C., Vretou E., Pasparakis D. and Caramerov A. Madessis: Fracture and epiphyseal deformities in β- Thalassemia. Clinical Orthopaedics and related research No. 189: 229-233, Oct 1984.
76. Ebong W.W., Kolawole T.M. Aseptic necrosis of the femoral head in Sickle disease. Br J Rheumatol 1986 Feb; 25[1]; 34-9.
77. Elke R., Morscher E. Total prosthesis arthroplasty in femoral head necrosis, Orthopade. 1990 Aug., 19(4), 236-41.
78. Epps, C.H., Jr. and Castro. Oswaldo: Complications of the Total hip replacements in Sickle cell disease. Orthop trans. 2 : 236-237 1978.
79. Emilio. S. Musso, Sharon N. Mitcheel, Marry Schink Ascani, C. Andrew Barett. Results of conservative management of osteonecrosis of the femoral head. CORR 1986, Vol. 207, 209-205.
80. Edward A, O'Hara: Roentgenographic osseous manifestation of the anaemias and the leukemias. Clinical orthpaedics and related research No. 52, May-June 1967, 63.
81. Ernest W. Smith and C. Lockord Conley. Clinical features of the genetic variants of Sickle cell disease. Bulletin - Johns Hopkins Hospital, 1954, Vol 94, 289-313.
82. Feingold B.F. and Case J.T. Roentgenologic skull changes in the anaemias of childhood. Amer. J. Roentgen., 29: 194, 1933.
83. Fleming A.F. Sickle cell disease. Churchill Livingstone, 23, 1982.
84. Goldberg,M.F.Retinal vaso-occlusion in sickling haemoglobinopathies. Birth defects, 12: 475,1976.
85. Goldenberg I.S. Sickle cell anaemia, Salmonella Enteritidis osteomyelitis and remote postoperative wound abscess. Report of a Case. Surgery, 38: 758, 1955.
86. Golding J.S.R. Conditions of the hip associated with haemoglobinopathies. Clinical Orthopaedics and Related Research. No. 90: 22-28, Feb'73.
87. Golding J.S.R. The bone changes in Sickle cell anaemia. Hunterian Lecture. Ann. Roy. Coll. Surg. Eng., 19: 296-314, 1956.

88. Golding J.S.R., MacIver J.E. and Went L.N. The bone changes in Sickle cell anaemia and its genetic variants. J. Bone Joint Surg. (Brit.), 41-B: 711-718, 1959.

89. Graham G.S. Case of Sickle cell anaemia with necropsy. Arch Intern. Med. (Chicago). 34: 778, 1924.

90. Gray R.H. Clinical features of homozygous SS disease in Jamaican children. W. Indian Med. J. 20: 60, 1971.

91. Gray R.H. (Symposium) : International symposium on Sickle cell anaemia. University of W. Indies. Kingston, Jamaica. "British Medical Journal", 373-374, Feb'69.

92. Green M., Nyham W.L. and Fousek M.D. Acute haematogenous osteomyelitis. Paediatrics, 17: 368, 1956.

93. Greenwald J.H. and Widen A.L.: E. coli osteomyelitis complicating haemoglobin Sickle cell disease. Amer J. Med., 116: 210, 1963.

94. Grinnan A.G. Roentgenologic bone changes in Sickle cell and erythroblastic anaemia. Report of Nine Cases. Amer. J. Roentgen., 34: 297, 1935.

95. Genin P, Vouge M, Bloch P: Osteonecrosis of the femoral head caused by Sickle cell anaemia in benign epidimiologic and radiological aspect. Bull. Asso. Pathol. Exot. Filiales 1985; 78(2); 249-55.

96. Gregory J. Hanker, Van Nuys, and Herlan C. Amstutz. Osteonecrosis of the hip in the Sickle cell disease. JBJS Vol. 70-A, No.4, April 1988. Page 499-506

97. Harden A.S. Jr. Sickle cell anaemia. Changes in the vessels and in the bones. Amer. J. Dis. Child., 54: 1045, 1937.

98. Harman J.V. and Ragaz F.J. The pathogenesis of experimental fat embolism. Amer. J. Path., 26: 551, 1950.

99. Hawker H., Neilson Hayes and Serjeant G.R. Haematological factors associated with avascular necrosis of the femoral head in homozygous Sickle cell disease. British Journal of Haematology. Vol.50: 29-34, 1982.

100. Henderson A.B. and Thornell H.E. Observations on the effect of lowered oxygen tension on sicklemia and Sickle cell anaemia among military flying personnel. J. Lab. Clin. Med., 31: 769, 1946.

101. Hendrickse R.G. and Collard P. Salmonella osteitis in Nigerian children. Lancet,1: 80, 1960.

102. Henkin W.A. Collapse of the vertebral bodies in Sickle cell anaemia. Amer. J. Roentgen., 62: 395, 1949.

103. Henriques C.Q. Osteomyelitis as a complication in urology with special reference to the paravertebral venous Plexus. Brit. J. Surg., 46: 49, 1958.

104. Herrick. J.B. Peculiar elongated and sickle-shaped red blood corpuscles in a case of severe anaemia. Arch. Intern. Med. (Chicago). 6: 517, 1910.

105. Hewett B.V. and Nice C.M. Jr. Radiographic manifestations of Sickle cell anaemia. Radiol. Clin. N. Amer., 2: 249, 1964.

106. Hill M.C., Sang OH K., Bowerman J.W., Siegelman S.S., James A.E. Apnormal epiphyses in the Sickling disorders. American Journal of Roentgenology, Vol. 124: 34, May '75.

107. Hook E.W., Campbell C.G., Weens H.S. and Cooper G.R.: Salmonella osteomyelitis in patients with Sickle cell anaemia. New Eng. J. Med., 257: 403, 1957.

108. Howells T.H., Huntsman R.G., Boys J.E. and Mahmood A. Anaesthesia and Sickle cell haemoglobin. British Journal of Anaesthesia. 44: 975-987, 1952.

109. Hughes G.J. and Carroll D.S. Salmonella osteomyelitis complicating Sickle cell disease. Paediatrics,19: 184, 1957.

110. Hamberg A.E. Skeletal Changes in Sickle cell anaemia. J. Bone Joint Surg., 32-A: 893, 1950.

111. Hurwitz D. and Roth H. Sickle cell-Thalassemia presenting as arthritis of the hip. Arthritis & Rheumatism, Vol. 13, No. 4: 422-429, July-Aug 1970.

112. Herold H.Z. Avascular necrosis of the femoral head in children under the age of three. CORR 126, July-Aug 1977 Page 193-195

113. Haddad R.J. Jr : Sickle cell disease involvement of the hip and its surgical treatment. Clin. orthop, 55: 135-149, 1967.

114. Hanker G.J., Amstutz H.C. Osteonecrosis of the Hip in the Sickle cell diseases. J.B.J.S. (Am); 1988 Apr; 70(A); 499-506.

115. Hernigou P., Galacteros F., Bachir D. and Goutallier D. Deformities in the hip in adults who have Sickle cell disease and had avascular necrosis in childhood. J.B.J.S. (Am.) 1991 Jan., 73 (1), 81-92.

116. Hernigou P. Avascular necrosis of the femoral head in Sickle cell disease. Treatment of collapse by the injection of acrylic cement. JBJS (Br) 1993 Nov, 75(6), 875-80

117. Hernigou P., Bachir D., Galacteros F. Hip dysplasia, a complication of Sickle cell disease. Rev. Rhum. Ed. Fr. 1993 Jul-Sept; 60 [7-8]; 505-13.

118. Hernigou P., Galacteros F., Bachir D., Goutellier D. Natural history of hip necrosis in Sickle cell disease. Rev. Chir. Orthop. 1989; 75[8]; 542-57.

119. Hungerford D.S., Lennox D.W. The importance of increased intraosseous pressure in the development of osteonecrosis of the femoral head; Orthop. Clin. North. Am. 1985 Oct.; 16[4]; 635-54.

120. Ingram V.M. A specific chemical difference between the globins of normal human and Sickle cell anaemia haemoglobin. Nature (London). 178: 792, 1956.

121. Ingram V.M. Gene mutation in human haemoglobin. The chemical difference between normal and Sickle cell haemoglobin. Nature, 180: 326, 1957.

122. Ingram V.M. Haemoglobin and its abnormalities. Springfield, Charles C. Thomas, Publisher, 1961.

123. Ivy R.E. and Howard F.H.: Sickle cell anaemia with unusual bone changes. J. Pediat., 43: 312, 1953.

124. Iwegbu C.G., A.F.Fleming: Avascular necrosis of the femoral head in Sickle cell disease. JBJS (Br.) 67B, 1985, pp 29-32.

125. Jaster D., Kolp W. Skeletal changes in Sickle cell anaemia; Beitr Orthop Traumatol 1987 May; 34[5]; 224-30.

126. Jenkins M., Scott R.B., Baird, R.L. Studies in Sickle cell anaemia. XVL sudden death during Sickle cell anaemia crisis in young children. J.Paed. 56: 30, 1960.

127. Jimenez C.T., Scott R.V., Henry W.L., Sampson C.C. and Ferguson A.D. Studies in Sickle cell anaemia. American Journal of Diseases of Children, Vol.III: 497-501, May '66.

128. Johnson A., Jackson M.A., Ferguson A.D. and Scott R.B. Studies in Sickle cell anaemia. Journal of the National Medical Association. Vol. 58 No. 4: 239-244, July '66.

129. Joseph Song. Pathology of Sickle cell disease. Textbook printed by Charles C. Thomas. 1971.

130. Kate B.R.,Anthropometry of Sickled cell anaemia patients. J. Anat. Soc. India. Vol. 26, No. 2: 98-103, 1977.

131. Katz S.H., Lubin B. and Armstrong D. Growth of adolescents with Sickle cell trait. The Lancet 2, 814: Apr '74.

132. Keeley K. and Buchanan G.R. Acute infarction of long bones in children with Sickle cell anaemia. The Journal of Paediatrics. Vol. 101, No. 2: 170-175, Aug'82.

133. Klinefelter H.F. The heart in the Sickle cell anaemia. Amer. J. Med. Sci., 203, 34, 1942.

134. Kraft E. and Bertel G. Sickle cell anaemia. Case report with unusual Roentgen findings. Amer. J. Roentgen., 57: 224, 1947.

135. Krammer M.S., Rooks R.N. and Pearson H.A. Growth and development in children with Sickle cell trait. The New England Journal of Medicine, Vol. 299, No. 13: 686-689, Sep'78.

136. Krammer M.S., Rooks Y., Washignton L.A. and Pearson H.A. Pre and Postnatal Growth and development in Sickle cell anaemia. The Journal of Pediatrics. No. 5: 857-860, May'80.

137. Kanoley and Ahulum FID, Lancet, 999, 1970

138. Kan Y.W., Dozy A.M. Antenatal diagnosis of Sickle cell anaemia by DNA analysis of amniotic fluid cells. Lancet, 2 : 910, 1978.

139. Koren A. Avascular necrosis of bones in children with Sickle cell anaemia. Pediatr. Hematol. Oncol.; 1993 Oct-Dec; 10(4) 385-7.

140. Khermosh O. and Weissman S.L. Coxa vara, avascular necrosis and osteochondritis dessicans complicating solitary bone cysts of the proximal femur. CORR 1977, No. 126; 143-146.

141. Lifeso R.M. Total joint replacement in Sickle cell disease. Orthop trans, 9 : 453, 1985.

142. Landesman S.H., Rao S.P. and Ahonkhai V.I. Infections in children with Sickle cell anaemia. (Special reference to pheumococeal & salmonella infections). Am. J. Paed. Haematol.Vol.4, No. 4: 407-415, 1982.

143. Lanzer W., Szabo R.S. and Gelberman R. Avascular necrosis of the lunate and Sickle cell anaemia. Clinical Orthopaedics and Related Research. No.187: 168-171, July-Aug'84.

144. Lee R.E.J., Golding J.S.R. and Serjeant G R. The Radiological features of avascular necrosis of femoral head in homozygus Sickle cell disease. Clinical Radiology. 32: 205-214, 1981.

145. Legant O. and Ball R.P. Sickle cell anaemia in adults. Radiology, 51: 655, 1948.

146. Lehman H. and Cutbush M. Sickle cell trait in Southern India. B.M.J. 1: 404, 1952.

147. Lewald L.T. Roentgen Evidence of osseous manifestations in Sickle cell (Drepanocytic) anaemia and in Mediterranean (Erythroblastic) Anaemia. Radiology, 18: 792, 1932.

148. Lohmuller H.W. and Marshall J.F.: Haemoglobin C-S disease complicated by paracolon osteomyelitis. Arch. Intern. Med. (Chicago), 101: 761, 1958.

149. Lowry M.F., Desai P., Ashcroft M.T., Serjeant B.E. and Serjeant G.R. Heights and weights of Jamaican children with homozygous Sickle cell disease. Human Biology. Vol. 49, No. 3: 429-436, Sep '75.

150. Luban N.L.C., Leikin S.L. and August G.A. Growth and development in Sickle cell anaemia. The American Journal of Pediatric Haematology/Oncology, Vol. 4, No. 1: 61-65, Spring'82.

151. Lutzker L.G. and Alavi A. Bone and marrow imaging in Sickle cell disease Diagnosis of infarction. Seminars in Nuclear medicine. Vol.6, No. 1: 83-93, Jan'76.

152. Ijiyawa M., Pfudie S., Pitche V., N'Dakena K., Amedegnato M.D., Doury P. Coxofemoral pathology in rheumatology; Med. Trop. (March) 1994, 54(1), 38-42.

153. Middlemiss J.H. Sickle cell anaemia, Journal of Faculty of Radiologists, No.16-24, 1958.

154. Milner P.F., Kraus A.P., Sebes J.I., Sleeper L.A., Dukes K.A., Emry S.H., Bellebue R., Koshy M., Moohr J.W., Smith J. Sickle cell disease as a cause of osteonecrosis of femoral head, N Engl. J. Med. Nov. 1991, 325(21), 1476-81.

155. Moran M.C., Huo M.H., Garvin K.L., Pellicci P.M., Salvati E.A. Total hip arthroplasty in Sickle cell haemoglobinopathy. Clin. Orthop. 1993 Sept; [294]; 140-8.

156. Micheal A. Mont, Dean C. Maar, Marc W. Urquhart, Dennis Lennox, David S Hungerford; Avascular necrosis of the humeral head treated by core decompression. J.B.J.S. 1993, Vol. 75B, No. 5, 785-88.

157. Micheal C. Hili, Kook Sang O.H., Jack W. Bowerman, Stanley, S. Siegelman and A. Everete James Jr. Abnormal epiphysis in the sickling disorders. From the Department of Radiology and Radiologic Sciences, Laboratory for Diagnostic Radiological Reasearch, The Johns Hopkins Medical Institutions, Baltimore, Maryland Pg. 34

158. Mathew D. Mitchell, Harold L. Kundel, Marvin E. Steinberg, Herbert Y. Kressel, Abass Alavi, Leon Axel,: Avascular necrosis of the Hip; AJR 1986; 147; 67-71.

159. Mitchell D.G., Kressel H.Y., Arger P.H. et al. Avascular necrosis of the femoral head: Morphologic assesment by MR imaging, with CT correlation. Radiology 1986; 161 : 739-42.

160. Mitchell D.G., Rao V.M., Dalinka M.K. et al. Femoral head avascular necrosis:correlation of MR imaging, radiographic staging, radionuclide imaging, and clinical finding. Radiology 1987; 162: 709-15.

161. Musso E.S., Mitchell S.N., Schink-Ascani M., Basset C.A.L. Result of conservative management of osteonecrosis of the femoral head: a retrospective review. Clin. Orthop. 1986; 207: 209-15.

162. Macht S.H. and Roman P.W. Radiological Changes in the Sickle cell anaemia. Amer. J. Radiol., 51: 697, 1948.

163. Magid D., Fishman E.K., Finizio J.P., Siegelman S.S. Case Report 254, Skeletal Radiology. Skeletal Radiology.11: 60-64, 1984.

164. Malhotra V. Sickle cell diseases. Arch Intern Med. 133. 612, 1974.

165. Marquis J.R. & Khazem B. Sickle cell disease. Radiology Vol.98: 47-52, Jan'1971.

166. Mason V.R. Sickle cell anaemia. JAMA, 79: 1318, 1922.

167. McCormack M.K., Dicker L., Katz S.H., Caleb M., McDaniels J., Humphery A., Buchert E. and Lubin B: Growth patterns of children with Sickle cell disease. Human biology, Vol. 48, No. 3: 429-437, Sep'76.

168. McCormack M.K., Salapatek S.S., Polesky H., Thompson W., Katz S.H. and Barker W.S. A comparison of the physical and intellectual development of Black children with and without Sickle cell trait. Paediatrics.Vol. 56, No. 6: 1021-1025, Dec'75.

169. Middlemiss J.H. & Raper A.B. Skeletal changes in haemoglobinopathies. J B JS. 48B, No. 4: 693-702, Nov'66.

170. Moore C. The Bone changes in Sickle cell anaemia with note on similar changes observed in skulls on ancient Mayan Indians. J. Missouri Med. Ass., 26: 561, 1929.

171. Moseley J.E. and Manly J.B. Aseptic necrosis of bone in Sickle cell disease. Radiology, 60: 656, 1953.

172. Moseley J.E. Skeletal changes in the anaemias. Seminars in Roentgenology, Vol. 9, No.3: 169-184, July'74.

173. Murphy R.C. and Shapiro S. The pathology of Sickle cell disease. Ann. Intern. Med., 23: 376, 1945.

174. Murphy S.B. Difficulties in Sickle cell states. Arch. Itern. Med. 133: 612, 476.

175. Ndugwa C.M. Aseptic necrosis of the head of femur among Sickle anaemia patients in Uganda. East African Medical Jr. Oct. 1992, 69(10), 572-6.

176. N. Olatunji Olambiwonnu, Robert Penny, S. Douglas Frasier. Sexual maturation in subjects with Sickle cell anaemia. Studies of serum gonadotropin concentration, height,weight, and skeletal age. The Journal of Paediatrics. Vol. 87, No. 3: 459-464, Sep'75.

177. Oduro K.A. & Searle J.F. Anaesthesia in Sickle cell states:A plea for simplicity. British Medical Journal. 4: 596-598, Dec'72.

178. Ogunjumo D.O. The clinical pattern of chronic-pyogenic osteomyelitis in a Nigerian community. Journal of Tropical Medicine & Hygiene. Vol. 85: 187-194, 1982.

179. Onwubalili J.K. Sickle cell disease and infection. Journal of Infection. 7: 2-20, 1983.

180. O'Hara E.A. Roentgenographic osseous manifestations of the anaemias & leukemias. Clinical Orthopaedics & Related Research. No.52: 63-82, May-June'67.

181. Omojala M.F., Annobil S., Adzaku F., Addae S.K., Mohammad S. Bone changes in Sickle cell anaemia. East African Med. Jr. 1993 March 70 (3) 184-88.

182. Owen Dyer, News; BMJ 1995 Vol.11.

183. Onuba O.; Bone disorders in Sickle cell disease. Int. Orthop. 1993 Dec.; 17 [6]; 397-9.

184. Oladele Akinla: Pregnancy and the skeletal complication of Sickle cell disease. Postgraduate Medical Journal (April 1973) 49, 255-257.

185. Padmos M.A., Roberts G.T., Sackey K., Kulozik A., Bail S., Morris J.S., Serjeant B.E., Serjeant G.R.: Two different forms of homozygous Sickle cell disease occurring in Saudi Arabia; Br. J. Haematol. 1991 Sept.; 79[1]; 93-8.

186. Pande Ketan C., Babhulkar Sushrut S., K. Prasad S.R.S. Multifocal osteomyelitis in a case of Sickle cell disease, Jr. of Indian Medical Association, Vol. 93, No.3, March 1995, P-122.

187. Powers J.A. Magnetic resonance imaging in marrow diseases. Clin Orthop 1996 May; [206]; 79-85.

188. Parastavros C.S. Aseptic necrosis of the femoral head due to Sickle cell - Thalassemia disease. Delaware Med. J., 29: 94, 1957.

189. Pauling L., Itano H.A., Singer S.J. and Wells I.C.: Sickle cell anaemia, A molecular disease. Science, 110: 543, 1949.

190. Pauling L., Itano H.A. and Singer S.J. Sickle cell anaemia haemoglobin. Science III: 459, 1950.

191. Phebus C.K., Gloninger M.F. and Maciak B.J. Growth patterns by age and sex in children with Sickle cell disease. The Journal of Pediatrics, Vol. 105, No. 1: 28-33, July'84.

192. Pierce R.O. Jr. Aseptic necrosis of the hip in Sickle cell disease. Journal of the National Medical Association. Vol. 71. No. 1: 45-48, 1979.

193. Platt O.S., Rosenstock W. and Espeland M.A. Influence of Sickle haemoglobinopathics on growth and development. The New England Journal of Medicine, Vol. 311, No. 1: 7-12, July '84.

194. Pollen A.G. Bone changes in Haemoglobin Sickle cell disease. Proc. Roy. Soc. Med., 54: 882, 1961.

Ponder E. "Haemolysis and related phenomenon". Grune and Stratton, New York, 1948.

195. Rand C., Pearson T.C., Heatley F.W. Avascular necrosis of femoral head in sickle cell syndrome, Acta Haematol, 1987; 78(2-3), 186-92.

196. Rutt A., Kusswetter W. Sickle cell anaemia and its skeletal and joint changes as an orthopaedic problem. Z. Orthop. 1986 Mar-Apr; 124[2]; 140-3.

197. Rijke A.M., Pope T.L. Jr., Kent T.E. Bilateral protrusio acetabuli in Sickle cell anaemia, South Med. Jr. March 1990, 83(3), 328-9.

198. Rao V.M., Mitchell D.G., Rifkin M.D. et al. Marrow infarction in Sickle cell anaemia: correlation with marrow type and distribution by MRI, Magan Reson Imaging 1989; 7 : 39-44

199. Reynolds J., Pritchard J.A., Ludders D. & Mason R.A. Roentgenographic and clinical appraisal of Sickle cell beta-Thalassemia disease. Radiology Vol. 118, No. 2: 378-400, June'73.

200. Reynolds J.A. Re-evalution of the Fish Vertebra sign in Sickle cell haemoglobinopathies. American Journal of Roentgenology, Vol. 97, No. 3: 693-707, July'66.

201. Reynolds J. Radiologic manifestation of Sickle cell haemoglobinopathy. JAMA. Vol. 238, No. 3: 247-250, July'77.

202. Reynolds J. An evaluation of some Roentgenographic signs in Sickle cell anaemia and its variants. Southern Media J., 55: 1123, 1962.

203. Reich R.S. and Rosenberg N.J. Aseptic necrosis of bone in Caucasians with chronic haemolytic anaemia due to combined Sickling and Thalassemia traits. J.Bone Joint Surg.,35-A: 894-904, 1953.

204. Riggins R.S., DeNardo G.L., D'Ambrosia R. and Goldman M. Assessment of circulation in the femoral head by 18f scintigraphy. Journal of Nuclear Medicine. Vol.15, No.3: 183-186, Oct'73.

205. Roberts A.R. and Hilburg L.E. Sickle cell disease with Salmonella osteomyelitis. J. Paediat, 52: 170, 1958.

206. Robinson I.B. and Sarnat B.G. Roentgen studies of the Maxilla and Mandible in Sickle cell anaemia. Radiology, 58: 517, 1952.

207. Rose C. Some unusual X-ray findings in skulls. Radiology, 13: 508, 1929.

208. Rothschild B.M. and Sebes J.I.: Calcaneal abnormalities and erosive bone disease associated with Sickle cell anaemia. The American Journal of Medicine. Vol. 71: 427-430, Sept '81.

209. Rowe C.W. and Haggard M.E. Bone infarcts in Sickle cell anemia. Radiology. Vol. 68: 661-668, May'57.

210. Sain A., Sham R., Silver L. Bone scan in Sickle cell crisis. Clinical Nuclear Medicine. 3: 85-88, March'78.

211. Sanger R.G., Greer R.O., Averbach R.E. and Denver Colo. Differential diagnosis of some simple osseous lesions associated with Sickle cell anaemia. Oral Surgery. Vol. 43, No. 4: 538-545, April '77.

212. Sarles H.E. Osteomyelitis complicating a Sickle cell Thalassemia syndrome. Texas Rep. Biol. Med., 22: 356, 1964.

213. Schumacher H.R., Andrews R. and McLaughlin G. Arthropathy in Sickle cell disease. Annals of Internal Medicine. 78: 203-211, Feb'73.

214. Schumacher H.R.,Dorwart B.B., Bond J., Alavi A. and Miller W. Chronic synovitis with early cartilage destruction in Sickle cell disease. Annals of the Rheumatic Disease. 36: 413-419, Feb'77.

215. Schwartz A.M., Homer M.J. and McCauley R.G.K. "Step off" vertebral body-Gaucher's disease versus Sickle cell haemoglobinopathy. American Roentgen Ray Society. Am. Journal Roentgenology, 132: 81-85, Jan'79.

216. Scott R.B. and Kessler A.D. Studies in Sickle cell anaemia. Southern Medical Journal. 1187-1190, Nov'68.

217. Scott R.B., Hiatt H.H., Clark B.G., Kessler A.D. and Ferguson A.D. Growth and development of Negro infants. Pediatrics Jan'62, 65-81.

218. Sebes J.I., Brown D.L. Terminal phalangeal sclerosis in Sickle cell disease. American Journal of Radiology, 148: 763-765, April'83.

219. Sebes J.I. and Kraus A.P. Avascular necrosis of the hip in the Sickle cell haemoglobinopathies. Journal of the Canadian Association of Radiologists. Vol. 34: 136-139, June'1983.

220. Serjeant G.R., Serjeant B.E. and Milner P.F. The irreversibly Sickled cells, a determinant of haemolysis in Sickle cell anaemia. Br. J. Haematol. 17: 527, 1969.

221. Serjeant G.R. and Ashcroft M.T. Delayed skeletal maturation in Sickle cell anaemia in Jamaica. Johns Hopkins Medical Journal, Vol. 132: 95-102, Feb'73.

222. Serjeant G.R. Irreversibly sickled cells and Splenomegaly in Sickle cell anaemia. Br. J. Haematol, 19: 635, 1970.

223. Sherman M.: Pathogenesis of disintegration of the hip in Sickle cell anaemia. Southern Med. J., 52: 632, 1959.

224. Sherman I. Sickling phenomenon, with special reference to differentiation of Sickle cell anaemia from Sickle cell trait. Bull. Hopkins Hosp., 67: 309, 1944.

225. Sherman J.D. Erythrocyte sickling phenomenon in the Golden Hamster (Mesocricetus Auratus). Boston Med. Quart. 8: 109, 1957.

226. Shukla R.N. and Parande A.S. Occurrence of Sickle cell anaemia and cases of Sickle cell trait in Nagpur. "Indian Journal of Medical Science", Vol 10, No. 11, 892-95, 1956.

227. Shukla R.N., Solanki B.R. and Parande A.S. Sickle cell disease in India. Blood; Vol.13, No.6, 552-556; 1958.

228. Shukla R.N. and Solanki B.R. Sickle cell trait in Central India. Lancet, 1: 297, 1958.

229. Shupak W., Berniev V., Rabinovich S., Gordon D.A. and Wright T. Avascular necrosis of bone with rheumatoid vasculities. The Journal of Rheumatology. Vol. 10, No. 2: 261-266, Dec'82.

230. Silver H.K., Simon J.L. and Clement D.H. Salmonella osteomyelitis and abnormal haemoglobin disease. Paediatrics, 20: 439, 1957.

231. Smith W.S. Sickle cell anaemia and Salmonella osteomyelitis. Ohio. Med. J., 49: 692, 1953.

232. Stevens M.C.G., Hayes R.J. and Serjeant G.R. Body shape in young children with homozygous Sickle cell disease. Pediatrics Vol. 71, No. 4: 610-614, Apr '83.

233. Stewart D.Y. Multiple joint lesion in a young Negro adult exhibiting the Sickle cell trait. Clin. Orthop., 16 : 287, 1960.

234. Sydenstricher A.P., Mulherin W.A.R. and Houseal A.R. Sickle cell anaemia. Report of two cases in children and necropsy in one case. American Journal Dis. Child 26: 132, 1924.

235. Sydenstricker V.P. Elliptical human erythrocytes. JAMA, 81: 113, 1923.

236. Sadat Ali M.:Avascular necrosis of the femoral head in Sickle cell disease. An integrated classification. Clin. Orthop 1993 May, (290), 200-05

237. Shah A., Mukerjee, Moreau: Knee arthroplasties for Sickle cell disease. Acta. Orthop. Scand. April 1993; 64 [2]; 150-2.

238. Sennara H. and Gorry F.:Orthopaedic aspects of Sickle cell anaemia & haemoglobinopathies. CORR 1978, No. 130, 154-157.

239. Sebes J.I. Diagnostic imaging of bone and joint abnormalities associated with Sickle cell haemoglobinopathies.: AJR Am. J. Roentgenol. 1989 June; 152[6]; 1153-9.

240. Smith E.W. and Conley C.L. Clinical features of genetic variants of Sickle cell disease. Bull. Johns Hopkins Hosp. 94, 289-1954.

241. Sebes Jeno I. Diagnostic imaging of bone in joint abnormalities associated with Sickle cell haemoglobinopathies, AJR Am. J. Roentgenol., 1989 June, 152(6), 1153-9.

242. Sebes Jeno I, Alfred P. Kraus: Avascular necrosis of the hip in the Sickle cell hemoglobinopathies. Journal of the Canadian Association of Radiologists, Vol. 34, June 1993 Page 136.

243. Soloman L., Mechanism of idiopathic osteonecrosis; Orthop. Clinic. North Am. 1985, Oct 16(4); 655-67.

244. Taylor P.W., Thorpe W.P., Trueblood M.C. Osteonecrosis in Sickle cell trait. J. Rheumatol. 1986 Jun; 13[3]; 643-6.

245. Theis J.C., Owen R. Skeletal complications in Sickle cell disease in the UK. J.R. Coll. Surg. Edinb. 1988; 33: 306-10.

246. Totty W.G., Murphy W.A., Ganz W.I. et al.: Magnetic resonance imaging of the normal and ischemic femoral head. AJR 1984; 143: 1273-80.

247. Todd R.C., Freeman M.A.R. and Piric C.J. Isolated trabecular fatigue fractures in the femoral head. JBJS Vol. 54-B No.4 Nov 1972 Page 723-728

248. Tanaka K.R., Clifford G.O. and Axelrod A.R. Sickle cell anaemia (Homozygous S) with aseptic necrosis of femoral head. Blood Vol.11: 998-1008, May'56.

249. Tanner J.M. and Whitehouse R.H.: Clinical longitudinal standards for height, weight, height velocity, weight velocity and stages of puberty. Archives of Disease in Childhood, 51: 170-179, 1976.

250. Tiagi G.K., Cooley's anaemia in India. Proc. Indian Association of Pathology; 1; 62, 1953

251. Tori G., Clinical and radiological observations on 102 cases of Sickle cell anaemia. Radiol. Clin., 23: 87, 1954.

252. Trueta J. True haematogenous osteomyelitis: Its pathology and treatment. Bull Johns Hopkins. Hosp. Joint Dis., 14: 5, 1953.

253. Veal J.R. and McFertridge E.M. Paratyphoid osteomyelitis. Report of two additional cases. J. Bone Joint Surg., 16: 445, 1934.

254. Verghese K.P., Scott R.B., Peixeira G. and Ferguson A.D. Physical growth of North American Negro children. Pediatrics, Vol 44, No. 2: 243-247, Aug'69.

255. Victor A.B. and Imperiale L.E. Pulmomary and small bone changes in infants with Sickle cell anaemia. New York, J. Med., 57: 1403, 1957.

256. Vogt E.C. and Diamond L.K.: Congenital anaemias, roentgenologically considered. Amer. J. Roentgen., 23: 625, 1930.

257. Watson J., Burko H., Megas H. and Robinson M. The Hand-foot Syndrome in Sickle cell disease in Young Children. Pediatrics, 31: 975, 1963.

258. Washburn R.E. Peculiar elongated and sickle-shaped red blood corpuscles in a case of severe anaemia. Virginia Med. Semi monthly, 25: 490-493, 1910.

259. Weil I.F. and Lerner H.H. A case of long.standing Sickle cell anaemia with marked changes. Amer. J. Roentgen., 60: 251, 1948.

260. Weinberg A.G. & Currarino G. Sickle cell dactylitis: Histopathologic observations. American Journal of Clinical Pathology. Vol.58: 518-523, Nov'72.

261. Weinberg.:Severe sclerosis of the long bones in Sickle cell anaemia. Radiology, 145: 41-43, Oct'82.

262. Wethers D.L. & Grover R. Pitfalls in diagnosis of osteomyelitis in children with Sickle cell disease. Clinical Paediatrics. Vol. 22, No. 9: 614-618, Sept'83.

263. Whitten C.F. Growth status of children with Sickle cell anaemia. Amer. J. Dis. Child., 101: 355-364, 1961.

264. Widen A.L. and Cardon L. Salmonella Typhimurium osteomyelitis with Sickle cell haemoglobin-C disease. A review and case report. Ann. Intern. Med., 54 : 510, 1961.

265. Wigh R. and Thompson H.J.Jr. Cortical fissuring in osteomyelitis complicating Sickle cell anaemia. Radiology, 55: 553, 1950.

266. Winsor T. and Burch G.E. The habitus of patients with Sickle cell anaemia. Human Biology. 16: 90, 1944

267. Worrall V.T. & Butera V. Sickle cell dactylitis. Journal of Bone & Joint Surgery. Vol. 58A, No. 8: 1161-1163, Dec'76.

268. Ware H.E., Brooks A.P., Toye R., Berney S.I. Sickle cell disease and silent avascular necrosis of the hip. J.B.J.S. (Br.) Nov. 1991, 73B, 947-9.

269. Washington E.R., Root L. Conservative treatment of Sickle cell avascular necrosis of the femoral head. J. Paediatr. Orthop. 1985 Mar.-Apr., 5, 192-4.

270. Wayne Alen S., Steven B. Zelicof, Clement B. Sledge. Total hip arthroplasty in Beta Thalassemia. CORR 1993, 294, 149-54.

Subject Index

A

E

F

G

Q

R

S

T

U

V

W

X

Z

Author Index